The Prevention and Treatment of Pressure Ulcers

Edited by

Moya J Morison BA BSc(Hons) MSc PhD PGCE RGN

Reader in Health and Nursing, School of Social and Health Sciences,
University of Abertay, Dundee, UK

Foreword by

Lia van Rijswijk RN BSN CWCN COCN

Nurse Consultant and Graduate Student, School of Nursing, La Salle University,
Philadelphia, USA

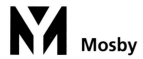 Mosby

EDINBURGH   LONDON   NEW YORK   PHILADELPHIA   ST LOUIS   SYDNEY   TORONTO   2001

MOSBY
An imprint of Harcourt Publishers Limited

© Harcourt Publishers Limited 2001

First published 2001

ISBN 0 7234 3158 2

British Library Cataloguing in Publication Data
A catalogue record for this book is available from the British Library

Library of Congress Cataloging in Publication Data
A catalog record for this book is available from the Library of Congress

Note
Medical knowledge is constantly changing. As new information
becomes available, changes in treatment, procedures, equipment and
the use of drugs become necessary. The editor, contributors and the
publishers have taken care to ensure that the information given in this
text is accurate and up to date. However, readers are strongly advised
to confirm that the information, especially with regard to drug usage,
complies with the latest legislation and standards of practice.

The
publisher's
policy is to use
**paper manufactured
from sustainable forests**

Printed in China

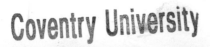

Contents

Contributors

Patricia R Boynton MS RN CS CWCN
Gerontological Clinical Nurse Specialist; Certified
Wound Care Nurse, Bryan, Ohio, USA

Michael Clark PhD
Honorary Senior Research Fellow, Wound
Healing Research Unit, University of Wales
College of Medicine, Cardiff; Senior Research
Fellow, School of Electronics, University of
Glamorgan, Pontypridd, UK

Mark E Collier BA(Hons) RGN ONC RCNT RNT
Nurse Consultant and Senior Lecturer – Tissue
Viability, The Centre for Research and
Implementation of Clinical Practice, Thames
Valley University, Wolfson Institute of Health
Sciences, London, UK

Jo Corlett BA MSc RGN RNT
Lecturer in Nursing, School of Social and Health
Sciences, University of Abertay, Dundee, UK

Mary Dyson PhD FCSP FAIUM LHD(Hon)
Emeritus Reader in Biology of Tissue Repair,
King's College London; Centre for
Cardiovascular Biology and Medicine, GKT,
Guy's Hospital Campus, London, UK

Peter J Franks BSc MSc PhD
Co-Director, The Centre for Research and
Implementation of Clinical Practice, Thames
Valley University, Wolfson Institute of Health
Sciences, London, UK

Yvonne Franks BSc(Hons) RGN
Senior Nurse, Outpatient and Diagnostic
Services, Queen Mary's Hospital, London, UK

Finn Gottrup MD DMSci
Professor and Head of Copenhagen Wound
Healing Centre, Bispebjerg University Hospital,
Copenhagen, Denmark

Sue M Green RN BSc MMedSci PhD
Lecturer in Nursing, University of Hull,
Kingston upon Hull, UK

Jane Harris BN MSc RGN RM RHV DN PWT DNT
Lecturer in Nursing, School of Social and Health
Sciences, University of Abertay, Dundee, UK

Bo Jørgensen MD
Senior Registrar, Copenhagen Wound Healing
Centre, Bispebjerg University Hospital,
Copenhagen, Denmark

Tim Kilner BN RGN PGCE Dip IMC RCS Ed
Lecturer in Nursing, University of Birmingham,
Birmingham, UK

Courtney H Lyder ND GNP FAAN
Professor, Yale University School of Nursing,
New Haven, USA

Amanda McGough BSc RGN MSc (yet to be awarded)
R&D Adviser and Teaching Fellow, Department
of Health Sciences and Clinical Evaluation,
Alcuin College, University of York, York, UK

Susan M McLaren BSc PhD RGN
Professor of Nursing, Faculty of Healthcare
Sciences, Kingston University and St George's
Hospital Medical School, Kingston-upon-Thames,
UK

Moya J Morison BA BSc(Hons) MSc PhD PGCE RGN
Reader in Health and Nursing, School of Social
and Health Sciences, University of Abertay,
Dundee, UK

Jane Nixon BSc(Hons) MA RGN
Research Fellow, University of York, York, UK

Liza G Ovington PhD CWS
Clinical Education Manager, Skin and Wound
Care, Johnson & Johnson Medical, Arlington,
Texas, USA

Barbara Pieper PhD RN CS CETN FAAN
Associate Professor and Nurse Practitioner,
College of Nursing, Wayne State University,
Detroit, Michigan, USA

Linda Russell BSc(Hons) RGN
Tissue Viability Nurse Specialist, Queen's
Hospital, Burton Hospitals NHS Trust, Burton
upon Trent, UK

Jens Lykke Sørensen MD PhD
Consultant, Department of Plastic and
Reconstructive Surgery, Roskilde County
Hospital, Roskilde, Denmark

Nancy A Stotts RN EdD
Professor, School of Nursing, University of
California, San Francisco, California, USA

Lia van Rijswijk RN BSN CWCN COCN
Nurse Consultant and Graduate Student, School of
Nursing, La Salle University, Philadelphia; Clinical
Editor *Ostomy/Wound Management*, USA

Charlotte Woollaston RGN Dip Adult Nursing
Project Sister, Pressure Sore Prevention, Chelsea
and Westminster Hospital, London, UK

Foreword

Science is built up of facts, as a house is built of stones:
But an accumulation of facts is no more a science than
a heap of stones is a house.

Henri Poincaré (1854–1912)

We can all look back at a century of learning about pressure ulcer prevention and care. Some learning led to facts that fit our house of knowledge. Some 'facts' became fallacies shortly after they appeared. Many are still lying around like unused bricks, and only time and future research will determine their value, if any. One of the biggest strengths of *The Prevention and Treatment of Pressure Ulcers* is that the stones that built our current house of pressure ulcer knowledge are carefully examined. Existing facts are put in perspective *and* in the right context. This is as valuable for practising clinicians as it is for researchers and those interested in the economic implications of pressure ulcers. Despite an ancient history, the science of pressure ulcer prevention and care is relatively young. If you have practised during the time most pressure ulcer facts were gathered, this book provides an excellent summary of what we have learned thus far. If you are new to this area of patient care, it is a comprehensive source which will provide the knowledge needed to deliver optimal care. For the research-oriented reader, contributing authors have not only identified gaps in our collective knowledge, but many also provide useful information about pressure ulcer study designs.

It has been my privilege to care for and learn from patients who worry about pressure ulcers in very different health care environments, cultures and countries. And if there is only one thing that has become clear to me, it is that all patients and providers speak the same language. Pressure ulcers are a universal concern, as evidenced by the diversity of contributors to this book and the literature from which they draw to substantiate their recommendations and support their ideas. This is good news because it enables us to use our collective resources and knowledge at a time of increased concerns about rising health care costs. As we continue to find the appropriate place for our science facts and are able to secure them with the mortar that is the art of care, our house of knowledge will gain in strength and, eventually, patients all over the world will receive the care they need and deserve.

Lia van Rijswijk

Acknowledgements

We would like to express our appreciation of the help and encouragement of our families, friends and colleagues, without whose support and forbearance this book could not have been written.

1 *Moya J Morison*

Introduction: issues and paradoxes

INTRODUCTION

Pressure ulcers are commonly encountered in both hospital and community settings and, with inappropriate care, can develop into complex lesions of the skin and underlying tissues. Most pressure ulcers are avoidable and their prevention and management is regarded by most health care professionals as largely a nurse's responsibility, although other members of the health care team may be involved at one time or another.

The last 20 years has seen a burgeoning of knowledge relating to pressure ulcer prevention and management, a proliferation of wound care products and pressure-relieving devices, and a number of national and international initiatives to establish and disseminate best practice in the form of policy documents and clinical guidelines. There is, however, disturbing evidence that many health care professionals are ill informed about basic aspects of care in this context (Beitz et al 1998), that some textbooks continue to disseminate misinformation (Anthony 1996) and that some researchers are failing to take cognisance of what is already known when designing studies aimed at extending our knowledge. This text book aims to address these deficits.

PRESSURE ULCERS AS INDICATORS OF QUALITY OF CARE

Health care providers, quality-assurance managers and consumers are increasingly interested in rating facilities on outcomes of patient care (Berlowitz et al 1996). Outcome indicators used to date include the incidence of falls and injuries, bacteraemias and pressure ulcers. Pressure ulcer development is an important outcome measure because it is a common complication, it is largely preventable, and it can be costly both to patients and to health care providers (Department of Health 1993). In the USA, poor ratings can be used to limit reimbursements, thereby acting as a catalyst to organizational change aimed at improving patient care.

Based on a review of the literature completed in 1990, the United States Agency for Health Care Policy and Research (AHCPR) found pressure ulcer incidence in hospital settings to range from 2.7 to 29.5% and prevalence to range from 3.5 to 29.5% in the adult hospitalized population, rising from 60% to 66% in high-risk populations such as hospitalized quadriplegic patients and elderly patients admitted with a fractured neck of femur (AHCPR 1992) (Ch. 2). However, prevalence and incidence data needs to be viewed with caution. Prevalence is calculated on the total number of individuals who have a condition at a particular time (or during a particular time period) divided by the population at risk of having the condition at this time (or mid-way through the time period). One of the many difficulties is defining the population 'at risk' for the denominator. Another relates to the identification and grading of the pressure damage itself (Reid and Morison 1994, Collier 1999). Other consequences of the lack of standardization of pressure ulcer grading include difficulties in interpreting and comparing clinical trials of pressure-relieving equipment, the efficacy of local wound care products and studies to test the sensitivity and specificity of risk assessment tools. This is compounded by inter-observer variation in the assessment of skin ulceration (Buntinx et al 1996).

Many of these problems can be overcome by scrupulous attention to study design, as in Bergstrom et al's (1998) multisite study of the predictive validity of the Braden Scale (see Ch. 6). In this study, research staff were trained in the use of the scale and in grading ulcers. Inter-rater reliability between the investigators and the research staff was evaluated at regular intervals and maintained at 95% or better. To minimize misclassification of grade I ulcers this was coded only when ulcers were noted on two consecutive observations. Risk assessment on admission was found to be highly predictive of pressure ulcer development, but not as predictive as the assessment completed 48–72 h after admission.

HIGH-RISK POPULATIONS

Immobility, altered consciousness, greater age and nutritional deficiencies are important risk factors for pressure ulcers (Ch. 3). The particular vulnerability of those with spinal cord injuries and the elderly admitted with a fractured neck of femur is well known, but there are other high-risk groups, such as the previously healthy critically injured survivors of serious trauma (Baldwin & Ziegler 1998), patients undergoing lengthy surgery, such as cardiac surgery (Lewicki et al 1997), the terminally ill (Sopata et al 1997) and children in intensive care (Olding & Patterson, 1998). Wound healing in the neonate and in the elderly is qualitatively different from that of the 'normal' adult (Desai 1997a,b), and in all age groups it is impaired by medical conditions such as diabetes mellitus (Silhi 1998). It is the variety of factors that can lead to delayed healing that can make planning the care of patients with pressure ulcers so challenging (Ch. 9).

THE EDUCATIONAL NEEDS OF PROFESSIONAL AND LAY CARERS

The prevention and management of pressure ulcers is often covered very early on in under-graduate nursing programmes since it is regarded as 'basic care'. The topic may not be revisited when students are more experienced and knowledgeable. Such an approach underestimates the gulf between expert and novice nurses' knowledge (Lamond & Farnell 1998) and the decision-making skills required to care for high-risk patients and those with pressure ulcers. Furthermore, research suggests that registered nurses are often unaware of the deficits in their knowledge (Beitz et al 1998). The European Pressure Ulcer Advisory Panel (EPUAP 1998) is explicit in what needs to be included in educational programmes, and research suggests that staff education can have a significant effect in reducing the incidence of pressure ulcers and their associated costs (Moody et al 1988).

Much has been written about the theory–practice gap (Rolfe 1996), and what is becoming increasingly clear is that the implementation of evidence-based practice is the responsibility of managers as well as individuals. There are many published examples of the implementation of evidence-based practice guidelines within organizations (e.g. Hopkins et al 1998) (Ch. 15). Tremendous benefits can accrue when health care professionals collaborate to develop interdisciplinary patient care plans. Dzwierzynski et al (1998) found that the implementation of a pathway for surgical reconstruction of pressure ulcers decreased the length of hospital stay, and the use of medication, laboratory tests and radiology services, saving almost $11 000 per patient.

Clinical nurse specialists in tissue viability clearly have an important role to play as advanced practitioners, researchers and educators (Hutton 1997). One of their roles is effectively to liaise with other professionals such as physiotherapists (McCulloch 1998), dietitians (Liebmann 1998) and occupational therapists (Aldersea 1997). However, a role that is often neglected is the education and support of patients and lay carers (Ch. 14). For every person aged 65 years and older admitted to some form of institutionalized care there are twice as many people of equal disability living at home, whose carers are intimately involved in every aspect of care giving, often with little or no professional support (Baharestani 1994).

PATIENT SUPPORT SYSTEMS: KNOWLEDGE DEFICITS AND PARADOXES

It is perhaps timely to make explicit some of the gaps in our knowledge and some of the paradoxes that have been brought to light through research, using patient support systems by way of example.

Although many guidelines recommend that any individual in bed who is assessed to be at risk of developing pressure ulcers should be regularly repositioned, there remain many unanswered questions relating to the effectiveness of this practice, the frequency with which repositioning should be undertaken and the positions in which patients should be placed (Clark 1998) (Ch. 7). Furthermore, local practice is very variable, with regular repositioning by nurses having been supplanted, in many cases, by the use of pressure-redistributing support surfaces.

Clark & Cullum (1992) conducted a series of pressure ulcer prevalence surveys within one health district over a 4-year period. The prevalence of pressure ulcers increased from 6.8% (1986) to 14.2% (1989), while the available stocks of pressure-relieving mattresses increased from 69 (1987) to 186 (1989). These results appear to question the common assumption that successful pressure ulcer prevention can be achieved through expanding the stocks of pressure-relieving mattresses and beds. Price et al (1999) have challenged the assumption that low-unit-cost support systems are ineffective for very high-risk patients, and health economists and others are encouraging managers to be more sophisticated in their decision making when purchasing equipment, by including considerations of efficiency, reliability, depreciation and operating costs (Conine and Hershler 1991, Price 1999).

INNOVATIONS IN LOCAL WOUND ASSESSMENT AND MANAGEMENT

In relation to local wound assessment there have been many recent innovations, such as MAVIS, a non-invasive instrument for measuring the area and volume of wounds (Plassmann & Jones 1998).

However, sophisticated techniques such as photoplethysmography are not always available and a number of other methods have proved useful to clinicians in practice (Ch. 8).

Having assessed the wound, deciding on the most appropriate local wound management regimen is far from straightforward. Over the last 20 years there has been a proliferation of new primary wound dressing products (Ch. 10), many with similar physical and therapeutic properties. The place of antiseptics in wound management has been the subject of intense debate (Moore 1992, Lawrence 1998), while certain historical approaches, such as the use of larval therapy and honey, are experiencing a resurgence of interest and are being re-evaluated for both efficacy and clinical effectiveness (Thomas et al 1998, Cooper & Molan 1999, Naylor 1999). New challenges are being presented by the epidemic methicillin-resistant *Staphylococcus aureus* (EMRSA) in hospital settings (Perry 1996) and there is almost certainly the potential for further restricting the use of topical antibiotics in chronic wounds (Tammelin et al 1998), which led to the rapid emergence of MRSA in the 1980s.

Of the new generation of products, growth factors are currently stimulating intense interest because of their potential to actively stimulate wound healing by modulating endogenous repair processes (Graham 1998a,b). Until the processes involved in normal and abnormal wound healing are more fully understood their use can, however, be somewhat haphazard.

Local wound management products are an adjunct to, rather than a replacement for, therapeutic regimens aimed at tackling the underlying causes of the wound and the threats to the tissue's tolerance of pressure. Assessing and where necessary correcting more general patient factors that can delay wound healing, such as malnutrition (Ch. 13), are likely to be more cost-effective than the application of costly local therapeutic agents, until such time as these agents have been rigorously tested for clinical effectiveness. Other therapies that are proving of value today include vacuum-assisted wound closure (Kalailieff 1998, Banwell 1999) and ultrasound

(Hart 1998) (Ch. 12). Surgical reconstruction may be the treatment of choice for some patients (LaRossa & Bucky 1997) (Ch. 11).

While science and technology have so much to offer wound care it would be a pity if increasingly sophisticated treatment at the molecular level should become so much the focus of interest that well known and well tried basic principles are lost sight of.

PATIENT-CENTRED CARE

While rejoicing in the technical advances that there have been over the last 20 years, it is important not to lose sight of the prime focus of our care and concern and that is the patient. For many, pressure ulcers are associated with pain and discomfort, lowered self esteem and altered body image (Rintala 1995) (Ch. 4) and for some, complications such as sepsis and osteomyelitis can be life-threatening. Baharestani (1994) found that consequences for carers included increased fatigue, limited socialization and often financial hardship. The social support required by elderly patients and their carers living in the community

has been underestimated (Keeling et al 1997), as has the role of health care professionals as patient advocates in relation to tissue viability services. Patient advocacy can highlight a number of ethical, legal and contractual dilemmas for the individual practitioner. For example, in what circumstances should a health care professional report concerns about the care environment or the competence of colleagues, or inform patients or their families that a duty of care has been breached and that redress could be sought through a civil action?

Whether at a molecular, organ, individual, interpersonal or organizational level, pressure ulcers can present health care professionals with enormous technical and personal challenges.

I would like to conclude with some advice given to new recruits by their Senior Nurse Tutor, in the 1930s:

… you will see many changes in both technology and medicine, which you will learn to apply to the benefit of your patients. I want you to remember that it is every bit as important that you should turn his pillow and find time for a friendly word as it is to give him his medication. … You must never forget to care.

(Baker 1999, p. 33)

REFERENCES

Agency for Health Care Policy and Research 1992 Pressure ulcers in adults: prediction and prevention: clinical practice guideline number 3 (AHCPR No. 92–0047). US Department of Health and Human Services, Rockville

Aldersea P 1997 Sore points. Nursing Times 93(40):63–66

Anthony D 1996 The treatment of decubitus ulcers: a century of misinformation in the textbooks. Journal of Advanced Nursing 24(2):309–316

Baharestani M M 1994 The lived experience of wives caring for their frail home-bound elderly husbands with pressure ulcers. Advances in Wound Care 7(3):40–52

Baker M 1999 The hard old days. Nursing Times 95(31):32–33

Baldwin K M, Ziegler S M 1998 Pressure ulcer risk following critical traumatic injury. Advances in Wound Care 11(4):168–173

Banwell P E 1999 Topical negative pressure therapy in wound care. Journal of Wound Care 8(2):79–84

Beitz J M, Fey J, O'Brien D 1998 Perceived need for education vs. actual knowledge of pressure ulcer care in a hospital nursing staff. Medical Surgical Nursing 7(5):293–301

Bergstrom N, Braden B, Kemp M, Champagne M, Ruby E 1998 Predicting pressure ulcer risk: a multisite study of the predictive validity of the Braden Scale. Nursing Research 47(5):261–269

Berlowitz D R, Ash A S, Brandeis G H, Brand H K, Halpern J L, Moskowitz M A 1996 Rating long-term care facilities on pressure ulcer development: importance of case-mix adjustment. Annals of Internal Medicine 124(6):557–563

Buntinx F, Beckers H, Briers A, et al 1996 Inter-observer variation in the assessment of skin ulceration. Journal of Wound Care 5(4):166–170

Clark M 1998 Repositioning to prevent pressure sores – what is the evidence? Nursing Standard 13(3):58–64

Clark M, Cullum N 1992 Matching patient need for pressure sore prevention with the supply of pressure-redistributing mattresses. Journal of Advanced Nursing 17:310–316

Collier M 1999 Blanching and non-blanching hyperaemia. Journal of Wound Care 8(2):63–64

Conine T A, Hershler C 1991 Effectiveness: a neglected dimension in the assessment of rehabilitation devices and equipment. International Journal of Rehabilitation Research 14:117–122

Cooper R, Molan P 1999 The use of honey as an antiseptic in managing *Pseudomonas* infection. Journal of Wound Care 8(4):161–164

Department of Health 1993 Pressure sores – a key quality indicator: a guide for NHS purchasers and providers. Department of Health, London

Desai H 1997a Ageing and wounds. Part 1: foetal and postnatal healing. Journal of Wound Care 6(4):192–196

Desai H 1997b Ageing and wounds. Part 2: healing in old age. Journal of Wound Care 6(5):237–239

Dzwierzynski W W, Spitz K, Hartz A, Guse C & Larson D L 1998 Improvement in resource utilization after development of a clinical pathway for patients with pressure ulcers. Plastic and Reconstructive Surgery 102(6):2006–2011

European Pressure Ulcer Advisory Panel 1998 Pressure ulcer prevention guidelines. EPUAP Review 1(1):7–8

Graham A 1998a The use of growth factors in clinical practice (part 1). Journal of Wound Care 7(9):464–466

Graham A 1998b The use of growth factors in clinical practice (part 2). Journal of Wound Care 7(10):536–540

Hart J 1998 The use of ultrasound therapy in wound healing. Journal of Wound Care 7(1):25–28

Hopkins A, Gooch S, Danks F 1998 A programme for pressure sore prevention and management. Journal of Wound Care 7(1):37–40

Hutton D J 1997 The clinical nurse specialist in tissue viability services. Journal of Wound Care 6(2):88–90

Kalailieff D 1998 Vacuum-assisted closure: wound care technology for the new millennium. Perspectives 22(3):28–29

Keeling D, Price P, Jones E, Harding K G 1997 Social support for elderly patients with chronic wounds. Journal of Wound Care 6(8):389–391

Lamond D, Farnell B 1998 The treatment of pressure sores: a comparison of novice and expert nurses' knowledge, information use and decision accuracy. Journal of Advanced Nursing 27:280–286

LaRossa D, Bucky L P 1997 Surgical management. In: Parish L C, Witkowski J A, Crissey J T (eds) The decubitus ulcer in clinical practice, Springer Verlag, Berlin, pp. 84–113

Lawrence J C 1998 The use of iodine as an antiseptic agent. Journal of Wound Care 7(8):421–425

Lewicki L J, Mion L, Splane K G, Samstag D, Secic M 1997 Patient risk factors for pressure ulcers during cardiac surgery. AORN Journal 65(5):933–942

Liebmann L J 1998 Patterns of nursing home referrals to consultant dieticians. Geriatric Nursing 19(5):284–285

McCulloch J M 1998 The role of physiotherapy in managing patients with wounds. Journal of Wound Care 7(5):241–244

Moody B L, Fanale J E, Thompson M, Vaillancourt D, Symonds G, Bongsoro C 1988 Impact of staff education on pressure sore development in elderly hospitalized patients. Archives of Internal Medicine 148:2241–2243

Moore D 1992 Hypochlorites: a review of the evidence. Journal of Wound Care 1(4):44–53

Naylor I L 1999 Ulcer care in the Middle Ages. Journal of Wound Care 8(4):208–212

Olding L, Patterson J 1998 Growing concern. Nursing Times 94(38):74–79

Perry C 1996 Methicillin-resistant *Staphylococcus aureus*. Journal of Wound Care 5(1):31–34

Plassmann P, Jones T D 1998 MAVIS: a non-invasive instrument to measure area and volume of wounds. Medical Engineering and Physics 20(5):332–338

Price P 1999 The challenge of outcome measures in chronic wounds: a review of measures of efficacy, efficiency and effectiveness. Journal of Wound Care 8(6):306–308

Price P, Bale S, Newcombe R, Harding K 1999 Challenging the pressure sore paradigm. Journal of Wound Care 8(4):187–190

Reid J, Morison M J 1994 Classification of pressure sore severity. Nursing Times 90(20):46–50

Rintala D H 1995 Quality of life considerations. Advances in Wound Care 8(4).28.71–28.83

Rolfe G 1996 Closing the theory practice gap: a new paradigm for nursing. Butterworth-Heinemann, Oxford

Silhi N 1998 Diabetes and wound healing. Journal of Wound Care 7(1):47–51

Sopata M, Luczak J, Glocwacka A 1997 Managing pressure sores in palliative care. Journal of Wound Care 6(1):10–11

Tammelin A, Lindholm C, Hambraeus A 1998 Chronic ulcers and antibiotic treatment. Journal of Wound Care 7(9):435–437

Thomas S, Andrews A, Jones M 1998 The use of larval therapy in wound management. Journal of Wound Care 7(10):521–524

2 *Lia van Rijswijk*
Epidemiology

INTRODUCTION

Knowledge of the epidemiology of pressure ulcers, their 'incidence, prevalence, distribution, and the sum of factors that control their presence or absence' (Merriam-Webster 1994) is an important first step toward meeting the challenge of preventing them. For centuries, pressure ulcers have troubled, frustrated, challenged and intrigued health care professionals, patients, and families alike. The pressure ulcers of a priestess of Amen of the XXIth Dynasty (2050–1800 BC) were found to be carefully covered with pieces of soft leather before embalming (Thompson 1961), probably in an attempt to restore physical integrity. In the nineteenth century, following observations that one must 'deplore the wretched condition of those who, being bedridden through accident or infirmary, have contracted sores of a very painful and dangerous kind' (Haberden 1815), Charcot suggested that these sores were 'inevitable' and the result of trophic disturbances. This resulted in what has been characterized as the 'era of trophic fatalism' or 'therapeutic nihilism' (Parish et al 1997). Until unprecedented numbers of individuals sustained spinal cord injuries and pressure ulcers during World War I, the inevitability of pressure ulcers was rarely questioned. However, traditions take a long time to change and, as Munro (1940) observed; 'Like Mark Twain's weather, everybody talks about bed sores associated with spinal cord injuries but no one does anything about them'. More than 40 years after Munro's observations, clinicians were still wondering why pressure ulcers were so maligned, their existence denied or punishment for their occurrence contemplated (Parish et al 1988). Health care providers tend to receive and confer blame. For example, family caregivers have been made to feel guilty by physicians and nurses for providing poor care as 'evidenced' by the presence of pressure ulcers (Baharestani 1994).

It is still not uncommon to hear that 'most of our pressure sores occur prior to admission' or that, 'human beings are left in the same position for so long that their flesh wears away to the bone' (National Citizens' Coalition for Nursing Home Reform 1999). Indeed, whether viewed as a 'visible mark of caregiver sin', evidence of a 'failing body', or a sign of vulnerability, the topic of pressure ulcers continues to invoke emotions (van Rijswijk 1997). Pressure ulcer-related lawsuits may focus on issues of risk, risk documentation and the use of appropriate prevention strategies (Dimon 1994, Soloway 1998), but at the heart of most cases is their historical legacy and the emotions they summon.

Neither emotional responses, nor denial or blame will help prevent pressure ulcers. Understanding their epidemiology, their 'incidence, prevalence, distribution, and the sum of factors that control their presence or absence' (Merriam-Webster 1994) on the other hand, may not only reduce the prevalence of these wounds but may also help reduce patient and caregiver anxiety, stress and feelings of guilt. A clear picture of their epidemiology will help health care professionals, caregivers and patients focus on practical methods to meet the challenge of preventing pressure ulcers, without feeling accused or defensive.

INCIDENCE AND PREVALENCE

To gauge the extent of the pressure ulcer problem, studies to ascertain their incidence (the rate at which their development occurs), point prevalence (number of individuals who have a pressure ulcer at a particular time) and period prevalence (number of individuals known to have a condition at any time during a specific time period) are conducted. Unfortunately, the challenge of preventing pressure ulcers starts with problems documenting their prevalence and incidence. First, there is no universal, standard, pressure ulcer classification system that has undergone extensive reliability and validity testing (see Ch. 3). When populations are assessed using different instruments, both the prevalence and incidence of the condition assessed is likely to vary considerably. Second, data collection methods and training of the persons who perform the assessment may affect the results of prevalence and incidence studies. For example, administrative databases can be very helpful to determine the extent of the pressure ulcer problem. However, the limitations of this method, such as data completeness, accuracy, reliability, and validity, have to be taken into account (Berlowitz et al 1997). With respect to methods, there is evidence to suggest that studies using well-trained data collectors will report a higher pressure ulcer rate than those using untrained data collectors (Allcock et al 1994). This may be particularly true for assessing non-blanching hyperaemia and could explain the reported low prevalence of these lesions in persons with darkly pigmented skin (Meehan 1994, Barczak et al 1997). Indeed, when nurses trained to assess darkly pigmented skin conducted a study, the incidence of non-blanching hyperaemia among Black and Latino/Hispanic older patients admitted to an acute care facility was higher than generally reported (Lyder et al 1998).

Despite these limitations and the resultant variations in reported prevalence and incidence rates,

patterns of their distribution have emerged. Based on a literature review completed in the summer of 1990, the United States Agency on Health Care Policy and Research found a pressure ulcer incidence range of between 2.7% and 29.5%, with pressure ulcer prevalence ranging from 9% in 'general' to 66% in 'high risk' populations (Panel for the Prediction and Prevention of Pressure Ulcers in Adults 1992). When reviewing the results of subsequent research (see Tables 2.1 and 2.2), it is obvious that pressure ulcers remain a common condition in different care environments all over the world, and that reported incidence and prevalence rates still vary widely. The challenge of reducing pressure ulcer rates by applying pressure ulcer aetiology and risk factor knowledge in clinical practice is confounded by the 'greying' of many populations. As with all conditions that are epidemic, that 'affect a disproportionately large number of persons in a population' (Merriam-Webster 1994), continuous prevalence and incidence monitoring is crucial.

HIGH-RISK POPULATIONS

Before discussing high-risk populations and applying epidemiological data to individual patients, it is important to understand the limitations of this approach. First, issues that limit the generalizability of pressure ulcer prevalence and incidence studies also apply to risk factor research. Second, risk factors derived from different populations do not necessarily apply to a particular individual. Third, when reviewing the presence of risk factors, clinicians can gauge the magnitude, but not the specific nature of that risk (McNees et al 1998). While some of these issues continue to be addressed, clinicians can, and should, base their risk assessment and prevention strategies on the most currently available data and assessment of each individual patient.

At first, 'general' prevalence and incidence studies appear to indicate that persons in long-term care facilities have a higher risk of developing pressure ulcers than those admitted to acute care facilities or home care agencies (see Tables 2.1 and 2.2). However, these numbers simply reflect

Table 2.1 Reported pressure ulcer prevalence

Patient care setting	Country	Study method (n)	Prevalence (including non-blanching hyperaemia)	Reference
Acute care	USA	Point prevalence, multicentre, not including maternity/obstetrics & gynaecology (39 874)	10.8%	Barczak et al (1997)
Acute care	Germany, Italy, UK, The Netherlands	Point prevalence, multicentre – Germany (8678), Italy (945), The Netherlands (1136), UK (8123)	Germany 7%, Italy 9% The Netherlands 15%, UK 18%	O'Dea (1995)
Acute care	UK	Point prevalence, one hospital, not including obstetrics, acute psychiatry, day surgery and metabolic unit (714)	32.1% (Includes blanching hyperaemia)	Allcock et al (1994)
Acute care community	UK	Point prevalence, mail survey (149)	Acute care 12.2%, community 2.5%	Hallett (1996)
Acute care extended care, community	Canada	Point prevalence, multisite, not including Pediatrics (2384)	25.7%	Foster et al (1992)
Acute care, extended care, community	The Netherlands	Point prevalence, multisite (2031)	Acute care 10.1%, extended care 83.6%, community care 12.7%	Bours et al (1999)
Acute care, community	UK	Point prevalence, multisite, five annual surveys (1992–1996)	Acute care range 8.5–14.7%; community care range 3.0–6.1%	Torrance & Maylor (1999)
Extended care	USA	Period (3 months) prevalence, sample of minimum data set plus data state facilities (15 121)	12%	Spector & Fortinksy (1998)
Community	Japan	Point prevalence, mail survey (23 500)	14.6% (inclusion of non-blanching hyperaemia unknown)	Kanagawa et al (1998)
Community	USA	Point prevalence, convenience sample of home health care patients, visited by trained nurse (103)	29%	Oot-Giromini (1993)

general differences in population characteristics. Understanding the effect of these population characteristics on pressure ulcer risk may help individual facilities, and different units within them, target prevention practices.

Demographic variables

Most studies show that in all patient care environments pressure ulcers are more common in older than in younger patients (Kemp et al 1990, Allman et al 1995, Bergstrom et al 1996, Perneger et al 1998) (see Fig. 2.1). In general, persons who do not develop or do not have a pressure ulcer have been found to be an average of 10 years younger than those who do (Maklebust & Magnan 1994, Tourtual et al 1997, Bergstrom et al 1998). Age has been found to affect the risk of developing pressure ulcers in general, as well as specific population studied. For example, in one study, the risk of developing a pressure ulcer following surgery was found to be five times greater in persons more than 70 years of age than in persons less than 60 years of age (Papantonio et al 1994).

In contrast to the effect of age, the influence of race on pressure ulcer risk is less clear, in part because many studies do not include sufficient numbers of patients of varying race to find any effect of this demographic variable. While patients

Table 2.2 Reported pressure ulcer incidence

Patient care setting	Country	Study method (n)	Prevalence (including non-blanching erythema unless indicated otherwise)	Reference
Acute care	Switzerland	Three surveys followed by observation (2373)	10.3%	Perneger et al (1998)
Acute care (university affiliated), veterans administration medical centre (VAMC), long-term care	USA	Random selection upon admission, trained observers – maximum follow-up 4 weeks – acute care (306), VAMC (282), long-term care (255)	Acute care 8.5%, VAMC 7.4%, long-term care 23.9%	Bergstrom et al (1998)
Acute care	USA	Prospective, cohort (286)	12.9%	Allman et al (1995)
Community	USA	Convenience sample of home health care patients, visited by trained nurse (103)	16.5%	Oot-Giromini (1993)
Community	USA	Retrospective cohort study, all individuals > 60 years of age, record review (1711)	3.2% (not including non-blanching erythema)	Bergquist & Frantz (1999)
Acute care	UK	Admission records and floor surveys collected weekly (8834)	4%	Clark & Watts (1994)
Extended care	USA	Prospective, multicentre, facility-based assessments for 3 months (10% audited) (4232)	12.9%	Brandeis et al (1994)
Rehabilitation facility	USA	Retrospective chart review, all admissions (170)	6%	Schue & Langemo (1999)
Acute care, rehabilitation facility, skilled nursing care nursing home, home health agency, hospice agency	USA	Prospective, all adults admitted, facility-based skin assessments, follow-up: 2–4 weeks (acute care and nursing home, respectively) acute care (74), rehabilitation (40), nursing home (30), home health care (30), hospice (20)	Overall 9%; acute care 14%, rehabilitation 0%, nursing home 28%, home care 0%, hospice 0%,	Langemo et al (1991)

with darkly pigmented skin have been found to have higher proportions of severe pressure ulcers than those with light-coloured (Fuhrer 1993, Barczak et al 1997), this may be related to problems assessing non-blanching hyperaemia in darkly pigmented skin (Lyder et al 1998). As a result, prevention strategies may be less than optimal in this population. Studies that do include a sufficient number of individuals in different categories either show no effect of race (Allman et al 1995, Tourtual et al 1997), or that being white is a

risk factor for developing pressure ulcers (Manley 1978, Bergstrom & Braden 1992, Brandeis et al 1994, Bergstrom et al 1996). An increased awareness of the importance of examining this relationship and training health care providers to assess hyperaemia in patients with darkly pigmented skin may provide much needed data. In the meantime, available evidence suggests that the effect of race on pressure ulcer incidence is either not as important as other variables, or that being white is a risk factor for developing pressure ulcers.

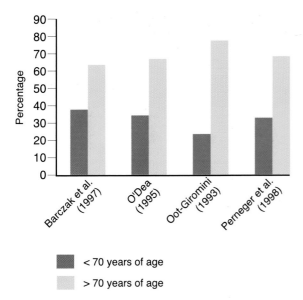

Figure 2.1 Reported pressure ulcer prevalence and incidence by age group.

In general, gender does not appear to affect the development of pressure ulcers. Most studies do not report any effect, but some suggest that being male increases the risk of developing a pressure ulcer (Brandeis et al 1994) whereas others report that women are more likely to develop them (Bergstrom et al 1996).

In summary, while increased age is often correlated with an increase in other pressure ulcer risk factors (e.g. limited mobility and medical diagnosis), the elderly are clearly more likely to develop pressure ulcers. With respect to clinical practice, individuals more than 65 or 70 years old in all patient care environments should be considered at high risk for developing these wounds.

Patient variables and diagnoses

Regardless of age and care environment, patient populations with mobility limitations are at high risk for developing pressure ulcers. For example, individuals with spinal cord injuries have been reported to have a pressure ulcer prevalence of 50–60% (Munro 1940; Panel for the Prediction and Prevention of Pressure Ulcers in Adults

1992). More recent studies show that the incidence of pressure ulcers in this population is between 20% and 30% during hospitalization (Carlson et al 1992, Curry & Casady, 1992). However, these numbers are still considerably higher than the incidence reported in non-spinal cord injured hospitalized individuals (Table 2.2). Furthermore, in this population, a prevalence rate of 33% has been documented following discharge (Fuhrer et al 1993) and approximately 50–60% of paralyzed individuals report having had at least one pressure ulcer (Knutsdottir 1993, Salzberg et al 1998).

Even in populations with limited mobility such as paralyzed individuals, level of mobility (e.g. limited versus none and level of dependence on others in activities of daily living) may affect the risk of pressure ulcer development (Fuhrer et al 1993, Salzberg et al 1998). Some studies have suggested that more complete or higher levels of injury are associated with a higher incidence of pressure ulcers (Carlson et al 1992, Curry & Casady 1992).

All patients with conditions that reduce mobility (e.g. surgery, hip fracture or stroke) are consistently found to be at increased risk of developing pressure sores (Berlowitz & van Wilking 1989, Spector 1994, Perneger et al 1998). For example, 13 out of 15 prevalence and incidence studies conducted in the community, acute care, long-term care and rehabilitation facilities show a relationship between mobility levels and pressure ulcers (see Fig. 2.2).

The next most commonly reported variable is nutritional status. Whether studied and reported as low albumin levels (Berlowitz & van Wilking 1989, Lewicki et al 1997, Tourtual et al 1997, Zulkowski 1998, Schue & Langemo 1999), depleted triceps skin fold and low body weight (Allman et al 1995), difficulty in feeding oneself (Spector 1994) or being malnourished (Maklebust & Magnan 1994), a consistent relationship exists between nutritional deficiencies and the development of pressure ulcers.

The presence of incontinence, diabetes mellitus, decreased mental status and a history of pressure ulcers seems most commonly to affect the risk of developing pressure ulcers in long-term care

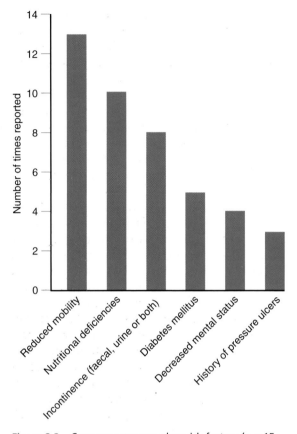

Figure 2.2   Common pressure ulcer risk factors (*n* = 15 studies).

facilities. In many acute care facilities, relationships have been found between pressure ulcers and the number of medical conditions (Lewicki et al 1997), a diagnosis of respiratory disease (Papantonio 1994, Tourtual et al 1997), cancer (Maklebust & Magnan 1994, Tourtual et al 1997) or peripheral vascular disease (Maklebust & Magnan 1994, Tourtual et al 1997) and the patient's length of stay (Tourtual et al 1997, Baldwin & Ziegler 1998).

Immobility and nutritional deficiencies clearly increase the risk of developing pressure ulcers. Specifically, decreasing levels of mobility, assessed separately or as part of the Braden Scale, are associated with an increased incidence and prevalence of pressure ulcers in all patient care environments. In addition, health care professionals should be concerned about pressure

ulcers in all patients who have a less than optimal nutritional status, are incontinent, have a history of pressure ulcers, a decreased mental status, or multiple medical conditions including diabetes mellitus and cancer.

KEY POINT

◆ All individuals with mobility limitation and nutritional deficiencies are at high risk of developing pressure ulcers.

Within facility variations and physiological factors

Prevalence and incidence rates of different populations in acute care facilities vary widely. While some of these variations may be explained by mobility levels and admission diagnoses, a patient's overall health condition also influences the risk of developing pressure ulcers.

Based on their review of the literature, the Agency on Health Care Policy and Research identified the following high-risk populations in acute care facilities: elderly patients admitted with femoral fracture, orthopaedic patients with fractures, hospitalized quadriplegic patients and those admitted to critical care units (Panel for the Prediction and Prevention of Pressure Ulcers in Adults 1992). Subsequent acute care studies have also shown a relationship between pressure ulcer rates and populations of immobile (e.g. fractures, orthopaedic patients) and/or acutely ill (critical care units) patients. During three biannual prevalence studies conducted in a teaching hospital in the USA, the number of pressure ulcers per occupied bed on the oncology, orthopaedics and general medical/surgical units was consistently lower than on the cardiology, urology, coronary care or medical intensive care/stepdown units (O'Brien et al 1998). Data from other countries also show considerable variations among different hospital units. Studies conducted in the UK (Torrance & Maylor 1999), Canada (Foster et al 1992), Japan (Sanada 1997) and Switzerland (Perneger et al 1998) all show that departments with older (e.g. elderly medical), immobile (e.g. rehabilitation) and more critically ill (e.g. intensive/critical care unit) patients have a higher pressure ulcer prevalence and incidence. While immobility and other risk factors affect patients admitted to critical care units, their overall health condition (e.g. problems with perfusion and immune system disorders) also increase their susceptibility to complications such as pressure ulcers. For example, in one acute care study the incidence of pressure ulcers was found to be correlated with increased acuity levels, death, infections and patient complaints (Reed et al 1998). (See also Ch. 3.)

Other risks

When trying to define high-risk populations, psychological and social issues, although not well understood at this time, should be considered. While some studies do not suggest that they affect the development of pressure ulcers, other studies, involving spinal cord injured patients, have found associations between pressure ulcers and life satisfaction, quality of life, level of self esteem and social support (Rintala 1995).

Finally, patient care environment and staff factors need to be considered. Differences between pressure ulcer rates between different facilities (e.g. rural versus urban) have been observed even when known pressure ulcer risk factors, patient acuity level and case-mix are taken into account (Berlowitz et al 1996, Spector & Fortinksy 1998). Consistent variations between different units in acute care facilities that cannot be explained by patient Braden Risk (see Ch. 6) scores have also been documented (O'Brien et al 1998). In this respect, results from studies showing an inverse relationship between the number of hours of care delivered by registered nurses and the incidence of pressure ulcers (American Nurses Association 1997, Blegen et al 1998) warrant attention and further research.

SUMMARY

When reviewing the epidemiology of pressure ulcers, their 'incidence, prevalence, distribution,

and the sum of factors that control their presence or absence' (Merriam-Webster 1994), it is easy to understand why pressure ulcers continue to trouble, frustrate and challenge patients and caregivers alike. Worldwide studies paint a relatively clear picture of their incidence, prevalence and distribution. Unfortunately, this cannot be said for the 'sum of factors' that cause their development. Because the latter is crucial in the implementation of effective prevention strategies, risk factor research in a variety of populations needs to continue.

In the meantime, health care professionals can integrate individual patient assessment information and existing knowledge about high-risk populations and risk factors. There are three, mostly independent, patient variables that should always draw the attention of health care professionals: immobility; increased age; and nutritional deficiencies. Other variables that may increase the risk of developing pressure sores include: high acuity level, increased length of stay, decreased mental status, incontinence, a history of pressure sores, and the presence of medical conditions such as diabetes mellitus and problems with perfusion. Additional research

CASE STUDY 2.1

Mrs M is admitted to an acute care facility after falling and breaking her hip. She is 78 years old, has a slight build, and is in good health. Upon admission, she tells you that 'The only time I have seen the inside of a hospital was when I visited others'. She does not have diabetes mellitus, her blood pressure is 155/95 and her only complaint is pain from the fracture. She lives alone and fell when standing on a chair to retrieve some plates from her cupboard. She is proud of her independence and only needs help 'to get some food in the house once-in-a-while'. An order for pain medication is obtained, and surgery is scheduled for the next morning. At 02.30 hours, the nurses hear Mrs M talk. She is trying to get out of bed, does not seem to remember she is in the hospital and complains about having to change her sheets because she couldn't get to the bathroom in time.

◆ Was Mrs M at risk for developing a pressure ulcer upon admission or should she be considered at risk now?

is needed to confirm suggested relationships between pressure ulcer rates and 'external' variables such as social support, type of facility, caregiver knowledge, skill and availability. Although practiced for hundreds of years, there is no research to suggest that blame, guilt or denial help reduce the prevalence of pressure ulcers:

historical evidence suggests that the opposite may be true. Emotional responses interfere with research efforts as well as objective patient assessments and the initiation of timely prevention strategies. This neither helps individual patients, nor increases our much-needed understanding of pressure ulcer risk factors.

REFERENCES

Allcock N, Wharrad H, Nicolson A 1994 Interpretation of pressure-sore prevalence. Journal of Advanced Nursing 20:37–45

Allman R M, Goode P S, Patrick M M, Burst N, Barolucci A A 1995 Pressure ulcer risk factors among hospitalized patients with activity limitation. Journal of the American Medical Association 273:865–870

American Nurses Association 1997 Implementing nursing's report card: a study of R N staffing, length of stay and patient outcomes. American Nurses Publishing, Washington DC

Baharestani M M 1994 The lived experience of wives caring for their frail, homebound, elderly husbands with pressure ulcers. Advances in Wound Care 7(3):40–52

Baldwin K M, Ziegler S M 1998 Pressure ulcer risk following critical traumatic injury. Advances in Wound Care 11:168–173

Barczak C A, Barnett R I, Child E J, Bosley L M 1997 Fourth national pressure ulcer prevalence survey. Advances in Wound Care 10(4):18–26

Bergstrom N, Braden B 1992 A prospective study of pressure sore risk among institutionalized elderly. Journal of the American Geriatric Society 40:747–758

Bergstrom N, Braden B, Kemp M, Champagne M, Ruby E 1996 Multi-site study of incidence of pressure ulcers and the relationship between risk level, demographic characteristics, diagnoses, and prescription of preventive characteristics. Journal of the American Geriatric Society 44:22–30

Bergstrom N, Braden B, Kemp M, Champagne M, Ruby E 1998 Predicting pressure ulcer risk. Nursing Research 47(5):261–269

Berlowitz D R, van B Wilking S 1989 Risk factors for pressure sores: a comparison of cross-sectional and cohort-derived data. Journal of the American Geriatrics Society 37:1043–1050

Berlowitz D R, Ash A S, Brandeis G H, Brand H K, Halpern J L, Moskowitz M A 1996 Rating long-term care facilities on pressure ulcer development: importance of case-mix adjustment. Annals of Internal Medicine 124(6):557–563

Berlowitz D R, Brandeis G H, Moskowitz M A 1997 Using administrative databases to evaluate long-term care. Journal of the American Geriatrics Society 45:618–623

Bergquist S, Frantz R 1999 Pressure ulcers in community-based older adults receiving home health care: prevalence, incidence, and associated risk factors. Advances in Wound Care 12:339–351

Blegen M A, Goode C J, Reed L 1998 Nurse staffing and patient outcomes. Nursing Research 47(1):43–50

Bours G J J W, Halfens R J G, Lubbers M, Haalboom J R E 1999 The development of a national registration form to measure the prevalence of pressure ulcers in The Netherlands. Ostomy/Wound Management 45(11):28–40

Brandeis G H, Oois W L, Hossain M, Morris J N, Lipsitz L A 1994 A longitudinal study of risk factors associated with the formation of pressure ulcers in nursing homes. Journal of the American Geriatrics Society 42:388–393

Carlson C E, King R B, Kirk P M, Temple R, Heinemann A 1992 Incidence and correlates of pressure ulcer development after spinal cord injury. Rehabilitation Nursing Research 1(1):34–40

Clark M, Watts S 1994 The incidence of pressure sores within a National Health Service Trust hospital during 1991. Journal of Advanced Nursing 20:33–36

Curry K, Casady L 1992 The relationship between extended periods of immobility and decubitus ulcer formation in the acutely spinal cord-injured individual. Journal Neuroscience Nurs 24(4):185–189

Dimon B 1994 Pressure sores: a case to answer. British Journal of Nursing 39(14):721–727

Foster C, Frisch, S R, Denis N, Forler Y, Jago M 1992 Prevalence of pressure ulcers in Canadian institutions. J Can Ass Ent Ther 11(2):23–31

Fuhrer M J, Garber S L, Rintala D H, Clearman R, Hart K A 1993 Pressure ulcers in community-resident persons with spinal cord injury: Prevalence and risk factors. Arch Phys Med Rehab 74:1172–1177

Haberden W 1815 Some account of a contrivance which was found of singular benefit in stopping the excoriation and ulceration consequent upon continued pressure in bed. Medical Transactions of the College of Physicians London, 5:39–40

Hallett, A 1996 Managing pressure sores in the community. Journal of Wound Care 5(3):105–107

Kanagawa K, Emiko S, Tadaka E et al 1998 Prevalence of pressure ulcers of patient in home visiting nursing service. Nippon Koshu Eisei Zasshi 45(8):758–767

Kemp M G, Keithley J K, Smith D W, Morreale B 1990 Factors that contribute to pressure sores in surgical patients. Research in Nurs & Health 13:293–301

Knutsdottir S 1993 Spinal cord injuries in Iceland 1973–1989. A follow up study. Paraplegia 31:68–72

Langemo D K, Olson B, Hunter S, Hanson D, Burd C, Cathcart-Silberberg T 1991 Incidence and prediction of pressure ulcers in five patient care settings. Decubitus 4(3):25–36

Lewicki L J, Mion L, Splane K G, Samstag D, Secic M 1997 Patient risk factors for pressure ulcers during cardiac surgery. AORN-Journal 65(5):933–942

Lyder C H, Yu C, Stevenson D, Mangat R, Empleo-Frazier O, Emerling J, McKay J 1998 Validating the Braden scale for the prediction of pressure ulcer risk in Blacks and

Latino/Hispanic elders: A pilot study. Ostomy/Wound Management 44(3A):42S–50S

McNees P, Braden B, Bergstrom N, Ovington L 1998 Beyond risk assessment: Elements for pressure ulcer prevention. Ostomy/Wound Management 44(3A):51S–58S

Maklebust J A, Magnan M A 1994 Risk factors associated with having a pressure ulcer: A secondary data analysis. Advances in Wound Care 7(6):25–42

Manley M T 1978 Incidence, contributory factors and costs of pressure sores. South African Medical Journal 53:217–222

Meehan M 1994 National pressure ulcer prevalence survey. Advances in Wound Care 7(3):27–38

Merriam-Webster 1994 Merriam-Webster's collegiate dictionary, 10th edn. Merriam, Springfield

Munro D 1940 Care of the back following spinal-cord injuries: A consideration of bed sores. New England Journal of Medicine 223(11):391–398

National Citizens' Coalition for Nursing Home Reform. Statement before the Maryland Task Force on Quality of Care in Nursing Homes. August 5, 1999. *http://www.nccnhr.org/Updates/md-task-force.htm*. Accessed Sept. 17, 1999.

O'Brien S P, Wind S, van Rijswijk L, Kerstein M 1998 Sequential biannual prevalence studies of pressure ulcers at Allegheny-Hahnemann University hospital. Ostomy/Wound Management 44(3A):78S–89S

O'Dea K 1995 The prevalence of pressure sores in four European countries. Journal of Wound Care 4(4):192–195

Oot-Giromini B A 1993 Pressure ulcer prevalence, incidence and associated risk factors in the community. Decubitus 6(5):24–32

Panel for the Prediction and Prevention of Pressure Ulcers in Adults 1992 Pressure ulcers in adults: prediction and prevention. Clinical practice guideline #3. AHCPR Publication No. 92–0047. Agency for Health Care Policy and Research, Public Health Service, US Department of Health and Human Services, Rockville

Papantonio C J, Wallop J M, Kolodner K B 1994 Sacral ulcers following cardiac surgery: incidence and risk factors. Advance in Wound Care 7(2):24–36

Parish L C, Witkowski J A, Millikan L E 1988 Cutaneous torsion stress: alias the decubitus ulcer: A felony. International Journal Dermatology 27(6):375

Parish L C, Witkowski J A, Crissey J T 1997 Bedsores over the centuries. In: Parish L C, Witkowski C, Crissey J T (eds) The decubitus ulcer in clinical practice. Springer Verlag, Berlin

Perneger T V, Héliot C, Rae A C, et al 1998 Hospital-acquired pressure ulcers. Archives of Internal Medicine 158:1940–1945

Reed L, Blegen M A, Goode C S 1998 Adverse patient occurrences as a measure of nursing care quality. Journal of Nursing Administration 28(5):62–69

Rintala D H 1995 Quality of life considerations. Advances in Wound Care 8(4):28–71–28–83

Sanada H 1997 The effect of support surfaces on pressure ulcers. Journal of Sleep and Environments 4(1):2–9

Salzberg A, Byrne D W, Cayten G, Kabir R, van Niewerburgh P, Viehbeck M, Long H, Jones E C 1998 Predicting and preventing pressure ulcer in adults with paralysis. Advances in Wound Care 11:237–246

Schue R M, Langemo D K 1999 Prevalence, incidence, and prediction of pressure ulcers on a rehabilitation unit. Journal of Wound Ostomy Continence Nursing 26:121–129

Soloway D N 1998 Civil claims relating to pressure ulcers: A claimants' lawyer's perspective. Ostomy/Wound Management 44(2):20–26

Spector W D 1994 Correlates of pressure sores in nursing homes: Evidence from the National Medical Expenditure Survey. Journal of Investigative Dermatology 102:42S–45S

Spector W D, Fortinksy R H 1998 Pressure ulcer prevalence in Ohio nursing homes. Journal of Ageing and Health 10(1):62–80

Thompson, J 1961 Pathological changes in mummies. Proceedings of the Royal Society of Medicine 54:409–415

Torrance C, Maylor M 1999 Pressure sore survey: part one. Journal of Wound Care 8(1):27–30

Tourtual D M, Riesenberg L A, Korutz C J, Semo A H, Asef A, Talati K, Gill R D F 1997 Predictors of hospital acquired heel pressure ulcers. Ostomy/Wound Management 43(9):24–40

van Rijswijk L 1997 The language of wounds. In: Krasner D, Kane D (eds) Chronic wound care: a clinical source book for health care professionals, 2nd edn. Health Management Publications Wayne, pp. 5–8

Zulkowski K 1998 MDS+ RAP items associated with pressure ulcer prevalence in newly institutionalized elderly. Ostomy/Wound Management 44(11):40–53

3 *Jane Nixon*

The pathophysiology and aetiology of pressure ulcers

INTRODUCTION

Pressure ulcers are defined as 'a lesion on any skin surface that occurs as a result of pressure and includes reactive hyperaemia as well as blistered, broken or necrotic skin' (Parish et al 1983). They are complex lesions of the skin and underlying structures and vary considerably in size and severity. The principal causative factor is the application of localized pressure to an area of skin not adapted to the magnitude of such external forces, although the pathology and aetiology are complex.

This chapter outlines both normal and abnormal physiological processes which protect the skin and underlying structures from pressure-induced damage, the pathological mechanisms which lead to skin breakdown and aetiological factors, including the intensity and duration of pressure and the tolerance of the skin (Braden & Bergstrom 1987).

A clear distinction is made between the pathology and aetiology of pressure ulcer development. Pathology is 'the sequence of events that occurs from the time of first injury to the time when the disease expresses itself in functional and structural terms' (Woolf 1998, p. 4), while aetiology is the science of causation (Woolf 1998). Both areas of knowledge support nursing practice by improving our understanding of the complex processes involved, establishing general principles for practice and identifying risk factors relevant to the individual patient.

THE ANATOMY AND PHYSIOLOGY OF THE SKIN

Anatomy of the skin

The tissues involved in pressure ulcer development are the skin, subcutaneous fat, deep fascia, muscle and bone. Skin in particular plays an important role. It is described as the largest organ of the body (Woolf 1998) and is a dynamic structure in which cellular replacement and modification in response to local need is a continual process throughout life (Barton & Barton 1981). It is relatively resistant to water, chemicals and bacteria and provides some protection for the body against mechanical damage. Structurally, it consists of three layers: the epidermis, the dermis and subcutaneous tissue (Fig. 3.1).

Epidermis

The epidermis consists mainly of stratified squamous epithelium (keratinocytes) and a small number of melanocytes (for melanin synthesis), Langerhans cells (antigen-presenting cells) and Merkel cells (neuroendocrine function). The squamous epithelium cells are arranged in four layers: the stratum corneum, granular layer, stratum spinosum and stratum germinativum (or basal layer). The stratum corneum consists of cells which have no nuclei or cytoplasmic organelles, contain little water, are tightly packed and provide a physical barrier against water, bacteria and chemicals. These cells are constantly being shed and replaced by cells from the deeper layers.

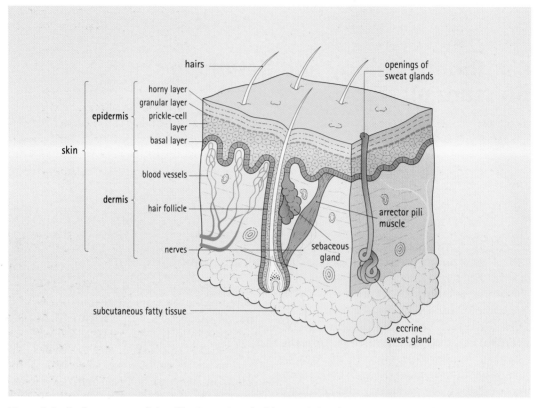

Figure 3.1   Basic structure of the skin. Reproduced with permission from Morison et al (1997), A Colour Guide to the Nursing Management of Chronic Wounds, 2nd edn, Mosby.

Basement membrane

A basement membrane separates the basal layer from the underlying dermis and the basal cells are attached to the membrane by structures known as hemidesmosomes (Fig. 3.2). This basal lamina region consists of four zones: the plasma membrane of the epidermal cells, which contain hemidesmosomes; an electron-lucent area (lamina lucida), which contains the protein laminin; an electron-dense area (lamina densa), consisting of type IV collagen; and extensions of the lamina densa, providing attachments to the underlying dermis (Woolf 1998).

Dermis

The dermis consists of two layers, the papillary dermis and reticular dermis. The former is configured in a series of papillae which are separ-

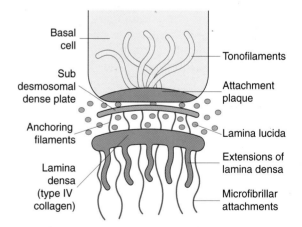

Figure 3.2   The dermoepidermal basement membrane. Reproduced with permission from Woolf (1998), Pathology Basic and Systemic, WB Saunders & Co Ltd.

ated by projections of the epidermis, known as rete pegs (Scales 1990). The collagen/elastin matrix of the papillary dermis is 'loose', and orientated at right angles to the epidermis. It supports loops of blood vessels, known as the papillary (nutritional) capillaries and nerve fibres responsive to touch, pain and temperature (Fagrell 1995, Woolf 1998).

The reticular dermis is beneath an imaginary line joining the tips of the rete pegs and consists of thick collagen bundles orientated parallel to the overlying epidermis (Woolf 1998). It supports blood vessels referred to as the subpapillary (or non-nutritional) vascular bed (Fagrell 1995) as well as sweat glands, sebaceous glands and hair follicles.

It is the collagen and elastin connective tissues which provide the skin with its characteristic recovery following stretching (Scales 1990). Collagen is synthesized in connective tissue fibroblasts, secreted from the cells and stabilized by the formation of cross-linkages which vary in permanence. It constitutes 99% dry weight dermis (Hall 1984). The collagen fibres form a series of layers with fibres in adjacent layers aligned at a fixed angle. When external pressure is applied, the fibres, which are inextensible, rotate relative to one another until they approach a parallel alignment. Tension increases as the fibres move nearer to a parallel alignment, and when external pressure is removed the collagen is restored to its former, open structure by elastic fibres which are intertwined around the collagen bundles (Hall 1984). The process of extension and recoil by rotation and alignment is an important aspect of the property of the collagen/elastin matrix because as well as buffering internal structures of the body it also protects the interstitial fluids and cells of the dermis from external pressure (Krouskop 1983).

Subcutaneous layer

A subcutaneous layer separates the dermis from the deeper structures of deep fascia, muscle and bone. It varies in thickness (depending upon body type, gender and the location on the body) due to the presence of a large number of fat cells, which provide mobility to skin and padding to dissipate pressure. The fat cells are arranged in lobules

which are separated by bands of connective tissue known as interlobular septa (Woolf 1998).

Deep fascia

The deep fascia beneath is a dense essentially avascular, inelastic membrane which covers muscle and muscle groups and over bony prominences may merge with the outer layer of the bone. It is resistant to pressure and it is the last line of protection of vulnerable muscle tissue.

Summary

In summary the skin is characterized by a number of structures which afford protection from mechanical disruption. Tissues beneath, including the layers of subcutaneous fat and deep fascia, also contribute toward protection of the skin's underlying structures. Despite these characteristics pressure ulcers do develop mainly as a result of disruption to the vascular network of arteries, arterioles and capillaries. With continued reference to the anatomical structures described, the following section provides a detailed account of the vascular system and capillary blood flow and briefly highlights vulnerable aspects.

The vascular system

A network of vascular and lymph vessels ensures the supply of necessary nutrients and oxygen to support cell metabolism and epidermal mitosis, blood flow to facilitate temperature regulation and the removal of waste products from the skin.

The arteries supporting the skin pierce the deep fascia and form a network of arterioles in the subcutaneous tissues with capillary branches supplying the hair follicles and sebaceous and sweat glands within the dermis.

Arterioles

The arterioles are highly muscular, which enables changes to their diameter, and branch into a network of metarterioles that have a structure midway between arterioles and capillaries. They do not have a continuous muscle coat, but smooth muscle fibres encircle the blood vessel at intermediate points (Guyton 1992).

Capillaries

The metarterioles further subdivide into capillaries, some of which are large and are called preferential channels and others which are small and are known as true capillaries (Guyton 1992). Smooth muscle cells at the origin of the capillaries act as precapillary sphincters and are important in the control of blood flow (Fig. 3.3).

The capillaries are composed of a single layer of highly permeable endothelial cells surrounded by a basement membrane (Fig. 3.4). Between

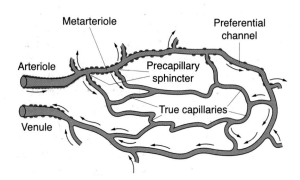

Figure 3.3 The microcirculation. Reproduced with permission from Guyton (1992), Human Physiology and Mechanisms of Disease, 5th edn, WB Saunders & Co.

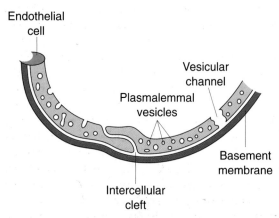

Figure 3.4 Structure of the capillary wall. Reproduced with permission from Guyton (1992), Human Physiology and Mechanisms of Disease, 5th edn, WB Saunders & Co.

each endothelial cell is a small channel referred to as an intercellular cleft and within the endothelial cells are plasmalemmal vesicles. These structures are important in the exchange of nutrients and other substances between the blood and interstitial fluid (Guyton 1992).

After passing through the capillaries, blood enters the venule and returns to the general circulation. The structures including the metarterioles, capillaries and venules are known collectively as the microcirculation (Lamb et al 1980).

Blood flow control mechanisms

An important characteristic of the vascular system is the ability of each tissue to control local blood flow in proportion to need and various acute, and long-term autoregulatory mechanisms are evident to ensure that blood flow is directly related to local tissue demand (Guyton 1992).

Direct observation of the microcirculation by microscope reveals that there is an intermittent ebb and flow through the capillary network controlled by the opening and closing of the metarterioles and precapillary sphincters – a phenomenon known as 'vasomotion' (Kosiak 1961, Guyton 1992). Flow through the metarterioles

---

BOX 3.1 BLOOD FLOW CONTROL MECHANISMS

An important characteristic of the vascular system is the ability of each tissue to control local blood flow. Mechanisms enabling this include:

◆ Active vasomotion within the capillary bed

◆ Capillary-artery feedback (endothelium-derived relaxing factor)

◆ Autoregulation of microcirculation following changes in systemic blood pressure

◆ Veni-arteriolar response

◆ Various nervous and humoral mechanisms.

and capillaries is controlled by local metabolic needs by either the release of a vasodilator substance(s) or oxygen demand, although the exact mechanism is not known (Michel & Gillott 1990). An interplay of osmotic and hydrostatic pressures of plasma and interstitial fluid determine capillary permeability and reabsorption as well as directly affecting the use of lymph vessels in removing proteins, large waste particles and excess fluid (Guyton 1992).

An increase in blood flow through the capillary bed requires an increase in supply from the feeding artery. The local mechanisms which determine capillary blood flow also involve a feedback mechanism which can initiate dilatation of the larger arterial vessels. Rapid flow of blood through the arteries and arterioles causes shear stress on the endothelial cells of the artery wall resulting in the release of endothelium-derived relaxing factor (EDRF). The EDRF then relaxes the arterial muscle and the artery dilates, thus increasing the blood supply. In the long-term, if blood flow continues excessively for days, weeks or months the arterial vessels enlarge (Guyton 1992). Indeed, the size of arterial vessels appears to be readjusted throughout life so that blood flow velocity is never great enough to cause an inordinate amount of blood flow resistance (Guyton 1992).

An acute increase or decrease in arterial blood pressure will result in a surge or reduction in blood flow through a tissue, but within minutes an autoregulatory mechanism readjusts flow to values of approximately $\frac{3}{4}$ of the previous level. The mechanism involved is not clearly understood (metabolic or myogenic), but the resulting autoregulation of blood flow ensures protection of capillaries from excessive pressure and maintains blood flow despite changes in arterial pressure. Over a period of hours, days or weeks a long-term regulatory mechanism is apparent, with control established by changes in the vascularity of the tissue (Guyton 1992, Michel & Gillott 1990).

Similarly, an autoregulatory mechanism, known as the veni-arteriolar response, protects the microcirculation from increases in venous pressure (for example, during standing or venous occlusion). An increase in venous pressure triggers an axon reflex of sympathetic nerve fibres, causing contraction of arterioles and a reduction of flow (Henriksen 1977).

Other mechanisms involved in the control of blood flow include nervous and humoral mechanisms whereby various vasoconstrictor agents (for example, norepinephrine, epinephrine, angiotensin and vasopressin) and vasodilator agents (for example, bradykinin, histamine, prostaglandins and various ions) are released. Some result in systemic effects and others in localized changes to tissue/organ blood flow (Guyton 1992).

Factors affecting blood flow in the skin

Blood flow in the skin varies from individual to individual, is site dependent and is affected by a combination of systemic, local and disease-related factors. These require consideration in the use and interpretation of various technologies in assessing blood flow in the skin and in the identification of possible risk factors in pressure ulcer development.

Individual differences, site-specific variation in skin blood flow and the positive correlation between skin temperature and blood flow are well documented within the research literature (Felder et al 1954, Ek et al 1984, Schubert & Fagrell 1989).

As a consequence, measures of skin blood flow are most commonly used to explore stimulus response, where relative changes rather than absolute values are examined and the effects of the stimuli outweigh other factors influencing blood flow in the test area (Barbenel & Cui 1993).

An increase in blood flow is observed following localized skin trauma and/or infection. The classic response to local trauma is referred to as the triple response, which includes the red reaction, wheal and flare. The red reaction results from capillary dilatation, the wheal from oedema of the local area and the redness spreading out from the injury (the flare) is caused by arteriolar dilatation (Ganong 1999). Similarly, local inflammation of skin or underlying tissue due to infection, chemical trauma, sunburn, radiation damage, and so on, results in increased localized skin blood flow with associated heat, pain and swelling (Soter 1990, Russell et al 1994, Woolf 1998).

The wider literature illustrates disease pathologies which may increase baseline skin blood flow including diabetes mellitus (Tooke & Brash 1996), liposclerotic skin resulting from venous insufficiency (Cheatle et al 1991) and spinal cord injury (Schubert & Fagrell 1991a). Of particular note is that the increase to baseline skin blood flow affects the capacity of the skin to respond to thermal stimuli and localized trauma and a reduced hyperaemic response is observed. This increases the risk of skin damage (Tooke & Brash 1996, Cheatle et al 1991, Schubert & Fagrell 1991a).

The interplay of factors in the control and autoregulation of skin blood flow are clearly illustrated by Tooke & Brash (1996) who review microcirculatory function of 'the diabetic foot'. Early increased microvascular pressure and flow cause an endothelial 'injury response' leading to microvascular sclerosis. With increasing duration of diabetes the sclerotic process results in limitation of vasodilatation with reduced maximal hyperaemia and loss of autoregulation. The increased baseline skin blood flow results in higher skin temperature and it is unclear whether the blood flow is adequate to meet the increased metabolic tissue demand. The pathophysiology is further complicated by peripheral neuropathy, which affects the sympathetic nerve fibres and reduces both the veni-arteriolar and axon flare response. The consequence of these pathophysiological changes is a high prevalence of minor trauma-induced foot ulcers within the diabetic population.

Protective autoregulatory blood flow mechanisms in response to pressure

Of particular interest in pressure ulcer aetiology are autoregulatory mechanisms which affect blood flow during and following pressure assault, including raising of capillary pressure to maintain flow, intermittent flow at subcritical pressures, response to repetitive loading and the reactive hyperaemic response following full/partial occlusion.

When external pressure is applied to the skin, an autoregulatory process allows internal capillary pressure to rise correspondingly. Landis (1930) noted that within 1 minute from the time of external pressure application (60 mmHg) a rise in capillary pressure occurred and stabilized at approximately 10 mmHg higher than the external pressure.

Various researchers have demonstrated that a reduced blood flow is maintained at subcritical external pressures (Daly et al 1976, Romanus 1976, Bader & Gant 1988). Romanus (1976) demonstrated that subcritical pressure applica-

 KEY POINTS

Pressure intensity and pressure: Various autoregulatory mechanisms maintain or restore skin blood flow in response to external pressure:

- Raised capillary pressure in response to external load
- Intermittent blood flow is maintained during subcritical pressure application
- The effect of repetitive loads is reduced with each successive load application
- Critical closing pressures are likely to be in the diastolic/systolic range
- Reactive hyperaemia
- It is the effect of local or point pressure which causes pressure ulcers
- There is no universal pressure threshold above which capillary occlusion occurs
- Low pressure for long periods and high pressure for short periods both cause ulceration
- If both a critical pressure threshold and critical time value is exceeded then tissue damage will proceed at a similar rate regardless of the magnitude of the pressure applied.

tion resulted in temporary circulatory arrest, followed by variable periods of recirculation. Using intravital microscopy he determined that recirculation was characterized by an unevenly distributed, slow and jerky blood flow.

Also of importance is the effect of repetitive loading on skin tissue, as demonstrated by Bader (1990). In two studies involving healthy volunteers the application of external load resulted in a reduction of transcutaneous oxygen tension which partially recovered during the load period. Following load removal, tissue recovery to unloaded oxygen levels was rapid. With each further load application the effect on transcutaneous oxygen tension diminished, demonstrating an active vasomotor response mechanism.

Reactive hyperaemia

Partial or full arterial/capillary occlusion results in an anoxia and a build up of metabolites. Release of pressure produces a large and sudden increase in blood flow through the deprived tissue, a response known as reactive hyperaemia. This was first described by Lewis & Grant (1925) who reported that during occlusion the supplying blood vessels became dilated, providing a reservoir of blood and a rapid high flow following pressure release.

It is thought that there are two mechanisms involved in the post-occlusive reactive hyperaemic response: the immediate post-occlusive blood flow is determined mainly by myogenic mechanisms, and the recovery of blood flow to baseline levels is influenced by metabolic factors (Khan et al 1991). The dominant metabolic driver is undetermined and it is generally believed to be either oxygen deficit or metabolite release from anoxic tissue (Michel & Gillott 1990). It is known that the reactive hyperaemic response is independent of vasomotor control (Michel & Gillott 1990).

The reactive hyperaemic response following occlusion of skin blood flow has been studied by researchers using various techniques including transcutaneous oxygen tension, laser Doppler flow, tissue reflectance spectrophotometry and

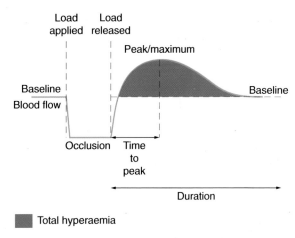

Total hyperaemia

Figure 3.5   Schematic diagram of reactive hyperaemia.

skin temperature. The hyperaemic response can be quantified in various ways and parameters compared within and between groups. A schematic diagram of the commonly used parameters is shown in Figure 3.5.

In normal healthy individuals the magnitude (maximum value), total hyperaemia and duration of the reactive hyperaemic response is related to the duration of the occlusion (Lewis & Grant 1925, Mahanty & Roemer 1979, Hagisawa et al 1994, Walmsley & Wiles 1990). The duration of the hyperaemic response is approximately $\frac{1}{2}$ to $\frac{3}{4}$ of occlusion time, although occlusion times studied are short (Lewis & Grant 1925, Khan et al 1991).

The maximum peak value is inversely proportional to the lowest values during occlusion and related to baseline skin blood flow and skin temperature (Ninet & Fronek 1985, Johnson et al 1986, Walmsley & Wiles 1990, Mayrovitz et al 1997).

Other factors affecting the reactive hyperaemic response are also associated with groups at high risk of pressure ulcer development (Ch. 6), including age and vascular disease. Evidence relating to spinal cord injury is inconclusive.

Comparison of the reactive hyperaemic response following short periods of occlusion in elderly and young subjects has identified lower peak perfusion values and faster time to peak in elderly groups, resulting in a much reduced total hyperaemia (Hagisawa et al 1991, Schubert & Fagrell 1991b). Indeed, mean total hyperaemia values reported by Hagisawa et al (1991) clearly illustrate the reduced hyperaemic response – younger subjects 7236 perfusion units, older subjects 1825 perfusion units.

Patients with symptomatic vascular disease have a reduced or absent hyperaemic response. Reactive hyperaemia is delayed, diminished and prolonged in patients with intermittent claudication, compared with young and elderly controls, and completely absent in many patients with critical ischaemia (Kvernebo et al 1988, Slagsvold et al 1991, 1992). Smokers have a reduced hyperaemic response (Hagisawa et al 1991), as do patients with medical conditions that result in vascular changes including diabetes mellitus (Tooke & Brash 1996), systemic sclerosis (Valentini et al 1991) and end-stage renal failure (Wilkinson et al 1989).

Reactive hyperaemia in the spinal cord injured requires consideration given their high risk of pressure ulcer development. Studies exploring reactive hyperaemia in spinal cord injured subjects have found no differences in the response when compared with able-bodied controls, supporting other evidence that reactive hyperaemia is independent of vasomotor control (Bidart & Maury 1973, Mahanty et al 1981, Hagisawa et al 1991). However, Schubert & Fagrell (1991a), who applied an external pressure known to be above occlusion pressure in the sample population reported significant differences in the percentage rise in skin blood flow over the sacrum and faster time to peak, lower peak and reduced percentage rise in skin blood flow over the gluteus muscle area. These are similar to the effects of ageing on the post-occlusive reactive hyperaemic response. Furthermore, Barbenel & Cui (1993) assessed the skin response of paraplegic subjects to thermal insulation. They found that in able-bodied subjects thermal insulation resulted in a significant rise in both skin temperature and skin blood flow, whereas paraplegic subjects only demonstrated a significant rise in skin temperature. The lack of thermally induced hyperaemia may have clinical consequences and reduce tissue tolerance during pressure assault.

PATHOLOGICAL MECHANISMS LEADING TO SKIN BREAKDOWN

A review of the literature suggests three types of pressure ulcer with possibly three mechanisms which lead to tissue breakdown. The three different types of pressure ulcer described by researchers are:

- necrosis of the epidermis or dermis which may or may not progress to a deep lesion (Groth 1942, Barton & Barton 1981, Witkowsky & Parish 1982)
- deep or 'malignant' pressure ulcers where necrosis is first observed in the subcutaneous tissue (muscle or fat) and tracks outwards (Barton & Barton 1981, Daniel et al 1981)
- full-thickness wounds of dry black eschar (Witkowsky & Parish 1982).

The mechanisms leading to tissue breakdown are not entirely clear from the limited research undertaken to date but at least three pathophysiological processes are evident from the literature:

- occlusion of skin blood flow and subsequent injury due to abrupt reperfusion of the ischaemic vascular bed
- endothelial damage of arterioles and the microcirculation due to the application of disruptive and shearing forces
- direct occlusion of blood vessels by external pressure for a prolonged period, resulting in cell death.

A limitation of research in the area of pressure ulcer pathophysiology is the difficulty in replicating the clinical situation. The majority of pathology research details the microvasculature response to a single pressure assault, whereas, in the clinical environment, patients are exposed to repetitive pressure complicated by friction and shearing forces. It is not possible to determine a dominant pathological mechanism; indeed it is possible that all three mechanisms play a role in the development of pressure-induced skin lesions.

There is also difficulty in determining the point at which the ischaemic assault becomes critical and results in tissue breakdown. Ischaemic conditions can develop even when partial flow is maintained (Xakellis et al 1991) and both clinical and pathological signs of localized trauma, including non-blanching erythema with associated induration and swelling, can resolve without superficial skin loss (Brooks & Duncan 1940, Lowthian 1994). The current research base cannot address this issue.

Occlusion of skin blood flow and tissue reperfusion

The majority of the pathophysiology literature outlines events following a period of critical ischaemia and subsequent reperfusion of skin, leading to pressure ulcer development. Visible changes/loss of skin are followed by deeper tissue destruction.

The application of local pressure resulting in complete occlusion of blood flow causes the squeezing out of blood from the microcirculation and a decrease in both glucose and adenosine triphosphate (ATP), indicating anaerobic cell metabolism (Romanus 1977). Following pressure release, the microvasculature rapidly refills with blood from both the arterioles and venules and a reactive hyperaemic response is observed (Brooks & Duncan, 1940, Husain 1953, Dinsdale 1973, Romanus 1977). The endothelial cells of the capillary wall swell (Dinsdale 1973, Brånemark 1976, Barton & Barton 1981), are infiltrated with leucocytes (Husain 1953) and increase in permeability, resulting in extravasion of red blood cells, white blood cells and plasma leakage into the interstitial space (Dinsdale 1973, Brånemark 1976, Romanus 1976, 1977, Witkowsky & Parish 1982, Romanus et al 1983). White blood cells are observed to adhere to the endothelial wall (Romanus 1976, 1977); red blood cells form rouleaux and thrombi but do not necessarily occlude the vascular lumen (Brånemark 1976, Romanus 1976, 1977, Witkowsky & Parish 1982).

The consequence of these events include localized oedema (Brooks & Duncan 1940, Husain 1953, Romanus 1976, 1977, Witkowsky & Parish 1982) and a significant decrease in blood flow through the microvasculature to either low or no flow (Brånemark 1976, Romanus 1977), resulting

from a combination of increased blood viscosity, obstruction within the vasculature by red and white cells and the reduced vascular lumen (Dinsdale 1973, Brånemark 1976). This response known as the 'no-flow phenomenon' extends the ischaemic assault (Ames et al 1968, Brånemark 1976, Romanus 1977, Lefer & Lefer 1996).

Much of the research pertaining to the pathophysiology of pressure ulcer development was undertaken over 20 years ago. However, the similarities between these early studies of pressure ulcer-related pathological events and the recent literature describing reperfusion injury identifies a common sequence of events suggesting that pressure ulcer development may result from reperfusion injury, a phenomenon which provokes tissue injury due to the process of abrupt reperfusion of the ischaemic vascular bed (Michel & Gillott 1990, Lefer & Lefer 1996, Homer-Vanniasinkam et al 1997). Reperfusion injury is characterized by two distinct but related events: endothelial dysfunction and neutrophil adhesion (Lefer & Lefer 1996).

Altered microvascular permeability, cytoskeletal changes, endothelial cell swelling and neutrophil adhesion are characteristic of endothelial injury during reperfusion, resulting in tissue oedema, capillary plugging by neutrophil adhesion to the endothelium and reduced or no blood flow (Kerrigan & Stotland 1993, Lefer & Lefer 1996, Homer-Vanniasinkam et al 1997). The no-reflow is a consistent feature of reperfusion injury (Homer-Vanniasinkam et al 1997). Important similarities between pressure ulcer pathophysiology and reperfusion injury is that the no-flow phenomenon is not related to thrombus formation but is a combination of factors, including endothelial disruption and swelling, red blood cell rouleaux formation and neutrophil adhesion (Ames et al 1968, Brånemark 1976, Romanus 1976, Homer-Vanniasinkam et al 1997).

The metabolic events which initiate the cellular response of reperfusion injury have been investigated in the major organs of the body in attempts to develop preventative treatments. There are some differences in response between organs that are dependent upon their basic cellular structure and adaptation, but a number of common metabolic features are evident. Biochemical events are complex and a full review is outwith the scope of this chapter. Briefly, during the ischaemic assault, oxygen debt leads to anaerobic metabolism of ATP and a build-up of metabolites. When perfusion is restored biochemical events generate oxygen free radicals which cause cell membrane damage and cellular dysfunction. High levels of intracellular calcium ions, which increase during both ischaemia and reperfusion, also have a pivotal role in cell damage (Kerrigan & Stotland 1993, Homer-Vanniasinkam et al 1997, Ganong 1999).

While the cellular events of pressure ulcer development and reperfusion injury pathophysiology indicate broad similarities, biochemical events have not been explored in relation to the former and firm conclusions cannot, therefore, be drawn. However, from a clinical perspective three pathophysiological features are of potential importance including the initial reactive hyperaemic response, subsequent development of tissue oedema and the low flow–no flow phenomenon.

Subcutaneous tissue necrosis

Two research studies describe pressure-induced lesions which first develop in the muscle, subcutaneous fat or deep dermis and lead to eventual death of the dependent skin area, which sloughs off to reveal a cavity beneath (Barton & Barton 1981, Daniel et al 1981). These are described as 'Type II' pressure ulcers by Barton & Barton (1981) and clinical experience suggests that they are most frequently seen over the trochanter and the sacral areas.

The experimental models describe two processes, repetitive disruptive and shearing forces causing endothelial cell damage and activation of intrinsic clotting mechanisms, particularly in the dermis (Barton & Barton 1981), and a single pressure assault of relatively long duration, resulting primarily in muscle necrosis (Daniel et al 1981). These clearly link to the body sites affected – the sacrum to repetitive disruptive forces (for example, repeatedly slipping down in sitting/semi-recumbent position) and the

trochanter can be exposed to long periods of high external pressure.

Barton & Barton (1981) describe in detail the effect of disruptive and shearing forces in pressure ulcer development by inducing a gait disorder on the foot of the mouse. The external repetitive forces cause distortion of blood vessels, disruption of endothelial cells and activation of intrinsic clotting mechanisms. Platelets aggregate and occlude the affected vessels, causing ischaemic necrosis of dependent tissues. The epidermis was observed to remain intact for a number of days before sloughing off to reveal the extent of the tissue damage beneath (Barton & Barton 1981). Some similarities exist in the pathological events described by Barton & Barton (1981) when compared with reperfusion injury but an important distinction is that platelet aggregation was observed to cause blood vessel occlusion and ischaemia of dependent tissue. It is not clear, however, from the existing research whether two different mechanisms exist, or how applicable Barton & Barton's work is given the severity of repetitive forces induced by the gait disorder.

With respect to muscle damage there is also difficulty in determining the pathological events which lead to necrosis and whether reperfusion exacerbates the primary ischaemic assault. There is also difficulty in determining the point at which the ischaemic assault becomes critical, resulting in pressure ulcer development. Muscle necrosis has been observed even when skin ulceration does not occur (Husain 1953, Nola & Vistnes 1980, Daniel et al 1981). It would seem, however, that two critical components in the development of such sores are underlying bone, which magnifies the pressure by increasing interstitial pressure particularly in the muscle (Guttmann 1976), and that the duration of pressure required is far in excess of clinically accepted periods of immobility.

Prolonged ischaemia resulting directly in tissue necrosis

While areas of dry black eschar are observed clinically there is little evidence within the literature as to the pathological mechanisms involved. However, findings of Witkowsky & Parish (1982), who describe histological changes characteristic of eschar/gangrene, suggest that the mechanism is distinct from those previously described.

Histological changes were reported by Witkowsky & Parish (1982) as follows:

'Black eschar. This phase in the decubitus ulcer spectrum represents full-thickness destruction of the skin. The tissue appears basophilic. Although the general architecture of the dermis is preserved, the cellular details are obliterated. The epidermis is not present in the black eschar. Red blood cells and inflammatory cells are not evident; neither are the other changes previously described in blanchable and nonblanchable erythema and decubitus dermatitis.' (p. 1017)

'The black eschar usually occurs in areas where the skin is thin and bony prominences and tendons are close to the surface. It may occur on normal-appearing skin or be preceded by blanchable erythema, or decubitus dermatitis. In either event, it is usually surrounded by an inner zone of nonblanchable erythema and outer zone of blanchable erythema. The black tissue is grossly dehydrated and compressed. Its acellular, dry nature suggests that necrosis occurred without reperfusion of the skin, unlike what is thought to occur in the other phases of the decubitus spectrum.' (p. 1020).

Similar in description to the 'dry gangrene' most frequently seen in the lower limb in patients with severe atherosclerosis where arterial narrowing has progressed slowly over a long period (Woolf 1998), it suggests that pressure ulcers may, in some instances, arise from prolonged ischaemic assault and direct tissue necrosis. It is unclear which tissue layer has the primary ischaemic injury.

AETIOLOGY OF PRESSURE ULCERS

A review of the mechanisms which protect the skin microvasculature from ischaemic assault and restore local tissue perfusion following occlusion illustrates clearly that there is an interaction between the pressure assault and the capacity of the skin to maintain and effectively restore skin blood flow. A number of autoregulatory mechanisms exist to protect the skin from pressure assault and these processes break down

at pressure values which are highly variable both between and within individuals. The literature also suggests that three differing pathological processes exist and further underline that pressure ulcer development is multidimensional and complex.

Exploration of the aetiology or cause of pressure ulcers reflects the complexities of the factors involved. In order to provide structure within which the current knowledge base can be organized a conceptual schema for the study of the aetiology of pressure ulcers was developed by Braden & Bergstrom (1987) and this provides a useful framework. They identified the critical determinants of pressure ulcers development as the intensity and duration of pressure and the tolerance of the skin and its supporting structure to pressure. At an individual level, pressure ulcers develop as a result of the interaction between these two elements.

Intensity and duration of pressure

The primary cause of pressure ulcers is the application of pressure in areas of skin and tissue not adapted to external pressure assault. Hence, the prevalence of pressure ulcers is greatest among patients with limited mobility and activity (Barbenel et al 1977). While no critical threshold values can be determined in relation to intensity and duration of pressure, important principles can be established to support to nursing practice.

Local verses uniform pressure

The nature of the pressure assault is important in the development of pressure ulcers. An external pressure applied in a uniform or enveloping manner has little, if any, long-term effect upon tissue. For example, a deep sea diver may be subject to extreme (but uniform) external pressure without suffering tissue damage. Similarly, a limb deprived of its blood supply by the application of a tourniquet will not develop a 'pressure sore' as a consequence (Bliss 1993).

It is the effect of the application of a local or point pressure upon the skin which is of interest in pressure ulcer aetiology. Such localized pressure is complicated by shear forces, contact area, underlying bone, bone depth, pressure distribution, contact surface conditions and associated tissue distortion (Bennett & Lee 1985, Sacks 1989, Bliss 1993). This was first observed and discussed by a pioneer in the field of the biomechanical aspects of pressure ulcer formation (Husain 1953). A tourniquet applied to rats' tails produced no permanent changes, with the exception of those exposed to 800 mmHg for 6 h, whereas localized pressure on the leg area produced microscopic changes following 100 mmHg for 2 h. Husain (1953) emphasized the need to distinguish between evenly distributed pressure and localized or point pressure.

Critical pressure thresholds

It appears that the autoregulation processes which maintain skin blood flow during pressure assault break down at pressure values which are highly variable both between and within individuals and there is no universal capillary occlusion threshold value. Furthermore, ischaemic conditions can develop even when skin blood flow is partly maintained (Xakellis et al 1991).

The 'critical closing pressure' is the pressure within a vessel at which it collapses completely and blood flow ceases. It is determined by an interplay of forces, including intravascular pressure, muscle contraction and elastic forces of the blood vessel wall and externally applied pressure (Guyton 1992). In the skin and subcutaneous tissues the interplay of forces is further complicated by the presence of shear and frictional forces (Dinsdale 1974, Bennett & Lee 1985). That at least four variables are involved explains why no individual response is the same, although trends are apparent.

Various researchers report an association between the external pressure required to stop skin blood flow and systemic blood pressure values. Some report an association with diastolic values (Holstein et al 1979, Larsen et al 1979) and others systolic blood pressure (Bennett et al 1981, Holloway et al 1985). Occlusion pressures reported for normal individuals range from 63–138 mmHg (Larsen et al 1979), 100–120 mmHg (Bennett & Lee 1985), 259 (SD ± 97) mmHg (Schubert & Fagrell 1991b) and 400–1000 g (Xakellis et al 1991).

Further variations in occlusion pressures or differences in response to the same load are reported between body sites. Schubert & Fagrell (1991b) reported reduced occlusion pressures at the sacrum of both elderly subjects and elderly long-term hospitalized patients compared with the gluteus. Similar differences were found by Seiler & Stähelin (1979) who applied a localized pressure of $175 \, g/cm^2$ and measured skin oxygen tension over 'hard sites' (trochanteric area) and 'soft sites' (quadriceps area). Oxygen tension in the trochanteric region dropped to approximately one-quarter of the baseline but only to approximately seven-eighths of baseline in the quadriceps region.

Of most interest in relation to pressure ulcer pathophysiology are the low occlusion pressures reported within high-risk patient populations. Bader & Gant (1985, 1988), in studies involving 20 disabled patients and 10 elderly patients, found that the critical pressure load causing the transcutaneous oxygen tension to drop below 20 mmHg ranged from 27 to 108 mmHg. Bennett & Lee (1985) reported that two out of 14 geriatric and ill patients occluded at pressure values of less than 20 mmHg and other research has found reduced occlusion pressures in tetraplegic/paraplegic patients (Schubert & Fagrell 1991a). Similarly, Ek et al (1987) noted that in four hemiplegic patients blood flow ceased at pressures between 11 mmHg and 50 mmHg.

Such variation in individual critical closing pressures is evident in different patient responses to similar clinical conditions. In a study which measured skin blood flow using the laser Doppler technique on 16 patients positioned for 1 h on the same mattress support, four responses were reported – no change (4/16), skin blood flow increase greater than 150% (4/16), skin blood flow decrease by more than 50% (5/16) and no blood flow (3/16) (Frantz et al 1993).

There is also evidence that some patients are unable to respond to repetitive pressure loading of the skin even at comparatively low external pressures. Bader (1990) exposed both normal and debilitated patients to repetitive pressure of 30 mmHg and reported that some debilitated patients showed no recovery during the initial load application; following load removal, recovery was not fully achieved and subsequent loading had a cumulative effect on reducing transcutaneous oxygen. The same cumulative reduction in transcutaneous oxygen was observed for some debilitated patients positioned on a dynamic cushion support (Bader 1990) and intensive care unit (ICU) patients on alternating pressure mattresses (Neander & Birkenfeld 1990).

The manner of pressure application and associated shear forces which reduce the occlusion pressure are also important. Shear reduces the external pressure required to stop blood flow in the skin, and there is evidence that high levels of shear halve the occlusion pressure (Bennett et al 1979). Bennett and colleagues demonstrated that pressure was the primary force responsible for occlusion but that shear force is an important secondary factor. In a later study, Bennett & Lee (1988) also showed that shear forces increase the smaller the compressing object.

Parabolic intensity–duration curve

It is widely quoted that prolonged low pressure is as hazardous as short-term high pressure. Studies which examine the relationship between pressure and time and ulcer/no ulcer all report an inverse relationship between the amount and duration of pressure; that is, low pressure for long periods and high pressure for short periods both cause ulceration (Groth 1942, Kosiak 1959, Dinsdale 1973, Reswick & Rogers 1976).

Data obtained by Reswick & Rogers (1976) from observations in spinal injured patients led to their development of a parabolic intensity–duration curve (Fig. 3.6) which included a 'grey area' representing variations in the tolerance of the skin. Subsequent research described above, however, highlights that skin blood flow is occluded at pressure values lower than levels defined in the curve and direct application in terms of threshold values is inappropriate, but an important principle for practice is established.

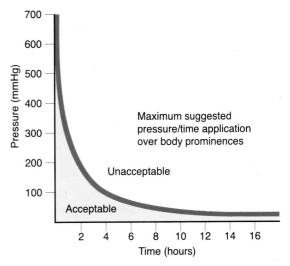

Figure 3.6 Parabolic pressure intensity–duration curve. Reproduced with permission from Reswick & Rogers (1976), Bedsore Biomechanics, Macmillan Press.

Critical time threshold

There is also evidence that once a critical pressure threshold and critical time value is exceeded, then tissue damage will proceed at a similar rate regardless of the magnitude of the pressure applied. This is established by studies which examine the pressure and time/extent of tissue damage relationship and was first demonstrated by Brooks & Duncan (1940), who concluded that the duration of pressure application was of greater importance than the degree of pressure.

Later, Husain (1953) described the effect of localized pressure of varying intensity and duration on skin and muscle tissue of rats, and raw data indicate that low and high pressures over a similar time span produced similar tissue changes. Pressures of 100 mmHg and 600 mmHg both produced patchy congestion when applied for 1–2 h and severe changes when applied for 6 h. The similarity in results was not highlighted by Husain (1953).

A similar omission was made by Kosiak (1961) who applied pressures ranging from 35 to 240 mmHg to the muscle of rats for periods of 1, 2, 3 and 4 h and examined the tissue microscopically. Results indicated that once above a

29

critical pressure (35 mmHg) and critical time value (1 h), as the time of applied pressure increased so did tissue damage. The extent of the tissue damage was the same, regardless of the pressure applied.

Tolerance of the skin to pressure

Braden & Bergstrom (1987) use the term 'tissue tolerance' to 'denote the ability of both the skin and its supporting structures to endure the effects of pressure without adverse sequelae'. They distinguish between extrinsic and intrinsic factors affecting tissue tolerance and describe intrinsic factors as 'those that influence the architecture and integrity of the skin's supporting structures and/or the vascular and lymphatic system that serves the skin and underlying structures.' This conceptual framework is used in the following text to discuss the large number of factors involved in the aetiology of pressure ulcers.

Extrinsic factors

Extrinsic factors associated with pressure ulcer development include friction, moisture and skin irritants, although the evidence base to these factors requires critical review.

Friction clearly increases the susceptibility of the skin to pressure ulceration. Dinsdale (1973), in a study exploring the pathogenesis of pressure ulcers using pigs, found that friction initially removes the stratum corneum and mechanically separates the epidermis above the basal cells. When pressure alone was applied, no pathological changes were observed for pressures of below 150 mmHg. When pressure plus friction was applied, pathological changes were observed for all pressures above 45 mmHg.

Similar findings were later reported in a further study by Dinsdale (1974) who explored pressure intensity and ulcer development. He compared pressure only with pressure plus friction, which were applied over tissues covering the iliac spines of paraplegic and normal pigs. In both instances, more ulcers developed on those exposed to pressure plus friction, with particu-

---

BOX 3.2   FACTORS AFFECTING SKIN TOLERANCE TO PRESSURE

Extrinsic factors

◆ Friction

◆ Incontinence

◆ Skin irritants.

Intrinsic factors – architecture of the skin

◆ Collagen

◆ Age

◆ Nutrition

◆ Spinal cord injury

◆ Steroid administration.

Intrinsic factors – perfusion

◆ Systemic blood pressure

◆ Extracorporeal circulation

◆ Serum protein

◆ Serum haemoglobin

◆ Haematocrit

◆ Smoking

◆ Vascular disease

◆ Vasoactive drug administration

◆ Increased body temperature

◆ Reduced peripheral temperature.

---

larly startling results among the normal pigs. Pressure alone required a level of 290 mmHg to produce ulceration, whereas pressure with friction produced ulcers at 45 mmHg. It was further established, using an isotope clearance technique, that friction did not produce ulcers by an ischaemic mechanism (that is, occlusion) but rather by mechanical disruption of the epidermis (Dinsdale 1974).

The contribution of moisture is linked to pressure ulcer development in numerous aetiological accounts, with particular reference to incontinence. The link was initially identified by early epidemiological studies, such as those conducted by Barbenel et al (1977) and Norton et al (1962). However, there has been further recent debate about the role of incontinence/moisture in pressure ulcer development and whether it is a primary causative factor, a symptom of illness or enhances local friction and shearing forces (Berlowitz & Wilking 1989, Bliss 1993). It is noteworthy that urinary incontinence is not identified by prospective cohort studies which identify key prognostic factors using multivariate statistical analyses (Ch. 6), suggesting that incontinence/ moisture is not a primary factor but a symptom or indicator of poor physical condition, particularly in elderly populations.

It is also suggested that skin irritants such as starch, soap and detergent residues (for example in sheets) are implicated in pressure ulcer development but have been little researched. It is suggested that surface lipids and sebum removed by soap allows dehydration, exposes the skin to water-soluble irritants and bacteria and increases frictional forces (Bettly 1960). It is also suggested that the use of plastic undersheets and skin dampness provide a combination which simulates the closed-patch test technique used by dermatologists and so potentiates the irritant material present (Alberman 1992). The significance of these factors, however, is still unknown.

Intrinsic factors

The complex pathology of pressure ulcer development is clearly reflected by the large number of intrinsic variables associated with pressure ulcer development. An overview is provided of factors affecting the architecture of the skin and tissue perfusion which reduce the capacity to respond to external pressure, friction and shearing forces, illustrating that no single 'causative' factor can be determined but common or recurrent themes are found within the evidence base.

Architecture of the skin   Many intrinsic variables associated with pressure ulcer development directly affect collagen, an important element within the structure of the skin and underlying tissues. There are five types of collagen in the body, each differing in amino acid composition. The adult dermis consists of Type 1 collagen (Hall 1984). Attention to this important structure has developed following observations which revealed that the collagen content of the dermis is reduced following spinal cord injury (Claus-Walker et al 1973).

It appears that collagen prevents disruption to the microcirculation by buffering the interstitial fluid from external load, thereby maintaining the balance of hydrostatic and osmotic pressures. A model of the aetiological events which probably occur when the collagen content of the skin is reduced has been developed by Krouskop (1983), (Fig. 3.7). It is known that as collagen is removed from tissue a larger fraction of an externally applied load is transmitted to interstitial fluids, which leaves the pressurized area (Reddy et al 1975) and, if sufficient, allows cell-to-cell contact and capillary bursting. Krouskop's model provides a framework which interrelates other predisposing factors such as age, nutrition and spinal cord injury which affect the synthesis, maturation and degradation of the connective tissue.

Age-related changes in the collagen content of the skin are particularly interesting. It has been shown that the total collagen content of the skin falls at a steady rate over the age range of 30–80 years (Hall et al 1974). It appears that such changes occur as a result of a gradual reduction in the synthesis of collagen from the ages of 20 to 60 years and a dramatic degradation of collagen in the 60 plus age group (Hall et al 1981). It has also been shown that the administration of steroids mimics the ageing process and leads to a reduction in the collagen content of the skin, which is reversible when treatment is withdrawn (Hall et al 1974).

The synthesis and maturation of connective tissues such as collagen require appropriate macro- and micronutrients and various studies identify an association between nutritional factors and pressure ulcer aetiology. Variables found to be associated with pressure ulcer development include reduced serum protein and albumin (Ek et al 1991, Bergstrom & Braden 1992, Cullum & Clark 1992), decreased body weight

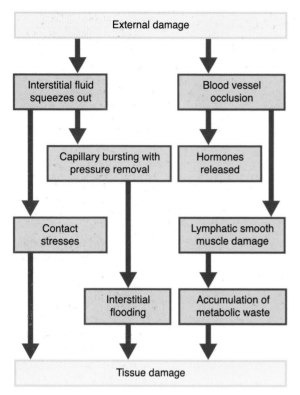

Figure 3.7   Integrated model of tissue damage. Reproduced with permission from Krouskop (1983), Medical Hypotheses, 11: 255–267.

(Allman et al 1995) and impaired food intake (Ek et al 1991, Bergstrom & Braden 1992, Berlowitz & Wilking 1989). However, studies have produced contradictory findings and the data in this area of the literature are complex.

For example, no association between serum albumin and pressure ulcer development was found by five studies (Berlowitz & Wilking 1989, Kemp et al 1990, Marchette et al 1991, Allman et al 1995, Nixon et al 2000). However, serum albumin is complicated by other variables, including age and systolic blood pressure (Dybkaer et al 1981, Phillips et al 1989). It is clear from analysis using multivariate techniques that nutritional factors are associated with pressure ulcer development (Ch. 6) and a full review of these issues is presented in Chapter 13.

Claus-Walker et al (1973) observed an associated breakdown of collagen in the spinal cord injured patient by examining excretion of elec-

trolytes in urine. In a further study, Rodriguez et al (1989) found significantly increased urinary concentration of a collagen metabolite (glucosyl-galactosyl hydroxylysine) in spinal cord injured patients compared to controls. Significant differences were also found between patients with and without skin complications.

Perfusion   A large number of intrinsic factors found to be associated with pressure ulcer development affect tissue perfusion, including systemic blood pressure, extracorporeal circulation (Kemp et al 1990), serum protein (Cullum & Clark 1992), smoking (Guralnik et al 1988, Hagisawa et al 1994), serum haemoglobin (Guralnik et al 1988), haematocrit (Papantonio et al 1994), vascular disease including diabetes and cerebrovascular accident (Berlowitz & Wilking 1989, Brandeis et al 1994, Hoshowsky & Schramm 1994, Nixon et al 2000), cool skin temperature (Nixon et al 2000), vasoactive drug administration (Papantonio et al 1994) and increased body temperature (Bergstrom & Braden 1992, Nixon et al 2000).

The literature again presents contradictory findings; for example, systolic/diastolic blood pressure is significantly associated with pressure ulcer development in three studies (Bergstrom & Braden 1992, Papantonio et al 1994, Nixon et al 2000) and non-significant in three other studies (Berlowitz & Wilking 1989, Cullum & Clark 1992, Allman et al 1995).

Low skin temperature and raised body temperature are also found to be significantly associated with pressure ulcer development (Nixon et al 2000), suggesting both metabolic and perfusion causality. The temperature of tissue affects its metabolic demands and early studies report the effects of increased skin temperature on the magnitude of the hyperaemic response (Catchpole & Jepson 1955) and the protection offered by tissue cooling (Romanus 1976). However, skin temperature is also an indicator of skin perfusion (Guyton 1992), although the relationship is not linear (Felder et al 1954).

The literature suggests an overall trend: that is, the tolerance of the skin is affected by perfusion-related variables but there is no single cause–effect factor. This can be linked to the physiology of blood flow and the interplay of factors which determine capillary blood pressure, exchange mechanisms between capillaries and interstitial fluid (Guyton 1992) and factors affecting the availability of essential nutrients (particularly oxygen) to the local tissue.

CONCLUSIONS

This review of the pathology and aetiology of pressure ulcer development details autoregulatory mechanisms which prevent tissue damage and restore skin perfusion and pathological mechanisms which lead to tissue damage. These processes are affected at an individual level by various aetiological factors particular to individual patients, which determine the ability of the skin to respond to external pressure and maintain skin integrity. While general principles can be established, the complexity of the processes and interplay of factors involved illustrate the multifaceted nature of tissue breakdown and highlight the individual nature of the skin's response to pressure.

CASE STUDY 3.1

Mrs Emery is a 72-year-old lady admitted to hospital following a cerebrovascular accident (CVA) resulting in right-sided hemiplegia. She has been an insulin-dependent diabetic for 10 years and has previously suffered foot ulceration with complete healing achieved by podiatry-led multidisciplinary team intervention.

She remains unconscious for 5 days following admission and has enteral nutritional support. She has been nursed on an alternating pressure mattress since admission and positioned in supine and left lateral positions on a 2–3-hourly basis. The skin on her sacrum, buttocks and hips show no signs of pressure-induced capillary occlusion. However, areas of non-blanching hyperaemia are present on both heels and the outer aspect of her left foot despite regular turning.

1 What are the risk factors for pressure ulcer development?

2 What specific problems are evident in relation to peripheral skin blood flow?

3 If Mrs Emery develops a heel pressure sore what is likely to be the dominant pathological process?

REFERENCES

Alberman K 1992 Is there any connection between laundering and the development of pressure sores? Journal of Tissue Viability 2(2):55–56

Allman R M, Goode P S, Patrick M M, Burst N, Bartolucci A A 1995 Pressure ulcer risk factors among hospitalized patients with activity limitation. Journal of the American Medical Association 273(11):865–870

Ames III A, Wright L, Kowada M, Thurston J M, Majno G 1968 Cerebral ischaemia. II. The no-reflow phenomenon. American Journal of Pathology 52(2):437–453

Bader D L 1990 The recovery characteristics of soft tissue following repeated loading. Journal of Rehabilitation Research and Development 27(2):141–150

Bader D L, Gant C A 1985 Effects of prolonged loading on tissue oxygen levels. In: Spence V A, Sheldon C D (eds) Practical aspects of skin blood flow measurements. Biological Engineering Society, London, pp. 82–85

Bader D L, Gant C A 1988 Changes in transcutaneous oxygen tension as a result of prolonged pressures at the sacrum. Clinical Physical and Physiological Measurement 9(1):33–40

Barbenel J C, Cui Z F 1993 Abnormal thermal hyperaemia in the skin in paraplegia. Physiol Meas, 14:231–239

Barbenel J C, Jordan M M, Nicol S M, Clark M O 1977 Incidence of pressure sores in the Greater Glasgow Health Board Area. Lancet, 2:548–550

Barton A A, Barton M 1981 Skin. The management and prevention of pressure sores. Faber, London, Ch. 2.

Bennett L, Lee B Y 1985 Pressure versus shear in pressure sore causation. In: Lee B Y (ed.), Chronic ulcers of the skin. McGraw Hill, New York, Ch. 3.

Bennett L, Lee B K 1988 Vertical shear existence in animal pressure threshold experiments. Decubitus 1(1):18–24

Bennett L, Kavner D, Lee B Y, Trainor F S 1979 Shear versus pressure as causative factors in skin blood flow occlusion. Archives of Physical Medicine and Rehabilitation, 60:309–314

Bennett L, Kavner D, Lee B Y, Trainor F S, Lewis J M 1981 Skin blood flow in seated geriatric patients. Archives of Physical Medicine and Rehabilitation, 62(8):392–398

Bergstrom N, Braden B 1992 A prospective study of pressure sore risk among institutionalized elderly. Journal of the American Geriatrics Society 40(8):747–758

Berlowitz D R, Wilking S V B 1989 Risk factors for pressure sores: A comparison of cross-sectional and cohort-derived data. Journal of the American Geriatrics Society 37(11):1043–1050

Bettly F R 1960 Some effects of soap on the skin. British Medical Journal 1:1675–1679

Bidart Y, Maury M 1973 The circulatory behaviour in complete chronic paraplegia. Paraplegia 11:1–24

Bliss M R 1993 Aetiology of pressure sores. Reviews in Clinical Gerontology 3:379–397

Braden B, Bergstrom N 1987 A conceptual schema for the study of the etiology of pressure sores. Rehabilitation Nursing 12(1):8–16

Brandeis G H, Ooi W L, Hossain M, Morris J N, Lipsitz L A 1994 A longitudinal study of risk factors associated with the formation of pressure ulcers in nursing homes. Journal of the American Geriatrics Society 42(4):388–393

Brånemark P-I 1976 Microvascular function at reduced flow rates. In: Kenedi R M, Cowden J M, Scales J T (eds) Bedsore biomechanics. Macmillan Press, London, pp. 63–68

Brooks B, Duncan G W 1940 Effects of pressure on tissues. Archives of Surgery 40:696–709

Catchpole B N, Jepson R P 1955 Hand and finger blood Flow. Clinical Science 12:33–40

Cheatle T R, Stibe E C L, Shami S K, Scurr J H, Coleridge-Smith P D 1991 Vasodilatory capacity of the skin in venous disease and its relationship to transcutaneous oxygen tension. British Journal of Surgery 78(5):607–610

Claus-Walker J, Campos R J, Carter R E, Chapman M 1973 Electrolytes in urinary calculi and urine of patients with spinal cord injuries. Archives of Physical Medicine and Rehabilitation 54:109–114

Cullum N, Clark M 1992 Intrinsic factors associated with pressure sores in elderly people. Journal of Advanced Nursing 17(4):427–431

Daly C H, Chimoskey J E, Holloway G A, Kennedy D 1976 The effect of pressure loading on the blood flow rate in human skin. In: Kenedi R M, Cowden J M, Scales J T (eds) Bedsore biomechanics. Macmillan Press, London, pp. 69–78

Daniel R K, Priest D L, Wheatley D C 1981 Etiologic factors in pressure sores: An experimental model. Archives of Physical Medicine and Rehabilitation 62(10):492–498

Dinsdale S M 1973 Decubitus ulcers in swine: Light and election microscopic study of pathogenesis. Archives of Physical Medicine and Rehabilitation 54:51–56 & 74

Dinsdale S M 1974 Decubitus ulcers: Role of pressure and friction in causation. Archives of Physical Medicine and Rehabilitation 55:147–152

Dybkaer R, Lauretzen M, Krakauer R 1981 Relative reference values for clinical, chemical and haematological quantities in 'healthy' elderly people. Acta Med Scandinavica 209:1–9

Ek A-C, Lewis D L, Zetterqvist H, Svensson P-G 1984 Skin blood flow in an area at risk for pressure sore. Scandinavian Journal Rehabilitation Medicine 16:85–89

Ek A-C, Unosson M, Larsson J, Von Schenck H, Bjurulf P 1991 The development and healing of pressure sores related to the nutritional state. Clinical Nutrition 10:245–250

Fagrell B 1995 Advances in microcirculation network evaluation: An update. International Journal of Microcirculation: Clinical and Experimental 15(Suppl 1):34–40

Felder D, Russ E, Montgomery H, Horwitz O 1954 Relationship in the toe of skin surface temperature to mean blood flow measured with a plethysmograph Clinical Scientist 13:251–257

Frantz R, Xakellis G C, Arteaga M 1993 The effects of prolonged pressure on skin blood flow in elderly patients at risk for pressure ulcers. Decubitus 6(6):16–20

Ganong W E 1999 Review of medical physiology, 19th edn. Appleton and Lange, Stamford

Groth K E 1942 Klinische beobachtungen und experimentelle studien uber die enstehung des dekubitus. Acta Chir. Scandinavica, 87, Supplement 76:198 (English summary)

Guralnik J M, Harris T B, White L R, Cornoni-Huntley J C 1988 Occurrence and predictors of pressure sores in the national health and nutrition examination survey follow-up. Journal of the American Geriatrics Society 36(9):807–812

Guttman L 1976 The prevention and treatment of pressure sores In: Kenedi R M, Cowden J M, Scales J T (eds) Bedsore biomechanics. Macmillan Press, London, pp. 153–59

Guyton A C 1992 Human physiology and mechanisms of disease, 5 edn. W B Saunders, Boston

Hagisawa S, Barbenel J C, Kenedi R M 1991 Influence of age on postischaemic reactive hyperaemia. Clinical Phys Physiol Meas. 12(3):227–237

Hagisawa S, Ferguson-Pell M, Cardi M, Miller D 1994 Assessment of skin blood content and oxygenation in spinal cord injured subjects during reactive hyperaemia. Journal of Rehabilitation Research and Development 31(1):1–14

Hall D A 1984 The Biomedical basis of gerontology. John Wright, London

Hall D A, Read F B, Nuki G, et al 1974 The relative effects of age and corticosteroid therapy on the collagen profiles of dermis from subjects with R. A. Age and Ageing, 3:15

Hall D A, Blackett A D, Zajac A R, Switala S, Airey C M 1981 Changes in skinfold thickness with increasing age. Age and Ageing 10(1):19–23

Henriksen O 1977 Local sympathetic reflex mechanism in the regulation of blood flow in the human subcutaneous adipose tissue. Acta Physiologica Scandinavica (Suppl.) 450:7–48

Holloway G A, Tolentino G, De Lateur B J 1985 Cutaneous blood flow responses to wheelchair cushion pressure loading measured by laser Doppler flowmetry. In: Lee B Y (ed.) Chronic ulcers of the skin. McGraw Hill, New York, Ch. 4

Holstein P, Neilson P E, Barras J R 1979 Blood flow cessation at external pressure in the skin of normal limbs. Microvascular Research 17:71–79

Homer-Vanniasinkam S, Crinnion J N, Gough M J 1997 Post-ischaemic organ dysfunction: A review. European Journal of Vascular and Endovascular Surgery 14:195–203

Hoshowsky V M, Schramm C A 1994 Intraoperative pressure prevention: An analysis of bedding materials. Research in Nursing and Health 17(5):333–339

Husain T 1953 An experimental study of some pressure effects on tissues with reference to the bed-sore problem. Journal of Pathology Bacteriology 66:347–358 plus 5 plates

Johnson J M, O'Leary D S, Taylor W F, Kosiba W 1986 Effect of local warming on forearm reactive hyperaemia. Clinical Physiology 6:337–346

Kemp M G, Keithley J K, Smith D W, Morreale B 1990 Factors that contribute to pressure sores in surgical patients. Research in Nursing and Health 13(5):293–301

Kerrigan C L, Stotland M A 1993 Ischaemia reperfusion injury: a review. Microsurgery 14(3):165–175

Khan F, Carnochan F M T, Abbot N C, Wilson S B 1991 The effect of oxygen supplementation on post-occlusive reactive hyperaemia in human forearm skin. International Journal of Microcirculation: Clinical and Experimental 10:43–53

Kosiak M 1959 Etiology and pathology of ischaemic ulcers. Archives of Physical Medicine and Rehabilitation 40:62–69

Kosiak M 1961 Etiology of decubitus ulcers. Archives of Physical Medicine and Rehabilitation 42:19–29

Krouskop T A 1983 A synthesis of the factors which contribute to pressure sore formation. Medical Hypotheses 11:255–267

Kvernebo K, Slagsvold C E, Gjolberg T 1988 Laser Doppler flux reappearance time (FRT) in patients with lower limb atherosclerosis and healthy controls. European Journal of Vascular Surgery 2:171–176

Lamb J F, Ingram C G, Johnston I A, Pitman R M 1980 Essentials of physiology. Blackwell Scientific Publications

Landis E M 1930 Micro-injection studies of capillary blood pressure in human skin. Heart 15:209–228

Larsen B, Holstein P, Lassen N A 1979 On the pathogenesis of bedsores: Skin blood flow cessation by external pressure on the back. Scandinavian Journal of Plastic and Reconstructive Surgery 13:347–350

Lefer A M, Lefer D J 1996 The role of nitric oxide and cell adhesion molecules on the microcirculation in ischaemia-reperfusion. Cardiovascular Research 32(4):743–751

Lewis T, Grant R 1925 Observations upon reactive hyperaemia in man. Heart 12:73–120

Lowthian P 1994 Pressure sores: A search for definition. Nursing Standard 9(11):30–32

Mahanty S D, Roemer R B 1979 Thermal response of skin to application of localized pressure. Archives of Physical Medicine and Rehabilitation 60(12):584–590

Mahanty S D, Roemer R B, Meisel H 1981 Thermal response of paraplegic skin to the application of localized pressure. Archives of Physical Medicine and Rehabilitation 62(12):608–611

Marchette L, Arnell I, Redick E 1991 Skin ulcers of elderly surgical patients in critical care units. Dimensions of Critical Care Nursing 10(6):321–329

Mayrovitz H N, Smith J, Delgado M, Regan M B 1997 Heel blood perfusion responses to pressure loading and unloading in women. Ostomy and Wound Management 43(7):16–26

Michel C C, Gillott H 1990 Microvascular mechanisms in stasis and ischaemia. In: Bader D L (ed.) Pressure sores clinical practice and scientific approach. Macmillan Press, London, pp. 153–164

Morison M, Moffatt C, Bridel-Nixon J, Bale S 1997 A colour guide to the nursing management of chronic wounds, 2nd edn. Mosby, London, p. 120

Neander K-D, Birkenfeld R 1990 Alternating-pressure mattresses for the prevention of decubitus ulcers: A study of healthy subjects and patients. Intensive Care Nursing 6:67–73

Ninet J, Fronek A 1985 Cuteneous postocclusive reactive hyperemia monitored by laser Doppler flux metering and skin temperature. Microvascular Research 30:125–132

Nixon J, McElvenny D, Mason S, Brown J, Bond S 2000 Prognostic factors associated with pressure sore development in the immediate post-operative period. International Journal of Nursing Studies 37(4):279–289

Nola G T, Vistnes L M 1980 Differential response of skin and muscle in the experimental production of pressure sores. Plastic and Reconstructive Surgery 66(5):728–735

Norton D, McLaren R, Exton-Smith A N 1962 An investigation of geriatric nursing problems in hospital. Churchill Livingstone, Edinburgh

Papantonio C T, Wallop J M, Kolodner K B 1994 Sacral ulcers following cardiac surgery: Incidence and risks. Advances in Wound Care 7(2):24–36

Parish L C, Witkowski J A, Chrissey J T 1983 The decubitus ulcer. Masson Pub., New York

Phillips A, Shaper G A, Whincup P H 1989 Association between serum albumin and mortality from cardiovascular disease, cancer and other causes. Lancet ii:1434–1436

Reddy N P, Krouskop T A, Newell P H 1975 Biomechanics of a lymphatic vessel. Blood Vessels 12:261–278

Reswick J B, Rogers J 1976 Experience at Ranchos Los Amigos Hospital with devices and techniques to prevent pressure sores. In: Kenedi R M, Cowden J M, Scales J T (eds) Bedsore biomechanics. Macmillan Press, London, pp. 301–313

Rodriguez G P, Claus-Walker J, Kent M C, Garza H M 1989 Collagen metabolite excretion as a predictor of bone- and skin-related complications of spinal cord injury. Archives of Physical Medicine and Rehabilitation 70(6):442–444

Romanus E M 1976 Microcirculatory reactions to controlled tissue ischaemia and temperature: a vital microscopic study on the hamster's cheek pouch. In: Kenedi R M, Cowden J M, Scales J T (eds) Bedsore biomechanics. Macmillan Press, London, pp. 79–82

Romanus M 1977 Microcirculatory reactions of local pressure induced ischaemia: A vital microscopic study in hamster cheek pouch and a pilot study in man. Acta Chirurgica Scandinavica 479(Supplement):1–30

Romanus M, Svensjö E, Ehira T 1983 Microvascular changes due to repeated pressure-induced ischemia: Intravital microscopic study on hamster cheek pouch. Archives of Physical Medicine and Rehabilitation 64:553–555

Russell N S, Knaken H, Bruinvis I A D, Hart A A M, Begg A C, Lebesque J V 1994 Quantification of patient to patient variation of skin erythema developing as a response to radiotherapy. Radiotherapy and Oncology 30:213–221

Sacks A H 1989 Theoretical prediction of a time-at-pressure curve for avoiding pressure sores. Journal of Rehabilitation Research and Development 26(3):27–34

Scales J T 1990 Pathogenesis of pressure sores In: Bader D L (ed.) Pressure sores clinical practice and scientific approach. Macmillan Press, London, pp. 15–26

Schubert V, Fagrell B 1989 Local skin pressure and its effects on skin microcirculation as evaluated by laser-Doppler fluxmetry. Clinical Physiology 9(6):535–545

Schubert V, Fagrell B 1991a Postocclusive reactive hyperaemia and thermal response in the skin microcirculation of subjects with spinal cord injury. Scandinavian Journal of Rehabilitation Medicine 23(1):33–40

Schubert V, Fagrell B 1991b Evaluation of the dynamic cutaneous post-ischaemic hyperaemia and thermal response in elderly subjects and in an area at risk for pressure sores. Clinical Physiology 11(2):169–182

Seiler W O, Stähelin H B 1979 Skin oxygen tension as a function of imposed skin pressure: Implication for decubitus ulcer formation. Journal of the American Geriatrics Society 27(7):298–301

Slagsvold C-E, Rosén L, Stranden E 1991 The relation between changes in capillary morphology induced by ischemia and the postischemic transcutaneous PO_2 response. International Journal of Microcirculation: Clinical and Experimental 10:117–125

Slagsvold C-E, Stranden E, Rosén L, Kroese A J 1992 The role of blood perfusion and tissue oxygenation in the postischemic transcutaneous PO_2 response. Angiology – The Journal of Vascular Diseases 43(2):155–162

Soter N A 1990 Acute effects of ultraviolet radiation on the skin. Seminars in Dermatology 9(1):11–15

Tooke J E, Brash P D 1996 Microvascular aspects of diabetic foot disease. Diabetic Medicine 13 Supplement:S26–S29

Valentini G, Leonardo G, Moles D A, Apaia M R, Maselli R, Tirri G, DEL Guercio R 1991 Transcutaneous oxygen pressure in systemic sclerosis: Evaluation at different sensor temperatures and relationship to skin perfusion. Archives of Dermatological Research 283:285–288

Walmsley D, Wiles P G 1990 Reactive hyperaemia in the skin of the human foot measured by laser Doppler flowmetry: effects of duration of ischaemia and local heating. International Journal of Microcirculation: Clinical and Experimental 9(4):345–355

Wilkinson S P, Spence V A, Stewart W K 1989 Arterial stiffening and reduced cutaneous hyperaemic response in patients with end-stage renal failure. Nephron 52:149–153

Witkowski J A, Parish L C 1982 Histopathology of the decubitus ulcer. Journal of the American Academy of Dermatology 6(6):1014–1021

Woolf N 1998 Pathology basic and systemic. WB Saunders, London

Xakellis G C, Frantz R A, Arteaga M, Meletiou S 1991 A comparison of changes in the transcutaneous oxygen tension and capillary blood flow in the skin with increasing compressive weights. American Journal of Physical Medicine and Rehabilitation 70(4):172–177

4 *Peter J Franks and Mark E Collier*

Quality of life: the cost to the individual

INTRODUCTION

Quality of life is a term which has entered the popular vocabulary over the last 20 years. Frequently, we hear of how people change their lifestyles to improve their 'quality of life' or how new inventions are likely to make our lives easier and so improve our 'quality of life'. This is a widely used phrase but one which is rarely adequately defined. One of the reasons for this may be an individual perspective of what constitutes 'quality' in life. To some, it may mean financial security, to others the freedom to do what one wants, be it freedom to express oneself or freedom to live one's life as one wishes. In this chapter, information will be presented on why quality of life (QoL) is a key factor in health care, how QoL tools are developed and how they may be used; their uses and limitations in evaluations of patients who suffer from pressure ulceration will also be indicated.

What do we mean by health?

Before considering quality of life as a construct, it is important to define what is meant by health. Investigations, which look at quality of life in relation to health require a definition of health. To many, health is considered to be the lack of disease. However, in 1946 the World Health Organization (WHO) wished to present a broader picture of health. It defined health as 'a state of complete physical, mental and social well-being and not merely the absence of disease' (WHO 1958). Thus, a state of 'ill' health may not be just the sensations of pain or discomfort directly related to one particular disease process but also loss of functioning and emotional state which may accompany deterioration in the patient's general condition. In the WHO definition, the patient is central to the concept of health since it is their own sense of well-being which is considered paramount, not simply a clinical or diagnostic procedure to establish the presence of disease. Within this the patient may 'feel' ill without clinical evidence of disease. In medicine, there is an ever-increasing reliance on technology to confirm diagnoses and indicate the severity of such disease, with little regard for how those diseases may affect the patient. However, there is now growing recognition that these techniques do not fully explain the impact of disease on the patient. There is a need to establish factors that are important to the patient in terms of impact on lifestyle and benefits of treatment.

Why measure quality of life?

Until the middle of the twentieth century medicine was widely perceived to be the fight against infectious diseases such as tuberculosis, cholera and typhoid. With changes in public health and the emergence of new anti-infective drugs such as penicillin, the fight against infection has been largely won in Western societies. However, with this reduction in infectious diseases came a corresponding increase in chronic diseases such as cancer and atherosclerosis, which had profound effects on the patients' lives. For infectious diseases, treatment led to clinical cure and hence to improvements in survival. With chronic diseases cure was rarely possible. Patients could live for many years with these diseases, which although less likely to lead to death in the short term, led to severe and chronic disability. The aims of treatment shifted from improving survival to the alleviation of symptoms, restoring function and returning the patient to their pre-disease levels of activity wherever possible. Quality of life research grew out of clinical trials of early cancer therapies. In these trials, patients were subjected to highly toxic therapies to improve their survival. It soon became clear, however, that patients experienced extreme side-effects from this treatment, with very little improvement in survival – often just a matter of a few additional weeks of life. From these studies it became clear that survival should not be the only consideration in evaluating health care interventions, but that quality of life could be as important as quantity of life.

HEALTH-RELATED QUALITY OF LIFE

Limitations of clinical outcomes in pressure ulceration

Pressure ulceration is rarely the principal cause of death in patients, so outcomes of treatment other than survival must be considered. Studies in pressure ulceration frequently use clinical cure (complete healing) as the outcome of interest. While this may be of value to the health care professional in a clinical trial of therapies, this is of limited value in evaluating the potential benefit to patients. Using clinical cure as the principal outcome makes the assumption that an outcome that is less than complete healing is of no benefit to the patient. In clinical studies of wound management it is frequently found that pain reduces significantly with effective treatment irrespective of whether the ulcer heals (Franks et al 1999a). Clearly, this benefit perceived by the patient cannot be evaluated when the outcome is a simple dichotomous variable. There is also evidence from other areas of health care that clinical cure may not be well correlated with the patient's perceived 'wellness'. Moreover, clinical cure makes the assumption that following healing, the

patient has achieved the maximum benefit from treatment. There is evidence that after healing it takes the patient some time to return to their previous levels of activity, a concept that cannot be described when using clinical cure as the only outcome of treatment. Clearly, the clinical outcomes of treatment are important but they may not fully describe the extent of the patient's perceived benefit of treatment.

Health-related quality of life

Despite acknowledging the need to assess quality of life there was and still is much debate over what constitutes quality of life. In the 1980s the term 'health related quality of life' (HRQoL) was offered as an alternative (Bullinger 1993). This is an easier concept to describe than quality of life, since it focuses on how health impacts on the patient's life. HRQoL is defined as 'the impact of a disease on patients' physical and mental well being, their ability to function socially and to describe their general health' (Bullinger 1993). This has a patient-based focus which attempts to assess the impact of disease on disability and activities of daily living. Fulfilment in HRQoL may be challenged not only by the disease process under study, but also the side-effects of treatment, other concurrent diseases and their treatment. These factors may have a profound effect on the patient suffering from pressure ulceration. While pressure ulceration may be an important contribution to the patient's ill health, the ulceration is rarely the principal reason for treatment. Pressure ulceration usually develops as a consequence of some other factors which cause temporary or longer-term restrictions in mobility, and other cofactors which put the patient at risk of pressure ulcer development. Thus, the pressure ulcer may contribute only part of the impact of health on the patient's life. The severe loss of function caused by stroke, dementia or multiple sclerosis is likely to have a greater overall impact on the patient than the pressure ulcer per se. The challenge in assessing HRQoL in these patients is attempting to tease out the factors that are likely to be influenced by the ulceration while acknowledging the broader holistic problems of the patient suffering from ulceration with many other pathologies.

What do we need to measure?

Health-related quality of life is an easier concept to describe than quality of life but there is still some debate over the precise domains that need to be assessed. Price (1996) reviewed the early work in the development of these tools and indicated that different researchers have developed models of HRQoL based on different domains that they believe to be important. For example, Fallowfield (1990) suggested four core domains: psychological, social, occupational and physical. Others have suggested up to six core domains, while Todd (1992) proposed that the domains of physical, social and psychological aspects are sufficient to describe the impact of disease on patients. In all these models there are a number of common themes key to the patient's life, namely physical, mental and social domains. These themes will be discussed in more detail in relation to the generic tools commonly used in HRQoL assessment later in this chapter.

ASSESSING HEALTH-RELATED QUALITY OF LIFE

Having established the need for assessments of health-related quality of life, the task then becomes to develop a tool to assess these. Psychologists and other health care professionals have worked together to develop tools which attempt to address the problems in patients' lives which poor health leads to. Initial studies in the development of these tools use qualitative methods to establish the areas of the patient's life which are affected by the disease either through one-to-one interviews or focus groups. Open-ended prompts may be used to lead patients to express their personal feelings about the problems they face, what is important to them and what they most hope and expect to achieve from treatment. A preliminary questionnaire is developed from the themes that appear to be common within these discussions. To confirm the relevance of these items the questionnaire is then tested on a different sample of patients suffering from the same disease. Questions that are found to be irrelevant, or themes which may have been missed are subtracted and added accordingly.

Within an HRQoL tool several conditions must be fulfilled before the tool is considered scientifically acceptable. The tool must be relevant to the patients suffering from the particular disease under investigation. This would normally be achieved through the questionnaire development procedure outlined above. Developing a tool through this qualitative method assures the health researcher of its relevance to the patient population under investigation. Moreover, the tool must also fulfil other scientific criteria:

- **validity** is the ability of the tool to measure what it purports to measure
- **repeatability** examines how robust the tool is under stable conditions; this is usually described in terms of the intra- and inter-observer agreement (or error)
- **sensitivity** to change describes the ability of a tool to detect changes when there is a real change in the patient's status.

While HRQoL tools may be of value in describing individuals, samples and populations, when evaluating health care treatments, we must be assured that when the patient's status changes this is reflected in changes in the tools which are used to measure HRQoL. Often, the use of HRQoL tools in outcome studies may fail to detect changes which are detected by changes in clinical outcomes. This need not mean that the HRQoL is insensitive, but may indicate that the change is not great enough to be detected by the patient. As already discussed, the patient who suffers from pressure ulceration is likely to suffer a number of other serious conditions, all of which may have a greater or lesser impact on their lives. These other disease processes may mask the benefit perceived by a change in the pressure ulcer. Another problem of evaluation using HRQoL tools in patients with pressure ulceration is the reliance on the patients to provide information. Patients who are susceptible to pressure ulcers can also be suffering from concomitant difficulties in expressing themselves. Problems such as stroke and dementia will often make the completion of questionnaires problematic. In a study of 75 patients suffering from pressure ulceration, 20% were unable to complete the questionnaire even with assistance from the research nurse (Franks et al 1999b). Some have advocated the use of proxies such as a close relative, friend or clinician in evaluating HRQoL issues in wound care (Rives et al 1997), but this remains controversial, particularly since one of the fundamental aspects of HRQoL is the personal nature of the experience of living with pressure ulceration.

Generic tools

In HRQoL research there are two broad questionnaire methods of patient evaluation. Generic tools, as their name suggests, are tools that are developed from population samples that relate to HRQoL in broad terms. They are valuable because they do not ask questions specific to particular diseases and may be used across a range of diseases and patient populations. Many are well validated within different countries and cultures and some have been translated for many languages. These 'off the shelf' tools are invaluable in comparing different populations and may be used to compare the impact of different diseases on HRQoL. The generic tools have been used in studies of leg ulceration both in descriptive studies (Lindholm et al 1993, Price & Harding 1996, Franks & Moffatt 1998), as outcome measures in evaluation studies (Franks et al 1994) and clinical trials (Franks et al 1999a). The most commonly used generic tools are the Nottingham Health Profile (NHP) (Hunt et al 1986) and MOS Short Form-36 (SF-36) (Ware et al 1993), both of which are highly validated tools which have been used in a variety of diseases and clinical situations. The generic tools may be valuable in patients who suffer from pressure ulceration because of their validity and the knowledge that these tools have been shown to be valuable in evaluating outcomes of wound treatment. In the following text the NHP and SF-36 are described in relation to three core areas of HRQoL: physical, social and psychological impact.

Physical problems

Lack of mobility is the key risk in the development of pressure ulceration, and assessment of mobility is an important part of the generic tools. Mobility does not merely mean the ability to walk but encompasses other aspects of daily living from which the patient needs movement to function. In the NHP for example, the domain of physical mobility is generated from eight questions (Hunt et al 1986). Some of these describe the process of walking and standing, but others relate to the ability to bend, reach for things and ability to dress oneself. In the SF-36, mobility is described in two scales, physical functioning and role-physical (Ware et al 1993). Physical functioning is the extent to which health limits physical activities, including self-care and walking, while role-physical examines the extent to which physical health interferes with work or other daily activities. Clearly, one would expect that patients suffering from pressure ulceration would have deficits in the ability to perform tasks and reduced mobility would interfere with the activities of daily life.

In addition to these factors directly related to physical problems, the NHP has scales for energy, pain and sleep, all of which are physical problems, but which may be associated with or heightened by the patient's psychological status. Similarly, the SF-36 has additional scales for pain, vitality and general health perception, again manifestations of physical problems associated with psychological status.

Social problems

It would not be unreasonable to expect that patients who suffer from pressure ulceration would experience deficits in their ability to socialize. Frequently, these patients are bed- or chair-bound, often being unable to leave their own homes. Within the NHP social isolation describes the ability of patients to interact with family and friends. Items such as the sense of loneliness, difficulty in getting close to others and the sense of being a burden to others are included within the five-item score. For the SF-36, social functioning is the extent to which physical or emotional problems interfere with normal social activities. Just two questions relate to this sense of social isolation.

Psychological problems

Understanding the psychological factors involved in health is important in obtaining a rounded sense of the patient's well-being. It is known for example that patients suffering from leg ulceration have heightened depression and hostility levels, which are reduced on ulcer healing (Franks et al 1994). The NHP evaluates psychological status of the patient within the emotional reactions sub-scale. This is a nine-question scale that looks at questions on the feelings of being down, on edge, worried and a sense of hopelessness. Within the SF-36 this is accounted for within the role-emotional and mental health scales. Role-emotional is the extent to which emotional problems interfere with everyday activities, while mental health looks at the specific characteristics of mental illness, such as depression, anxiety and emotional control.

Disease-specific tools

The generic HRQoL tools are valuable, but they have certain limitations in their use. The assumption when using generic tools is that the tool will be capable of detecting factors that affect the patient. However, when using such a broad tool there may be problems associated with the lack of sensitivity to factors that relate directly to the disease under investigation. In pressure ulceration, the development of a foul-smelling exudate may have a great impact on the patient, but this would not be detected as a problem within the generic tools. A disease-specific tool would be developed to look at factors that relate directly to the disease under investigation. As with the generic tools they are normally developed using the qualitative methods described previously. The disadvantages of the disease-specific tools are the need for extensive validation, which is often not performed adequately, and that the tools cannot be used to compare across different diseases. The methodology used to develop disease-specific tools underlines the role played by patients in its development and how their experiences shape the content of the tool. Despite the many advantages of these tools they have not been developed for all diseases because of the cost in both time and financial resources. At present, there do not appear to be any tools being developed that are specific to pressure ulceration.

Should generic or disease-specific tools be used?

In the previous sections the differences between generic and disease-specific tools were discussed. However, the challenge for the clinician is to make a considered opinion on which type of tool to use. To a certain degree, the type of tool chosen will depend on the study being performed. For comparative studies between diseases or between disease and population norms it is essential that generic tools should be the principal method of assessment. However, within a disease, whether it is a cross-sectional study or outcome study, one should consider the relevance of a disease-specific tool. Increasingly, researchers are choosing to use a generic tool and specific tool in combination. This allows for comparisons across populations and between diseases while retaining the sensitivity of the disease-specific tools. Within pressure ulceration we are limited in that, to date, no disease-specific tool has been developed. In leg ulcer disease there are a number of tools which are relevant: in particular the Exeter tool for the evaluation of patients with chronic leg ulceration (Hyland et al 1994), two questionnaires which have been designed for use in patients with chronic venous insufficiency (Launois et al 1996, Klyscz et al 1998) (of which chronic venous ulceration is the most severe form) and a questionnaire designed for use in patients with chronic venous ulceration (Smith et al 2000). While the evidence has been presented for the rational development of these tools, they have yet to be widely adopted in studies of patients with ulceration. Some of the issues described by patients with chronic leg ulceration will also be relevant to patients with pressure ulceration but there are clear areas of difference. As previously discussed, pressure ulceration is rarely

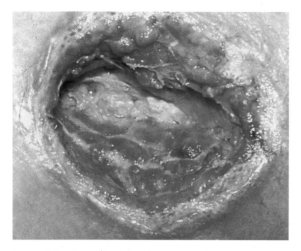

Figure 4.1 A grade IV sacral pressure ulcer.

the primary cause for patient care but is a consequence of another disease process leading to immobility, and other cofactors which increase the risk of pressure ulcer development. In leg ulceration, while the patient may have other pathologies, it is the ulceration which is usually the principal reason for care. For patients with pressure ulceration it is important to separate the effects of the ulceration and those of other processes (Fig. 4.1). The impact of pressure ulceration may be relatively small when compared with the overall health problems of the patients receiving community nursing care. It is expected that a tool specific to patients suffering from pressure ulceration would help to describe some of the subtle effects on the patients and allow one to evaluate the success of any intervention project proposed.

Economic impact on the individual

Health economists have attempted to determine the best treatments using economic models of health care and in particular the use of cost effectiveness and cost utility analysis (CUA). While the former may use quality of life as an outcome measure it is CUA which considers patients' quality as well as quantity of life. It derives utility scores which give a quality of life 'value' for the duration of follow-up studies, with perfect health equalling one and death having a

value of zero. This is a useful tool in that it combines quality and quantity of life in one measure. Thus, any change in the patient's status would be reflected as a change in their utility score. Changes in the pressure ulceration that do not benefit the patient's overall state would not be expected to change their utility. This is a useful tool in the health economist's armoury and is discussed in more detail in Chapter 5.

THE RIVERSIDE PRESSURE ULCER STUDY

In 1994, the Riverside Pressure Ulcer Study was established with the aims of evaluating care of patients being treated by community nurses (Franks et al 1999b). Within the study, patients with pressure ulcers were recruited together with patients who did not suffer from pressure ulceration, but who were receiving care for causes other than pressure ulceration, and who might be at risk of pressure ulcer development. During the 6-month recruitment period 75 patients suffering from a current pressure ulcer were recruited from the Riverside Community Nursing Service and were compared with 100 patients who were not suffering from a current pressure ulcer. While there were some differences between the two groups in terms of medical history and pressure ulcer risk derived from both the Waterlow and Braden scores, the similarity between the two patient groups is striking. Using the SF-36 it was possible to compare the patients with pressure ulceration with a UK normal population. In this analysis, age-specific values are not available, although data have been published on a random sample of the elderly. Comparison of the score in the patients with pressure ulceration and the 70–74-year-old normal population indicated that there were two scores within the SF-36 which were statistically different (Fig. 4.2). Both physical functioning (mean [95% confidence interval, CI] difference = −41 [−47 to −34], $P < 0.001$) and social functioning (difference = −35 [−44 to −25], $P < 0.001$) showed that patients suffering from pressure ulceration had a deficit in these two areas of their lives. However, when comparing patients with pressure ulceration and patients

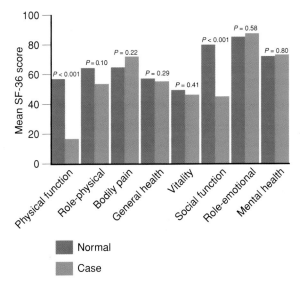

Figure 4.2 Comparison between cases (with pressure ulcers) and population normals.

with no ulceration being cared for by community nursing staff, these two differences largely disappeared. Instead, a significant difference was evident in the scale of role-physical (mean 54 versus 72, $P = 0.026$) (Fig. 4.3). This subscale gives

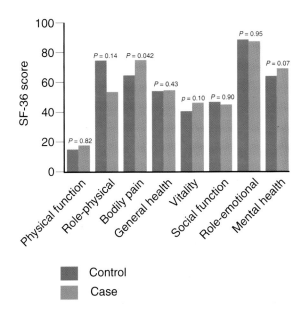

Figure 4.3 Comparison between cases (with pressure ulcers) and controls (without pressure ulcers) selected from community nursing caseloads.

an indication of how physical problems interfere with daily activities, in particular limiting and reducing the number of different activities being performed. Interestingly, while pain is perceived to be an important factor in pressure ulceration no significant differences were observed between patients suffering from pressure ulceration, their population norms or the controls. Indeed, the scores for bodily pain were higher in the patients with ulceration (indicating less pain) than both comparative groups. This would indicate that pain may be less of a problem than previously assumed, or that pain control was more effective in the patients suffering from pressure ulceration than in the other groups. Clearly, this is an area that deserves comprehensive investigation.

WHAT WE KNOW, WHAT WE NEED TO KNOW

In this chapter we have attempted to give an overview of the evidence behind quality of life assessments in patients suffering from pressure ulceration. One clear message is the general lack of studies that have tried to evaluate this. We have shown that generic tools may be inadequate to give a picture of patients suffering from this condition. While these tools do indicate certain deficits in patient's lives, this holistic approach generally fails to show the subtle differences between patients with and without ulceration who are receiving community nursing care. Thus, the overall chronicity of patients who receive care may be poorer than the general population. With this in mind, it is essential that researchers consider the development of a tool that is specific to patients suffering from pressure ulceration. There is now a demand for patient-led outcomes and HRQoL is an important measure both to assess the impact of the disease and as an outcome measure in clinical evaluations and trials. With an ageing population and increasing number of litigation cases, it is likely that pressure area care will become increasingly important in both community and acute care. The need to evaluate the impact of this problem on patients and to develop meaningful outcomes of treatment becomes greater by the day.

4

Mr and Mrs James were born in 1919 in Northumberland. They have known each other since childhood and married in 1939, just before Mr James joined the navy. After the war Jim became a coalface worker in the local pit, where he worked for the next 30 years. His wife Jessie never took up full-time employment, remaining at home to care for their three children. Jim retired from the mine on medical grounds at the age of 55. He had been diagnosed as suffering from severe, chronic bronchitis and osteoarthritis, for which he was prescribed non-steroidal anti-inflammatory and analgesic drugs on a daily basis. The orthopaedic surgeons considered him to be a poor candidate for surgery, and with Mr James' agreement it was decided that he should receive symptomatic relief only. Despite Jim's physical disabilities the couple enjoyed their life together and spent time in their garden; they were involved in a number of church-related activities. They enjoyed seeing their four grandchildren who visited weekly.

Two months ago all of this changed. As result of an awkward fall in the garden, Jim fractured his right hip. He was immediately admitted for surgery and underwent a dynamic hip screw operation under spinal anaesthesia. The operation was a success, but it was 5 days before Jim was able to mobilize. During this time he was nursed on a pressure-reducing (rather than pressure-relieving) mattress, as it was believed that an alternating pressure mattress would not be suitable for him. To compensate for the reduced pressure relief, a 2-hourly turning regimen was initiated, but owing to staff shortages he was often left for 4–6 h without turning, especially overnight. Jessie noticed what was happening and commented that his skin was looking red over bony prominences. She reported her concerns to the staff but they took no action. During this time of severely restricted activity, Jim had also lost his appetite

and his nutritional intake was poor. Routine blood tests showed that he was anaemic and his serum vitamin C levels were low. He was prescribed oral iron supplements, but vitamin C supplements were not considered to be necessary. Jim's rehabilitation was slow, but steady. However, in the third week after his operation he suddenly complained of severe pain in his sacral area. When he was examined by nursing staff a full-thickness grade IV pressure ulcer was discovered, which had broken through the skin from beneath. By this stage, the wound was cavernous and filled with sloughy and necrotic tissue. Treatment was initiated but his rehabilitation programme was severely curtailed and Jim spent much of the day in bed. Jim's ulcer caused him much pain, especially at dressing changes. Throughout this period Jessie visited him daily.

When eventually deemed fit for discharge 2 months later Jim was frail and had lost a good deal of weight. He was offered 2 weeks convalescence in a residential nursing home. He could only mobilize with the help of a Zimmer frame and had lost confidence, fearing another fall. Jessie feared that he would never live at home again.

1 Why was Mr James at particularly high risk of developing a pressure ulcer, following surgery? (See also Ch. 6.)

2 What factors may have contributed to the development of the pressure ulcer during the immediate period of his post-operative care? (See also Chs 3 and 7.)

3 Describe the impact that Mr James' pressure ulcer has had on the quality of his life and that of his wife. Plot the consequences for them both over time, from the scenario given. What are the likely consequences for them in the longer term?

1 Generic and disease-specific tools may both be indicated for use in patients who suffer from pressure ulceration. List the important features of both methods of assessment and determine their relative advantages and disadvantages in investigations of patients with pressure ulceration.

2 Pressure ulceration is likely to have a major impact on the lives of patients who suffer from this condition. Outline how you would attempt to develop a questionnaire that would evaluate this impact. From your own clinical experience, list 10 questions that you feel may be relevant to patients who suffer from pressure ulceration.

REFERENCES

Bullinger M 1993 Indices versus profiles: advantages and disadvantages. In: Walker SR, Rosser RM (eds), Quality of life assessment: key issues in the 1990s. Kluwer, Dortrecht

Fallowfield L 1990 The quality of life: the missing dimension in health care. Souvenir, London

Franks P J, Moffatt C J 1998 Who suffers most from leg ulceration? Journal of Wound Care 7:383–385

Franks P J, Moffatt C J, Connolly M, Bosanquet N, Oldroyd M, Greenhalgh R M, McCollum C N 1994 Community leg ulcer clinics: effect on quality of life. Phlebology 9:83–86

Franks P J, Winterberg H, Moffatt C J 1999b Quality of life in patients suffering from pressure ulceration: a case control study. Presented to the Symposium on Advanced Wound Care, Anaheim

Franks P J, Bosanquet N, Brown D, Straub J, Harper D R, Ruckley C V 1999a Perceived health in a randomised trial of single and multi-layer bandaging. European Journal of Vascular and Endovascular Surgery 17:155–9

Hunt S M, McEwan J, McKenna S P 1986 Measuring health status. Croom Helm, London

Hyland M E, Ley A, Thomson B 1994 Quality of life of leg ulcer patients: questionnaire and preliminary findings. J Wound Care 3:294–298

Klyscz T, Junger M, Schanz S, Janz M, Rassner G, Kohnen R 1998 Quality of life with chronic venous insufficiency (CVI). Results of a study using the newly developed Tubingen questionnaire for measuring quality of life in patients with CVI (TLQ-CVI). Hartarzt 49:372–81

Launois R, Reboul-Marty J, Henry B 1996 Construction and validation of a quality of life questionnaire in chronic lower limb venous insufficiency (CIVIQ). Quality of Life Research 5:539–54

Lindholm C, Bjellerup M, Christensen O B, Zederfeldt B 1993 Quality of life in chronic leg ulcers. Acta Dermato-Venereologica 73:440–443

Price P 1996 Defining and measuring quality of life. Journal of Wound Care 5:139–140

Price P, Harding K 1996 Measuring health-related quality of life in patients with chronic leg ulcers. Wounds 8:91–4

Rives J M, Pannier M, Castede J C et al 1997 Calcium alginate versus paraffin gauze in the treatment of scalp graft donor sites. Wounds 9:199–205

Smith J J, Guest M G, Greenhalgh R M, Davies A H 2000 Measuring the quality of life in patients with venous ulcers. Journal of Vascular Surgery 31:642–649

Todd C 1992 Quality of life and diabetes audit. Health Psychology Update 11:9–14

Ware J E, Snow K K, Kosinski M, Gandek B 1993 SF-36 Health Survey: manual and interpretation guide. Boston Health Institute, New England Medical Center, Boston

World Health Organization 1958 The first ten years. WHO, Geneva

5 *Peter J Franks*

Health economics: the cost to nations

INTRODUCTION

The cost of providing health care is rising year on year at a greater rate than the annual rise in inflation. Reasons for this are manifold, but include the need to provide care for an ever-ageing population, the increasing reliance on ever more sophisticated technologies and the rising expectations of health care provision from consumers. Despite increasing expenditure, the health care budget is still unable to cope with the complete demand for care. This leads to decisions being made on the allocation of funds to particular disease categories and treatment modalities in order to achieve the best 'value for money'.

While it is known that pressure ulcer treatment and prevention consume large quantities of resources in terms of disposables, equipment and nursing time, there is still little objective evaluation of the economic burden of pressure ulceration on the health services. Moreover, the economic burden of pressure ulceration may in itself be inadequate in describing the complete picture, since the burden of care falls increasingly outside the formal health services and on to patients and their families. Even the burden of disease does not describe the complete picture of health economics. It is not sufficient to just evaluate cost, there must be some measure of health gain to balance the equation. Cost effectiveness is therefore a balance between output (effectiveness) and input (resources). The best treatments are low cost per unit of health gain, but it is important to appreciate that the cheapest option is not necessarily the most cost effective. In this chapter we explore the different economic models used to evaluate the relative costs and effectiveness of treatment options, indicating where the largest burden of cost falls and how methods may be adapted to evaluate the cost and cost effectiveness of both treatment and prevention strategies in the USA and the UK. We will evaluate the evidence on the burden of pressure ulceration and the implications for adopting particular prevention and treatment programmes.

METHODS USED IN ECONOMIC APPRAISAL

Measuring the cost burden of pressure ulceration

When one thinks of the economic burden of a disease it is tempting to examine just the costs of providing the health services to patients suffering from the disease in question. However, this is a very narrow view of cost. Social appraisal requires that not only costs related to the health service should be considered but also costs to the patient and their family and the cost of the disease to the society within which the patient lives. Costs are divided into the 'direct' cost of treating the patient and the 'indirect' cost to society. Typically, direct costs would include health service costs as well as the costs of drugs and travel associated with the health care. Conversely, indirect costs would be derived from estimates of lost production by the patient or family members caused by the disease, losses to society caused by the patient being unable to function to their potential, and quality of life issues, particularly problems associated with pain, mobility, discomfort and distress. It is important that wherever possible the full impact of the disease is assessed by evaluating all aspects of the disease on the patient, the health services and society.

The need for outcomes in economic evaluation

While the burden of disease is an important evaluation, it must be acknowledged that this can only provide limited evidence for use by health scientists. Clearly, the treatment that provides the smallest cost burden to the health service is no treatment or care, i.e. not providing care to patients would be very cheap to health services. This does not take into account the financial burden placed on others, nor the outcome of treatment. At the extremes, a clinician may believe that the clinical outcome is all important, whatever the cost, while the accountant may believe that reduced cost is the aim whatever the clinical outcome. The aim of health economics is to try and steer a course between these two extremes.

Which measure of effectiveness?

In studies of acute life-threatening disease, survival would be the accepted measure of effectiveness. However, when dealing with chronic (generally) non-life-threatening diseases one must consider what our best outcome measure will be. In general, clinical measures of effectiveness are preferred since these are of direct relevance to the clinician. In pressure ulcer care one may consider the following outcomes:

- changes in ulcer area
- change in the severity of ulceration (such as depth of tissue involvement)
- subjective improvement in ulcer
- ulcer-free days
- complete ulcer healing (clinical cure).

The last outcome is most commonly used since it provides an unequivocal end point for clinical studies. However, it does have its limitations, since it assumes that complete ulcer healing is all that is valued by the patient. Thus, an ulcer which dramatically reduces in size, or leads to reduced pain is still considered a failure in these outcome studies. There is evidence from studies in other areas of health care that clinical cure is poorly correlated with the patients perceived health. This has led researchers to investigate how health-related quality of life may have a role in determining outcomes of treatment (see Ch. 4).

Methods of cost analysis

Because of the need to balance cost with effectiveness, different types of economic appraisals have been proposed. The choice of method will depend on the expectations of the treatment outcome and the level of funds available. The major cost evaluation methods are outlined in the following sections.

Cost minimization

This term is used to describe studies where the outcomes of treatment are expected to be the same, but the costs are likely to differ. This type of analysis becomes more important for the introduction of new therapies where the treatment is already highly effective. An example might be a comparison of hernia repair performed either laparoscopically or by the conventional open procedure. In this analysis the outcome is the same (hernia repaired) but the costs of treatment may vary considerably.

Cost effectiveness

While cost minimization may be useful in situations where the outcome is expected to be identical, frequently there is a balance between the effectiveness of a treatment and the cost of each procedure. There are four possible outcomes when introducing a new procedure into medical practice.

1. Outcome is better, cost is lower. This is the ideal situation, since by implementing the new procedure this improves the outcome and reduces cost. This new technique should be adopted.

2. Outcome is poorer, cost is higher. This situation is the worst possible, since not only is the new technique more expensive, but it gives poorer outcome. The new technique should be discarded immediately.
3. Outcome is better, cost is higher. This is a complicated problem since the patients have improved but at extra cost.
4. Outcome is poorer, cost is lower. As with 3, a decision has to be made about the relative reductions in outcome and the appropriate level of spending reduction.

Cost-effectiveness studies are designed to evaluate the last two models of care. This would normally be performed by examining the mean cost for each unit of outcome. In these analyses it is important that the outcome is the same for both treatment groups. In pressure ulcer management one may consider ulcer closure as the principal outcome of treatment. An analysis for outcome 3 given above is shown in Table 5.1. From this analysis, the new treatment is more cost effective than the standard treatment. While the cost is higher, the effectiveness is greater than that expected based on the increase in cost.

Cost benefit

As previously stated, cost-effectiveness studies rely on the outcomes of treatment being the same. Frequently, however, there may be multiple outcomes of interest, some of which may show benefit, while others may show deficit. Clearly, to evaluate the overall relative benefits of each treatment one must relate all outcomes to one common value. The common value most frequently used is that of a monetary unit (either dollars or pounds). All outcomes, be they ulcer-free years, medical complications avoided or improvements in social functioning are converted into a monetary equivalent. Analyses which use both the costs and consequences (outcomes) of treatment in monetary terms are called cost–benefit studies. Most studies called cost–benefit studies are actually cost-effectiveness studies!

Cost utility analysis

Early evaluation of treatment effectiveness revolved around the survival of patients suffering life-threatening diseases. However, the shift in focus from infectious to chronic diseases required a re-evaluation of the appropriate outcomes of treatment. While quantity of life was important, quality of life was also seen to be as important and led to the development of quality of life tools to evaluate this (see Ch. 4). Utilities are values placed on a health state which has a range that includes death (0) and perfect health (1). The principle of these analyses is that there is a trade-off between quality of life and survival. It makes the assumption that 1 year of perfect health can be traded off for longer periods of poorer health. Thus, 1 year of perfect health is equivalent to a health utility of 0.5 over 2 years. In these analyses it is possible to have negative scores which reflect health states that are considered to be worse than death. An example of this may be intractable pain, unrelieved by medication. The values of these utilities are derived from population studies where participants are asked to rate certain disease states to evaluate their potential worth on this scale. The utilities derived at different stages in a patient's life (or disease) may then be multiplied by the years of life within each state to derive a single index which incorporates both quality and quantity of life (the QALY, or quality-adjusted life year). This has the advantage of then being a single outcome measure which can then be used in economic assessment. The use of QALYs has many advantages in health economics since it allows for comparisons not only across different medical interventions for the same disease but also

Table 5.1 Cost-effectiveness study for outcome 3		
	Standard treatment	New treatment
Number of patients	100	100
Ulcers healed	25	50
Total cost of treating 100 patients (£)	200 000	250 000
Cost per ulcer healed (£)	8000	5000

between diseases. However, their use remains controversial and emotive, particularly with respect to the evaluation of the relative benefits of high-cost life-saving surgery to low-cost interventions which may help many more people. In particular, there is an issue of all life having the same value. This assumes that one QALY in a child is equivalent to that for someone aged over 85 years. This is a popular method of analysis for health economists and many policy decisions on health are made with it.

Limitations of economic evaluations

Economic evaluations have become increasingly important with improvements in technology and much greater expectations of health care by the population; however, it must be acknowledged that these studies may be limited. As previously mentioned, evaluations of outcome are critical, yet the methods used to quantify outcomes are frequently less than ideal. It is also impossible to make all decisions based purely on cost and cost-effectiveness arguments, as this excludes the wishes of the consumers of health care who may wish to influence the type of health care given and help set the health care agenda. Clearly, cost and cost-effectiveness arguments alone are insufficient to fulfil the broader aims of health services demanded by the public.

MEASURING COSTS

Direct versus indirect costs

We have examined the use of different methods to assess costs in the context of clinical outcomes; however, the collection of cost data remains problematic. In particular, there is often a bias in favour of collecting information which relates directly to health service use (the so-called direct costs) while ignoring the other direct and indirect costs of disease, such as lack of production due to time off for sickness. These other costs may be substantial and if not measured may lead to distortions of the true cost of a particular medical intervention. An example of this is earlier discharge from hospital. Other studies may choose to examine the health service cost difference between two systems of care, but may neglect the patient and community cost. This may be beneficial to the health services involved, but may exclude the costs to families who may have to give up work to care for the patient. Thus the reductions in cost to the health services may result in considerable losses to the patient and their carers. This would appear to be highly relevant to patients with pressure ulceration. While in the past care continued in hospital until the ulceration healed, patients are now being discharged into the community with active pressure ulceration. Thus, the cost to the hospital is lessened, but the cost to community nursing services and families is increased.

Recording the number of units used

Superficially, assessing the number of units of health care (in-patient days, GP visits, dressings used, etc.) would seem a relatively simple task. However, patients with pressure ulceration are a complex treatment group. The reason for admission to the health services is not usually the pressure ulcer itself, but the ulcer develops as a consequence of multiple pathologies. The work of Hibbs (1988) has been criticized for including all costs of treatment for the patient she studied. Theoretically, if analyses were done on a disease basis, the total cost of treatment would add up to greater than the total health care budget. Clearly, there is a need to determine the excess cost of treatment over and above that for the disease which caused the primary referral, which can then be ascribed to the pressure ulcer. For extended hospital stay, some researchers choose to examine the difference between the patients with pressure ulceration and the average duration of stay for particular conditions. However, this may give rise to inaccuracies, particularly since it does not take into consideration other features of the patient, particularly age and sex. An alternative method is to use a case control approach where patients with pressure ulceration may be matched with patients admitted for the same condition and other prognostic factors such as age and sex. The mean difference in hospital stay is then an indication of the excess stay used by patients suffering from pressure ulceration. This method has been used in the evaluation of excess hospital stay caused by patients developing nosocomial infections (Green et al 1982). Patients who developed infections were matched with patients of the same sex, age (to within 5 years) and surgical procedure. The difference in hospital stay could then be calculated and given as a mean difference. This approach can be used for all resources which may be consumed differently between patients suffering from pressure ulceration and those who do not. Preventative measures may also be analysed in this way, although the data may need to be interpreted with caution, since by the very nature of being 'at risk' the patient is likely to have many other prognostic factors and resources allocated to them.

Unit costs

Having recorded the number of resource units, it is now necessary to estimate the costs of each of the units used. Costs are generally divided into current, capital and marginal costs. Current costs would include costs of providing the services to patients and include the use of disposables and nursing time. Capital costs are the costs associated with providing the equipment and buildings which have been bought sometime previously, but which retain their value after usage. When estimating capital costs it is important to determine the lifetime of the products in order to estimate depreciation which occurs and the subsequent need for replacement in the future. Marginal costs reflect the additional services which may be required to treat additional patients. As an example, the marginal cost of admitting a patient to a ward which is fully staffed, but has only half its beds occupied, would be small (a theoretical concept only), whereas admitting a patient to a full ward may require additional staff and an extra ward bay being opened. A fuller description of these costs and how they may impact on economic analysis is given elsewhere (Brooks & Semlyen 1997).

Specific problems of economic appraisal in pressure ulceration

The key problem of attempting to understand the economics of patients suffering from pressure ulceration is that associated with multiple pathologies. While pressure ulcers may be frequently observed in hospitals and in patients within the community services, they are rarely the main reason for hospital admission or community nursing service visits; they are usually a consequence of some other disease process. It is known that patients with poor mobility are at risk of pressure ulcer development, which is accentuated by other factors such as poor nutrition and incontinence. The case control approach is a powerful tool in the health economist's armoury, but it is limited in its ability to assess differences in cost in patients matched for just a few clinical and demographic variables. In the example of nosocomial infections patients were matched by operation type, age and sex. For pressure ulceration one would need to match for these and other prognostic factors, particularly mobility status and incontinence. These factors are likely to lead to an increased utilization of resources without necessarily being associated with the pressure ulceration. This work becomes even more problematic when evaluating prevention strategies, since resources are allocated according to the perceived risk of ulcer development in the patient, which is based on factors such as the patient's mobility, nutrition and continence status.

BALANCING COST WITH EFFECTIVENESS

Is cost utility more appropriate than cost effectiveness?

So far we have discussed the general economic methods used to appraise effectiveness in its broadest sense and the cost consequences of such interventions. However, it is important to appreciate which methods may be the most appropriate for the study being performed. As previously described, cost effectiveness is used to evaluate one particular outcome in relation to the resources consumed. However, it may be less than clear which outcome measure is the most useful. Researchers may choose outcomes that will benefit one particular product, but which may not be the most clinically appropriate. In patients with many health problems we need to know whether concerted effort to treat the ulcer leads to a benefit to the patient as well as providing a useful end point for the clinician. It would be difficult to argue the case for an expensive treatment to heal the pressure ulcer when the patient perceives no benefit from it. In cost utility analysis the patient is seen holistically. Thus, improvements are noted which relate to the patient's overall health state and do not merely focus on the pressure ulcer. If healing the ulcer was perceived to be of no benefit by the patient then there would be no change in the patient's utility status. However, assuming that healing the ulcer leads to reduced treatment levels, this would provide an argument for intervention to heal the ulcer. In general, cost utility analysis would be the preferred method, although this is rarely performed in studies of pressure ulceration.

Evaluating products and their limitations within a wider economic strategy

Much of the evidence of economic analysis is related to evaluation of products, and in particular comparisons between products which are used in similar circumstances. There are a plethora of studies which have looked at comparisons of beds, mattresses and seating cushions, often with soft end points, which rely on subjective assessment, such as durability, clinical impressions, clinician-rated patient comfort, or indirect measures of effectiveness, such as pressure profiles. Frequently, these studies are used by companies to market their products, with very little hard evidence to support their use over and above other (often cheaper) products. In a systematic review of pressure ulcer treatments it was recommended that economic analysis should accompany any further randomized trials of pressure-relieving equipment (Cullum et al 1995). It was stated that if purchasers were to consider high-tech 'expensive' pressure equipment they should do so only in the context of a randomized clinical trial.

THE EVIDENCE

Evaluating the burden of pressure ulcer prevention and treatment

There have been many estimates of the burden of pressure ulcers in the UK, few of which have been substantiated by evidence (McSweeney 1994). In 1988, Waterlow quoted an annual cost of pressure ulcers of £300 million: a year later it was estimated at £200 million. In the document 'Health of the Nation' (Department of Health 1991) the cost of pressure ulceration was estimated to be at least £60 million, and in 1993 a figure of £420 million was suggested.

In an attempt to quantify the cost of a severe pressure ulcer, Hibbs (1988) followed up one patient with a necrotic sacral sore. Over a 1-year period over £25 000 was spent treating this patient, over 60% of which arose from staffing costs. Only 26% could be ascribed directly to the management of the pressure ulcer, 17.5% to bed hire and just 6% on wound care products. A similar pattern was observed in The Netherlands, where 65% of the excess cost was due to increased patient stay, 25% due to increased nursing staff and 10% on bed hire (Haalboom 1991). The Clinical Standards Advisory Group (1993) estimated the increase in length of stay caused by a minor ulcer to be, on average, 9 days, while a severe ulcer required an average stay of 140 days. Most of the additional costs of treating these patients are opportunistic costs – that is opportunities missed to treat other patients. This means that there are no additional costs per se, but the resources are being used to treat the patient with a pressure ulcer rather than other patients who have their treatment delayed or denied. As an example of this, if patients with a condition normally have a 10-day stay, then the addition of a severe pressure ulcer would deny 14 patients from receiving care over the same period.

While the cost data from hospitals are poor, information from community services is poorer still. One study was able to determine that 12% of patient contacts by community nursing staff were for pressure area care, one-third of these being daily visits to patients who were suffering from severe grades of pressure ulceration (McSweeney 1994).

Cost of prevention versus treatment of pressure ulcers

In 1993, the accountants Touche Ross & Co. published a report commissioned by the Department of Health on the cost of pressure sores. The panel derived figures for an 'average' 600-bed hospital comparing the strategies for treatment alone, or treatment within a larger prevention strategy. For each option, lowest and highest estimates were given. All data were derived from other published sources. A key finding of this report was that while the lowest estimated costs were similar for treatment versus prevention (£644 000/year), the highest estimated costs were doubled for treatment (£1153 000/year) and quadrupled for prevention (£2710 000/year). Thus, a high-cost prevention strategy could cost double that of providing treatment for pressure ulceration alone. The majority of this increase was accounted for in staff time (Fig. 5.1). While cost per patient was similar for treatment and prevention, the larger number of patients who required prevention was substantially higher, leading to a five-fold increase in staff costs. Clearly, accurate assessments of patients' risk of pressure ulcer development are essential to ensure that prevention strategies are targeted at those at high risk of ulcer development. Analysis such as this emphasizes the poor specificity (inability to detect patients who will not develop a pressure ulcer). A more detailed discussion of this is given in Chapter 6. While the overall cost of prevention may be higher than treatment, the authors concluded that there may be advantages in a prevention strategy, since treatment could require extended patient stay, plastic surgical intervention and additional dressing costs. These would be reflected as reduced opportunity costs, since the patient who stays longer in hospital will be preventing other patients from entering hospital. Overall, the

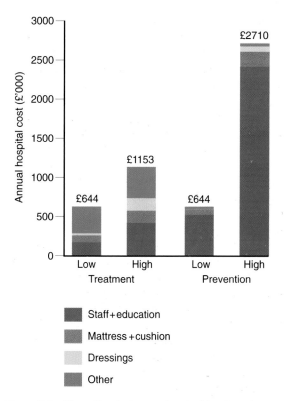

Figure 5.1 The estimated annual cost of treatment (£'000) and prevention in an average 600 bedded hospital for a high cost and a low cost hospital (redrawn from Touche Ross 1993).

Touche Ross report indicated that the cost of treatment for pressure ulcers would be in the range of £180–£321 million per year while the cost of introducing a prevention strategy would range from £180–£755 million per year. The authors acknowledged that this work was limited in that they felt unable to comment on the cost of community care for pressure ulceration owing to the paucity of good information, could not include the costs of self care and family care, and did not include the costs to the patient in terms of reduced health related quality of life.

How litigation may affect cost models

While the Touche Ross report identified the costs of treatment and prevention strategies, it also indicated the potential cost of pressure ulceration from litigation. Tingle (1997) reviewed recent judgements in cases of patients developing pressure ulcers on admission to hospital. He concluded that medico-legal cases of pressure ulcer development could easily have been avoided with little expense, provided that the staff had systematically assessed patients for pressure area care. The damages awarded in each case varied from £3500 to £12 500, although there have been cases which have led to damages in excess of £100 000 being awarded to patients (Touche Ross & Co. 1993).

CONCLUSION

In this chapter the methods used in economic evaluation of pressure ulcer prevention and treatment have been outlined, and the drawbacks and limitations of each method highlighted. While cost effectiveness is clearly the most clinician-friendly method, there is a clear issue on the best measure of effectiveness to consider clinical outcomes of treatment such as wound healing or examine improvements in the patients' quality of life as the main outcome of treatment. Cost utility analysis has many attractions, particularly in its holistic approach to the patient, but it is not easy to use and its interpretation remains controversial. While authors are keen to point out the economic cost of pressure ulceration to the health services, there is often little evidence on how these costs were derived. Moreover, the direct current costs of pressure

ulcer management are just a part of the overall equation. Most studies fail to appreciate the importance of the patients and families in the treatment process, and the indirect cost of pressure ulceration which leads to lower productivity for society.

Clearly the health care agenda is in a state of flux. Both the USA and the UK are struggling with ever-increasing costs of health care, with increases in new technologies and greater expectations from the public. Within this environment it is essential to provide quality 'effective' care. While earlier discharge from hospital reduces patient stays, this may lead to longer and more intensive care within the community setting, either through formal or informal carers. To evaluate the full impact of a new system of care it is essential to determine all costs to the health services, the individual and society. The literature would suggest that we have a long way to go before cost-effective pressure ulcer care becomes a reality. There is a clear need to evaluate the current protocols for pressure ulcer treatment and prevention, not only with regard to effectiveness but also to assess the cost effectiveness of treatment. Unlike pharmaceuticals, medical devices do not need to be evaluated in clinical trials prior to their launch on to the health care market. There is a clear need for health care managers to understand that cheaper does not necessarily mean better, and for clinicians to appreciate that more expensive does not necessarily mean better.

REFERENCES

Brooks R, Semlyen A 1997 Economic appraisal in pressure sore management. J Wound Care 6:491–494

Clinical Standards Advisory Group 1993 Prevention and treatment of pressure sores – guidelines for good practice. Middlesex University Health Research Centre, London

Cullum N, Deeks J, Fletcher A et al 1995 The prevention and treatment of pressure sores. Effective Health Care Bulletin 2:1. Churchill Livingstone, Edinburgh

Department of Health 1991 Health of the nation. HMSO, London

Green M S, Rubenstein E, Amit P 1982 Estimating the length of nosocomial infections on the length of hospital stay. Journal of Infectious Diseases 145:667–672

Haalboom J R 1991 The costs of decubitus. Nederlands Jijdschrift voor Geneeskunde 135(14):606–610

Hibbs P (ed.) 1988 Pressure area care for the City and Hackney Health Authority. City and Hackney Health Authority, London

McSweeney P 1994 Assessing the cost of pressure sores. Nursing Standard 8(52):25–26

Tingle J 1997 Pressure sores: counting the legal cost of nursing neglect. British Journal of Nursing 6(13):757–758

Touche Ross 1993 Pressure sores: a key quality indicator. Department of Health, London

Waterlow J 1988 Prevention is cheaper than cure. Nursing Times 83(25):69–70

6 *Jane Nixon and Amanda McGough*

Principles of patient assessment: screening for pressure ulcers and potential risk

INTRODUCTION

The purpose of baseline nursing assessment is to identify both actual and potential problems, which then inform individual planning and delivery of effective care. In the literature concerning the prevention and management of pressure ulcers baseline assessment is commonly associated with the term 'risk assessment' and there has been a focus toward the development and use of risk assessment tools to facilitate the identification of 'at risk' patients (AHCPR 1992, Effective Health Care 1995).

In the reality of practice, however, baseline nursing assessment aims to answer the following two clinically important questions:

1. Has the patient an existing pressure ulcer?
2. What is the patient's risk of pressure ulcer development?

A risk assessment tool is meaningless if a patient has an existing pressure ulcer, since the patient has a problem which requires treatment and that treatment will depend upon the severity of the lesion and the individual patient circumstance. The focus of patient assessment toward risk assessment of pressure ulcer-free patients (AHCPR 1992) is important but does not address the first clinical question. The practising nurse is therefore faced with three clinical management issues:

- Who to assess to determine the presence or absence of a pressure ulcer?
- Who to assess for potential risk of pressure ulcer development?
- How to assess for potential risk of pressure ulcer development?

In this chapter, it is advocated that assessment is a process of interactive decision making which includes the utilization of various levels of evidence including:

1. **Research evidence** which defines the characteristics of patients most likely to have pressure ulcers, identifies key prognostic or risk factors associated with pressure ulcer development, explores the validity of risk assessment scales and suggests factors important in improving the process and outcomes of care delivery.
2. **Patient-specific factors** derived from nursing assessment and specialty-based knowledge, including patient-specific risk factors; skin response to pressure; general condition and prognosis; local environmental factors (such as basic equipment provision) and relevant history.

There is much within the literature to support the assessment process, enabling informed decision making for both initial and ongoing care delivery.

SCREENING FOR PRESSURE ULCERS AND POTENTIAL RISK – FUNDAMENTAL PRINCIPLES

In order to determine whom to assess for the presence or absence of pressure ulcers and potential risk, it is useful to establish the high-risk groups and broad characteristics of patients most likely to present with or develop pressure ulcers within health care settings. The literature provides a clear framework for practice within the majority of clinical specialties, but some do require a greater level of clinical judgement or systems in place to prompt the screening process in more unusual clinical situations.

High-risk groups

Patient populations identified as high risk are described in Chapter 2 and include:

1. Elderly medical (Clark & Watts 1994, Bridel et al 1996)
2. Nursing home (Braden & Bergstrom 1994, Brandeis et al 1994)
3. Cardiovascular and vascular surgical (Kemp et al 1990, Nixon et al 2000)
4. Acute orthopaedic (Allman et al 1986, Versluysen 1986, Clark & Watts 1994)
5. Intensive care (Clough 1994, Robnett 1986, Bergstrom et al 1987b)
6. Spinal cord injured (Richardson & Meyer 1981)
7. The young disabled (Clark & Cullum 1992)
8. Terminally ill (Berlowitz and Wilking 1990, Bale et al 1995, Thomas et al 1996)

Of particular note in relation to screening for existing pressure sores is high prevalence rates reported on admission to health care facilities (Table 6.1). A common characteristic of patients admitted to health care facilities or residing in the community with existing pressure ulcers is that a high proportion have been transferred from other health care facilities (Brandeis et al 1994, Clough 1994, Guralnik et al 1988).

Characteristics of patients with pressure ulcers

The primary patient characteristic associated with existing pressure ulcers is reduced mobility. Observation of patient movement provided the first objective data demonstrating the importance of functional mobility in the development of pressure ulcers (Exton-Smith & Sherwin 1961). Early prevalence or cross-sectional data describing patients with existing pressure ulcers also identified reduced mobility as a key characteristic (Barbenel et al 1977, David et al 1983, Berlowitz & Wilking 1989). Barbenel et al (1977), in a prevalence survey involving a study population of 10 736, reported prevalence rates according to mobility category suggesting the probable importance of this factor in defining the pressure ulcer population (Table 6.2). Berlowitz & Wilking (1989) demonstrated a significant association between reduced mobility and the existence of a pressure ulcer on admission.

Pressure ulcers are also associated with increasing age. They are most prevalent in hospitalized patients of over 70 years (Barbenel et al 1977, 1980, Barrois & Colin 1995) and community residents of over 75 years (Collins 1988).

There has been little analysis of other factors associated with the presence of a pressure ulcer on admission to health care facilities. Only two studies have undertaken multivariate analyses to identify patient characteristics associated with the presence of existing pressure ulcers. Factors

Table 6.1 On-admission prevalence rates for different patient populations

Author	Patient population	Number of admissions	On admission prevalence
Versluysen (1986)	Fractured neck of femur	100	11% (11)
Berlowitz & Wilking (1989)	Chronic care hospital	301	33.22% (101)
Ek et al (1991)	Long-term medical care ward	495	14.1% (70)
Clough (1994)	Intensive care	638	12.8% (82)
Bale et al (1995)	Hospice	327	26.6% (87)
Bridel et al (1996)	Elderly medical	3742	6.15% (230)

Table 6.2 Summary report of prevalence by mobility category (Barbenel et al 1977)

	n	%
Totally/partially helpless bedfast	211/1164	18.1
Totally/partially helpless chairfast	363/1790	20.3
Not helpless bedfast/chairfast	132/1367	9.65
Semi ambulant	174/2446	7.1
Totally ambulant	64/3969	1.6

identified included altered level of consciousness, impaired nutritional intake, hypoalbuminaemia, faecal incontinence and fractures (Allman et al 1986, Berlowitz & Wilking 1989).

Characteristics of patients who develop pressure ulcers

Berlowitz & Wilking (1989) identified different risk factors when comparing cross-sectional and cohort data and emphasized the need to distinguish between characteristics of patients with pressure ulcers and risk factors associated with pressure ulcer development. However, a review of prospective cohort studies does identify similar themes.

A review of the literature has identified nine prospective cohort and two cohort studies, which have undertaken multivariate analyses to identify characteristics of patients who develop pressure ulcers (Table 6.3). Five key themes emerge: mobility, nutrition, perfusion, age and skin condition. Of most importance is that mobility-related factors are found to be significant and independent predictors of pressure ulcer development in 10 of the 11 studies detailed.

Who to assess: screening triggers

The high on-admission prevalence rates reported among acute elderly, fractured neck of femur, intensive care and chronic medical patients populations indicate the need for a comprehensive skin inspection and risk assessment of all patients admitted to these health care settings. Difficulties occur in local patient populations with diverse needs, such as general medical and surgical wards or a community setting. In such environments, decision support frameworks developed at a local level to reflect the health care facility patient population may be of value to support the decision-making process and establish minimum standards for practice.

The epidemiological literature allows the identification of the main prompts for baseline skin inspection to determine the presence or absence of a pressure ulcer and to identify patients who require assessment of potential risk. The main characteristic associated with both the presence of and development of pressure ulcers is reduced mobility, with increased occurrence found in high-risk groups, including elderly populations. It is suggested, therefore, that those patients require screening if one or more of the following criteria apply:

- mobility/activity restrictions – confined to bed or chair
- aged over 75 years
- high-risk group (for example, fractured proximal femur).

In specialized environments, more specific research literature and audit may be required to develop local guidelines for skin assessment in order to assist the practitioner through the decision-making process: For example, perioperative guidelines for pressure area assessment and care (vascular and gynaecology theatres) have been developed using a combination of research and audit data and by consensus agreement (Fig. 6.1) (Parkinson et al 1999). The guidelines provide a practical decision support tool within a theatre environment dealing with a diverse patient group.

This local guideline was developed and implemented underpinned by evidence generated through primary research and systematic literature review. Guidelines are 'more likely to be effective if they take into account local circumstances, are disseminated by an active educational intervention, and implemented by patient specific reminders relating directly to profes-

Table 6.3 Prospective cohort and cohort studies using multivariate statistical analyses

Study	Sample	Incidence	Prognostic factors	Statistical method
Clarke & Kadhom (1988)	88 Hospitalized (orthopaedic, elderly + ICU) bedfast/chairfast	29.5%	1 Change in condition of skin 2 Time on pressure area care 3 Appetite 4 Norton Score 5 Diagnosis 6 Method of manual pressure relief 7 Observed skin condition 8 Age	Discriminant analysis
	30 Community bedfast/chairfast	20%	1 Appetite 2 Condition of skin 3 Frequency of care 4 Norton Score 5 Age 6 Diagnosis	
Guralnik et al (1988)	5193 US nationwide cohort 55–75 years, 10-year follow-up	2.2%	1 Heart disease (negative association) 2 Activity level 3 Self-assessed health 4 Smoking 5 Neurological abnormality 6 Dry or scaling skin 7 Anaemia (Hb < 12)	Multiple logistic regression
Berlowitz & Wilking (1989) (record review)	185 Chronic medical	10.8%	1 Cerebrovascular accident 2 Bed or chair bound 3 Impaired nutritional intake	Multiple logistic regression
Kemp et al (1990)	125 Surgical > 20 years stratified by operating time	12%	1 Age 2 Time on operating table 3 Extracorporeal circulation	Discriminant analysis
Ek et al (1991)	495 Long-term medical LOS > 3 weeks	10.1%	1 Albumin 2 Mobility 3 Activity 4 Food intake	Multiple regression
Marchette et al (1991) (record review)	161 Postoperative ICU > 59 years	39.1%	1 Skin redness 2 Days on static air mattress for prevention 3 Faecal incontinence 4 Diarrhoea 5 Preoperative albumin	Discriminant analysis
Bergstrom & Braden (1992)	200 Nursing home > 65 years LOS > 10 days Braden Scale < 18	73.5%	1 Braden Scale 2 Diastolic blood pressure 3 Temperature 4 Dietary protein intake 5 Age	Logistic regression
Hoshowsky & Schramm (1994)	505 Surgical	16.8%	1 Time on operating table 2 Vascular disease 3 Age over 40 years 4 Preoperative Hemphill scale	Logistic regression
Brandeis et al (1994)	4232 Nursing home	12.9%	1 Ambulation difficulty 2 Faecal incontinence 3 Diabetes mellitus 4 Difficulty feeding oneself	Logistic regression

Table 6.3 *continued*

Study	Sample	Incidence	Prognostic factors	Statistical method
Allman et al (1995)	286 Hospitalized > 55 years, bed/chair > 5 days, hip fracture length of stay > 5 days	12.9%	1 Nonblanchable erythema of intact sacral skin 2 Lymphopenia 3 Immobility 4 Dry sacral skin 5 Decreased body weight	Multivariate Cox regression
Nixon et al (2000)	416 Surgical > 55 years, major general, gynaecology, vascular	15.6%	1 Intraoperative mattress 2 Number hypotensive episodes during surgery 3 Mean core temperature during surgery 4 Postoperative Braden mobility score	Logistic regression

sional activity' (Effective Health Care 1994). The guideline makes best practical use of the evidence available (Nixon et al 1998, 2000, Cullum et al 1999), while recognizing limitations in our knowledge base. The sensitivity and specificity is not of major concern because there is no real cost associated with assessment and preventative care. The main purpose was to establish a clear framework for assessment and preventative care in a multidisciplinary working environment that places conflicting demands upon practitioner time.

RISK ASSESSMENT – FUNDAMENTAL PRINCIPLES

When baseline skin assessment identifies that a patient has an existing pressure ulcer the patient has an actual problem which requires treatment and that treatment will depend upon the severity of the ulcer and the individual patient circumstance. Patients with existing pressure ulcers are also at risk of further pressure ulcer development and require active prevention. Detailed pressure ulcer assessment and care of patients with existing pressure ulcers are discussed in Chapters 8 and 9.

When baseline skin assessment determines that a patient is pressure ulcer-free, the purpose of further assessment is to identify any potential risk of pressure ulcer development in order that preventative measures can be adopted.

There is increasing debate within the literature about how to undertake risk assessment and, in particular, the role of risk assessment scales (Edwards 1996). It was recommended by the United States Agency for Health Care Policy and Research (AHCPR) that, 'A systematic risk assessment can be accomplished by using a validated risk assessment tool such as the Braden Scale or Norton Score' (AHCPR 1992).

In contrast the Effective Health Care Bulletin on the prevention and treatment of pressure ulcers concluded that, 'The evidence on the accuracy of pressure ulcer risk scales is confusing, and it is not clear that these scales are better than clinical judgement or that they improve outcomes' (Effective Health Care 1995).

Issues central to the debate include:

- How do nurses assess other aspects of patient need?
- Is it appropriate to summarize with a single score something which is multifaceted in nature?
- Have we enough evidence to develop predictive indexes?
- What are the key risk factors?
- Are existing risk assessment scales valid?

The research literature serves to underline the complexity of the processes involved in both nursing assessment of patient need and factors associated with pressure ulcer development. In

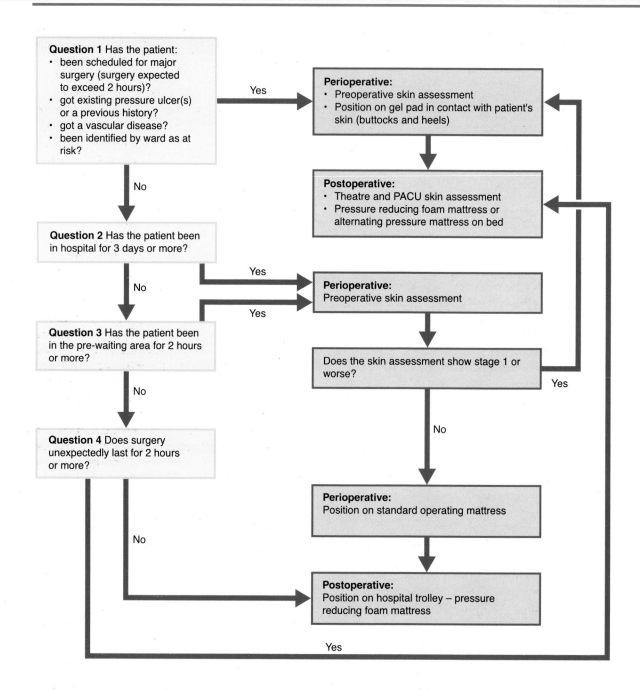

Question 1 Has the patient:
- been scheduled for major surgery (surgery expected to exceed 2 hours)?
- got existing pressure ulcer(s) or a previous history?
- got a vascular disease?
- been identified by ward as at risk?

Yes →

Perioperative:
- Preoperative skin assessment
- Position on gel pad in contact with patient's skin (buttocks and heels)

Postoperative:
- Theatre and PACU skin assessment
- Pressure reducing foam mattress or alternating pressure mattress on bed

No ↓

Question 2 Has the patient been in hospital for 3 days or more?

No ↓   Yes →

Perioperative:
Preoperative skin assessment

Yes →

Question 3 Has the patient been in the pre-waiting area for 2 hours or more?

No ↓

Does the skin assessment show stage 1 or worse?   Yes →

No ↓

Question 4 Does surgery unexpectedly last for 2 hours or more?

Perioperative:
Position on standard operating mattress

No ↓

Postoperative:
Position on hospital trolley – pressure reducing foam mattress

Yes

Other factors to inform clinical decision-making:
- Age > 55
- Hypotensive episodes
- Immobility time

Figure 6.1 Perioperative flow chart (vascular and gynaecology theatres) (Parkinson et al 1999). Reproduced with permission from The Leeds Teaching Hospitals NHS Trust, UK.

order to inform the debate at a clinical level the following sections review evidence relating to the cognitive processes involved in general nursing assessment, issues relating to the construction, limitations and validity of risk assessment scales and prospective cohort studies which identify prognostic factors associated with pressure ulcer development.

Nursing assessment – an overview

Nursing assessment is a dynamic decision-making process (Crow et al 1995). Its purpose is to provide an accurate picture of patients, including both their capacity to perform activities of daily living and the stability of their condition. Judgements are then made regarding the nursing care required and frequency of monitoring (Benner 1984, Crow et al 1995).

Various elements have been identified which are important in assimilation and interpretation of information by nurses while assessing patients. There is evidence that nurses develop knowledge structures for gathering and organizing information which enable them to select, weight and combine important factors. Nurses also distinguish between relevant and irrelevant information and cues, link past experiences and knowledge to the current situation and grasp the whole situation rather than distinguishing a series of subtasks (Benner & Wrubal 1982, Pyles & Stern 1983, Prescott et al 1989).

The quality of assessments and associated decisions about the nursing care that is required are related to underpinning theoretical knowledge, previous experience, specialty-based knowledge relating to usual patterns of recovery, perceptual awareness, recognition skills and knowing the patient (Benner & Wrubal 1982, Benner 1984, MacLeod 1994, Crow et al 1995).

Knowing the patient is increasingly understood to be a key component of excellent nursing practice (Jenny & Logan 1992, MacLeod 1993). Through a finely tuned knowledge of their patients, experienced nurses are able to note opportunities for action, to understand the meaningfulness and importance of ordinary occurrences and to act upon them, promoting patient recovery. The process of knowing the patient shapes caring activities and is integrally linked with patient outcomes (MacLeod 1994).

Crow et al (1995) in their critical review illustrate the dynamic and continuous nature of nursing assessment. Nurses continually update assessments of patients as their condition changes. They recognize their usual pattern of responses and use both their current status and judgements of the predicted future course of the patient to inform decisions about nursing care needs (Corcoran-Perry & Graves 1990, Yates 1990, Tanner et al 1993, MacLeod 1994). It follows that any shortcomings in the judgements nurses formulate will lead to decision errors (Crow et al 1995).

A review of the components involved in nursing assessment illustrates the complexity of the processes involved. The process is dynamic and continuous, with the nurse making judgements about immediate and future care needs, including the frequency of monitoring. In relation to pressure ulcer prevention it raises questions with regard to the appropriateness of summarizing with a single score something which is multifaceted (Deeks 1996), the development of clinical assessment skills (from novice to expert) and the role of risk assessment scales in nursing assessment of potential risk.

RISK ASSESSMENT SCALES
Construction and limitations

Measurement of health or illness testing in clinical practice can be grouped into three categories: discrimination (measuring a single point in time), prediction (of a future event) or outcome evaluation (measurement of change over time) (Kirshner & Guyatt 1985).

A predictive index is used to group patients into set categories when a gold standard is available and this type of index is used to screen patients to ascertain which patients have or will develop the illness or disease under scrutiny. In this way, a risk assessment scale designed to screen patients for risk of pressure ulcer development could be classified as a predictive index.

Using a risk assessment scale may eradicate the need for a more detailed assessment of a patient's susceptibility to the development of pressure ulcers. Larson (1986, p. 186) argues that such tools are useful given certain conditions:

'...(a) when there is an important health problem, (b) when the problem can be detected during an early stage, (c) when there is a useful treatment or intervention for the problem ... and (d) when the screening test is simple, convenient, reliable and cost-effective.'

In order to develop a predictive index, items need to be selected for inclusion in the index or scale. The most valid method of constructing predictive scales involves the use of statistical regression models to identify, rank and weight the factors which together best predict the development of a pressure ulcer (Effective Health Care 1995). Such studies are known as prognostic factor studies and they are generating increased methodological scrutiny and critique as statistical techniques advance within medical research (Simon & Altman 1994).

Simon & Altman (1994) describe three types of prognostic studies:

1. Early exploratory studies. Such investigations commonly examine issues such as the association of a factor with diagnosis and disease characteristics or the development of reproducible assays.
2. Studies to determine whether prognostic factors provide improved means of identifying patients at particularly high or low risk of disease progression or death.
3. Studies to determine which subsets of patients benefit from a given therapy.

They suggest that type 1 studies might be called Phase I prognostic factor studies and types 2 and 3 each include what might be called Phase II and Phase III factor studies. The Phase II studies are exploratory and generate hypotheses from extensive analysis of data. Phase III studies are large, confirmatory studies of prestated hypotheses and allow for more precise quantification of the effect (Simon & Altman 1994). Also detailed are methodological recommendations for the conduct of prognostic factor studies, including the use of inception

cohorts, < 15% patients lost to follow up, reproducible measures, blinding of outcome, standardized or randomized treatment, prestated hypotheses, sample size calculations, and so on.

An example of the potential for the development of predictive indexes using regression models is provided by Nixon et al (2000) who report the synthesis of a probability equation for the development of postoperative pressure sores. A clear benefit is that of the four elements within the model only mobility requires a score selection; the other three variables are actual values and the problem of inter-rater reliability is therefore minimized. Results are not generalizable since the hypothesis and sample size were not determined by the prognostic factor study and the end-point definition included persistent blanching erythema. The probability model derived is context specific and requires further confirmatory study but illustrates the potential application of prognostic factor research to assessment of risk.

Although there is a considerable pressure ulcer literature only nine prospective cohort studies and two cohort studies (medical record review) have been found which determine key prognostic factors associated with pressure ulcer development (Table 6.3). These can only be considered as Phase I prognostic factor studies. While themes can be identified, the small number of prospective studies worldwide and the diversity of health care settings and associated risks highlight that pressure ulcer prognostic factor research is very much in its infancy. Questions remain outstanding in relation to the magnitude of effect of generic and specialty-specific risk factors in different patient populations.

In a recent systematic review more than 40 pressure ulcer risk assessment scales were found detailed in the literature (McGough 1999). The review determined that the majority of risk assessment scales have been developed on the basis of expert opinion, literature review and/or adaptation of an existing scale, and only seven were original scales. Of the seven original scales only one had selected variables identified through a regression analysis of an inception cohort study (Salzberg et al 1996). Indeed, 61% were developed by modification of an existing scale and one scale, the Dutch Consensus Scale (Halfens 1997), is a fourth-generation modification of the original Norton Score (McGough 1999).

There is then no statistical basis to the majority of risk assessment scales either in relation to the selection of risk factors or the scores allocated to elements within the scales. In most risk assessment scales using a simple ordinal scoring system, the weighting within the scale is equally allocated between risk factors. Thus, any potential differences in the contribution or importance of one factor over another or the cumulative importance of two or more factors are not identified.

The absence of a statistical base is evident in the large number of variables found in risk assessment scales. McGough (1999) identified 23 different variables in 38 modified risk assessment scales, with most frequent inclusions being continence/moisture (36 scales), nutrition/appetite (32 scales) and mobility (30 scales). Given that only two out of 11 studies using multivariate analyses identified continence variables as important (both identified faecal incontinence), while 10 out of 11 identified mobility-related factors (Table 6.3) the validity of these scales in defining 'at risk' patients is immediately questionable.

Validity of risk assessment scales

In order to determine whether risk assessment scales are a powerful method of screening for risk, it is necessary to evaluate their accuracy in separating patients who are at risk from the patients who are not at risk: that is, the predictive validity. The use of sensitivity and specificity is widely accepted as a means of assessing the validity of risk assessment scales (Edwards 1996).

In simple terms the sensitivity is the accuracy of the tool in predicting those who develop the condition and the specificity is the accuracy of the tool in predicting those who do not develop the condition. The ideal scenario would be the achievement of 100% sensitivity and 100% specificity: that is, no over-prediction or under-prediction is observed (Bridel 1993); however, no agreed performance standard has been established (Edwards 1996).

The predictive validity of risk assessment scales has been shown to be variable both in comparison

of scales and in assessments of the same scale (Effective Health Care 1995), although a majority have not been subject to any testing prior to use in clinical settings. McGough's (1999) systematic review found that only six out of 43 risk assessment scales had been tested for their predictive validity (Table 6.4). Of these six scales, the Braden Scale (Fig. 6.2) has been subjected to the most testing across the greatest variety of clinical settings, both in the hospital and in the community. Although Bergstrom and colleagues have demonstrated that the predictive validity estimates for the Braden Scale have been high, other researchers have failed to replicate these findings (Langemo et al 1991, Barnes & Payton 1993, Ramundo 1995, Capobianco & McDonald 1996, Halfens 1997). Obviously, the different patient populations studied may partly account for the variation, as the incidence of pressure ulcers within each setting will vary. However, this cannot explain the difference in predictive validity values obtained in the same care setting such as a medical–surgical acute care unit (Bergstrom et al 1987a, Langemo et al 1991, Barnes & Payton 1993, Capobianco & McDonald 1996, Halfens 1997).

Principles established in research critique and evidence-based medicine add further to the debate with regard to the measurement and interpretation of predictive validity studies (Sackett et al 1997). As with prognostic factor studies, baseline standards are increasingly recognized for the conduct of research and the appraisal of research evidence (Sackett et al 1997). McGough (1999) identified six appraisal criteria, and of the 17 studies detailed in Table 6.4 the majority have methodological limitations in areas of non-random sample selection, an absence of sample size calculations and non-blinding of risk score to the caring nurse.

There also remain many outstanding questions in relation to the validity and effectiveness of risk assessment scales. Edwards (1996) doubts the appropriateness of applying measures of sensitivity and specificity to scales which from their conception were never based or tested on mathematical models. Difficulties in comparing the validity of different scales are highlighted by Deeks (1996) who points out that nursing care in the research environment will affect both

SENSORY PERCEPTION Ability to respond meaningfully to pressure related discomfort.	1. Completely limited: Unresponsive (does not moan, flinch or grasp) to painful stimuli, due to diminished level of consciousness or sedation OR limited ability to feel pain.	2. Very limited: Responds only to painful stimuli. Cannot communicate discomfort except by moaning or restlessness OR has a sensory impairment which limits the ability to feel pain or discomfort over 1/2 of body.	3. Slightly limited: Responds to verbal commands but cannot always communicate discomfort or need to be turned OR has some sensory impairment which limits ability to feel pain or discomfort in 1 or 2 extremities.	4. No impairment: Responds to verbal commands. Has no sensory deficit which would limit ability to feel or voice pain or discomfort.	
MOISTURE Degree to which skin is exposed to moisture.	1. Constantly moist: Skin is kept moist almost constantly by perspiration, urine, etc. Dampness is detected every time patient is moved or turned.	2. Very moist: Skin is often but not always moist. Linen must be changed at least once a shift.	3. Occasionally moist: Skin is occasionally moist, requiring an extra linen change approximately once a day.	4. Rarely moist: Skin is usually dry, linen only requires changing at routine intervals.	
ACTIVITY Degree of physical activity.	1. Bedfast: Confined to bed.	2. Chairfast: Ability to walk severely limited or non-existent. Cannot bear own weight and/or must be assisted into chair or wheelchair.	3. Walks occasionally: Walks occasionally during day but for very short distances, with or without assistance. Spends majority of each shift in bed or chair.	4. Walks frequently: Walks outside the room at least twice a day and inside room at least once every 2 hours during waking hours.	
MOBILITY Ability to change and control body position.	1. Completely immobile: Does not make even slight changes in body or extremity position without assistance.	2. Very limited: Makes occasional slight changes in body or extremity position but unable to make frequent or significant changes independently.	3. Slightly limited: Makes frequent though slight changes in body or extremity position independently.	4. No limitation: Makes major and frequent changes in position without assistance.	
NUTRITION Usual food intake pattern.	1. Very poor: Never eats a complete meal. Rarely eats more than 1/3 of any food offered. Eats 2 servings or less of protein (meat or dairy products) per day. Takes fluids poorly. Does not take a liquid dietary supplement OR is NPO and/or maintained on clear liquids or IVs for more than 5 days.	2. Probably inadequate: Rarely eats a complete meal and generally eats only about 1/2 of any food offered. Protein intake includes only 3 servings of meat or dairy products per day. Occasionally will take a dietary supplement OR receives less than optimum amount of liquid diet or tube feeding.	3. Adequate: Eats over half of most meals. Eats a total of 4 servings of protein (meat or dairy products) each day. Occasionally will refuse a meal but will usually take a supplement if offered OR is on a tube feeding or TPN regimen which probably meets most of nutritional needs.	4. Excellent: Eats most of every meal. Never refuses a meal. Usually eats a total of 4 or more servings of meat and dairy products. Occasionally eats between meals. Does not require supplementation.	
FRICTION AND SHEAR	1. Problem: Requires moderate to maximum assistance in moving. Complete lifting without sliding against sheets is impossible. Frequently slides down in bed or chair, requiring frequent repositioning with maximum assistance. Spasticity, contractures or agitation leads to almost constant friction.	2. Potential problems: Moves feebly or requires minimum assistance. During a move skin probably slides to some extent against sheets, chair, restraints or other devices. Maintains relatively good position in chair or bed most of the time but occasionally slides down.	3. No apparent problem: Moves in bed and in chair independently and has sufficient strength to lift up completely during move. Maintains good position in bed or chair at all times.		

Total Score [ ]

Figure 6.2 The Braden Scale. © Copyright Barbara Braden and Nancy Bergstrom 1988. Reproduced with permission of Barbara Braden.

Table 6.4 The predictive validity of risk assessment scales

Scale tested	Author(s)	Sensitivity (%)	Specificity (%)
Andersen	Andersen et al (1982)	88	87
Braden	Barnes & Payton (1993)	73	91
	Bergstrom & Braden (1992)	97	19
	Bergstrom et al (1987a)	100, 100	90, 64
	Bergstrom et al (1987b)	83	64
	Braden & Bergstrom (1994)	79	74
	Capobianco & McDonald (1996)	71	83
	Halfens (1997)	74	70
	Langemo et al (1991)	64 (acute)	87 (acute)
	Ramundo (1995)	100	34
Knoll	Towey & Erland (1988)	86	56
Norton	Norton et al (1962)	63	70
	Wai-Han et al (1997)	75	67
Mod. Norton	Stotts & Paul (1988)	16	94
Pressure sore prediction score	Lowthian (1989)	89	76
Waterlow	Edwards (1995) (see also Waterlow 1988)	100	10
	Wai-Han et al (1997)	88	28

sensitivity and specificity and that risk assessment scales will appear to be performing most poorly in the settings where preventative care is most effective. The testing of these scales is further compounded by the incipient nature of pressure ulcer development. Risk assessment scales are only a snapshot view and in acute or critical illness the score may not reflect the patient's condition at the time of pressure ulcer development.

Furthermore, there is no evidence that risk assessment scales are better than nurses' judgement in identifying patients at risk (Effective Health Care 1995, McGough 1999) and insufficient evidence to determine whether risk assessment scales are effective in reducing the incidence of pressure ulcers (McGough 1999).

Clinical utility of risk assessment scales

A review of the evidence challenges a central role for risk assessment scales as a valid method of screening for risk of pressure ulcer development. However, the literature highlights the complex nature of pressure ulcer development and the numerous factors potentially involved. Within a practice setting, awareness and assessment may be variable and risk assessment scales may be of use in providing a framework for assessment, highlighting key risk factors.

Risk assessment scales have been developed in an attempt to provide a structure and consistency in patient assessment; in a review of 138 pressure ulcer prevention policies, 90% recommended their use (Watts & Clark 1993). Their widespread use would suggest that clinical nurses value them and that their limitations are not necessarily important within the clinical environment. Evidence suggests that their introduction in conjunction with the establishment of skin care teams, education programmes and care protocols may reduce the incidence of pressure ulcers (McGough 1999). They can provide a number of important advantages which can be applied to practice (Box 6.1). However, the use of such scales as a single instrument to assess patient risk of pressure ulcer development cannot be supported on the basis of current evidence.

Practical benefits

1 Raise awareness of risk factors.
2 Provide a minimum standard of risk assessment.
3 Provide a prompt for risk assessment and improve documentation.
4 Provide a crude indicator of risk.
5 Provide a framework for care provision.

Practical limitations

1 Do not distinguish between:
   (a) actual problem (pressure ulcer)
   (b) potential problem (skin changes)
   (c) potential problem (at risk).
2 Do not distinguish between:
   (a) pressure factors
   (b) skin tolerance factors.
3 Are only a snapshot view.
4 Do not consider patient circumstances.
5 Do not predict skin response.

Key prognostic factors

From the 11 cohort studies using multivariate analyses detailed in Table 6.3, five key themes emerge: mobility, nutrition, perfusion, age and skin condition. These can be directly related to the aetiology of pressure ulcer development where the interaction between the intensity and duration of pressure (mobility) and the tolerance of the skin (nutrition, perfusion and age) determines the skin response (skin condition).

The studies cited have used a variety of possible risk factors, measured similar variables in different ways, included various population groups and do not use a common pressure ulcer definition. However, results do inform the risk assessment process.

Mobility

The important relationship between reduced mobility and pressure ulcer occurrence suggested by early prevalence surveys are confirmed by cohort studies which identify mobility-related factors to be significant and independent predictors of pressure ulcer development (Table 6.3). Of the 11 studies detailed in Table 6.3, 10 identify mobility-related factors as important determinants of pressure ulcer development. Interpretation broadly identifies mobility-related factors as all of the following:

- method of manual pressure relief
- activity level
- neurological abnormality
- bed or chair bound
- time on operating table
- mobility
- days on static air mattress for prevention
- ambulation difficulty
- immobility
- postoperative Braden mobility score.

The evidence fully supports the AHCPR guideline that 'bed- and chair-bound individuals or those with impaired ability to reposition should be assessed for additional factors that increase risk for developing pressure ulcers' (AHCPR 1992, p. 13).

Factors affecting skin tolerance

Studies using univariate analyses have identified a large number of factors affecting skin tolerance which are significantly associated with pressure ulcer development (Ch. 3). However, the three themes emerging from multivariate analyses both challenge and support some common assumptions made with regard to the relative importance of pressure ulcer risk factors.

Nutrition-related factors, including appetite, anaemia, impaired nutritional intake, albumin, dietary protein intake, difficulty feeding oneself, lymphopenia and decreased body weight, are identified by eight of the 11 studies, although the exact relationship remains unclear. It is likely that reduced dietary intake is a general indicator of morbidity, as well as directly affecting tissue perfusion and skin structures which reduce tolerance to pressure (Ch. 3). The wide range of factors identified within such a small number of research studies reflects the absence of recognized indicators of nutritional status. The influence of nutrition in patients with existing pressure ulcers is reviewed in Chapter 13.

Factors affecting tissue perfusion, including smoking, anaemia, cerebrovascular accident, extracorporeal circulation, blood pressure, vascular disease and diabetes mellitus, are identified by seven studies. This is the most diverse area of the literature, reflecting the large number of variables which affect tissue perfusion. The existing research base cannot identify key factors more specific than 'perfusion related' and there is a clear need for further exploration of these variables.

Four of the cohort studies determine age as associated with pressure ulcer development. Other studies suggest that in high-risk groups age is less important than associated morbidity (Berlowitz & Wilking 1989, Allman et al 1995, Nixon et al 2000). The relationship is likely to be multifactorial and related to both increased morbidity and disease, which affect mobility and age-related changes of the skin which reduce tissue tolerance (Allman 1997).

It is noteworthy that urinary incontinence is not identified by any of the studies using multivariate statistical techniques as being associated with pressure ulcer development. This challenges the common assumption that incontinence is an important risk factor in pressure ulcer development. It is likely that incontinence is strongly associated with both immobility and age and these factors emerge as more important in a multivariate model.

Skin response to pressure

Skin condition is identified as a risk factor associated with subsequent skin loss by all four studies which included this variable as a potential risk factor. It is an aspect of risk of increasing interest and the subject of current research.

Reactive hyperaemia and other skin changes are included in classification systems for the purposes of research, audit and clinical practice, and are considered to be clinically important (Lowthian 1994). Skin changes may vary from a normal hyperaemic response of short duration (5 min for example) to persistent non-blanching discoloration with localized swelling, heat and induration (Lyder 1991, Lowthian 1994, Bliss 1998).

Physiological differences between the clinical observations of blanching hyperaemia, non-blanching hyperaemia and non-blanching hyperaemia with associated induration, heat and pain have not been determined in relation to measures of skin perfusion or subsequent skin loss (Nixon et al 1999). However, cumulative research evidence is emerging which suggests that hyperaemia (particularly non-blanching) is an identifiable risk factor associated with subsequent pressure ulcer development and provides an indicator of the patient's individual response to pressure assault and care interventions. The central role of skin assessment in determining the individual nature of patient risk and informing care interventions and evaluation is recognized by experts in the field (Marchette et al 1991, AHCPR 1992, Edwards 1996).

Clarke & Kadhom (1988), in a prospective study involving 88 hospitalized and 30 community bedfast or chairfast patients, reported that 'skin changes are apparent before an actual skin break occurs'. Skin condition variables were identified by discriminant analysis as factors associated with pressure ulcer outcome. The study involved nursing staff and carers completing diary sheets on each occasion that pressure area care was given. It is not clear from the research report how 'the state of the skin at the site' was recorded: that is, whether there were description or category options and there is no descriptive data reporting the skin conditions observed. This study is, however, important in providing research evidence linking visible changes in skin condition to subsequent skin loss.

Further evidence is provided by the US National Health and Nutrition Survey 10-year follow-up, which found that individuals with physician-diagnosed dry or scaling skin at baseline were 2.5 times as likely to develop pressure ulcers during the 10-year follow-up period (Guralnik et al 1988). Results cannot be applied directly to practice owing to the limitations associated with the survey methodology, but together with other research are further evidence of an association between skin condition and the occurrence of pressure ulcers.

Marchette et al (1991), in a retrospective record review of 161 surgical intensive care patients, reported 'a significant relationship between the incidence of redness and skin ulcers ($P = 0.00001$)', although actual conversion rates were not reported. Discriminant analysis also identified skin redness as one of a combination of five factors which predicted 93% of the patients that developed pressure ulcers. The study methodology of record review is limited and there is no definition of the term redness (whether blanching or non-blanching, or both).

Allman and colleagues (1995), in a prospective cohort study of hospitalized patients with activity limitations and aged over 55 years, identified non-blanchable erythema of the sacrum at baseline assessment as one of five predictors of pressure ulcer development using Kaplan–Meir survival analysis and Cox regression analysis. A pressure ulcer was defined as epithelial loss or skin breakdown over a bony prominence. The risk ratio of pressure ulcer development associated with the presence of non-blanchable erythema at baseline assessment was 7.52 ($P = 0.05$). Non-blanchable erythema observed during hospital follow up (not included in the primary analysis) was also determined as significantly associated with pressure ulcer development with conversion of 11 out of 19 (57.9%) hospital acquired non-blanchable skin areas to a pressure ulcer ($P < 0.001$). The presence of blanching erythema was not recorded, neither was detail regarding other skin changes such as induration, swelling, heat or pain at the non-blanching sites.

The emerging evidence of the association between skin changes and subsequent pressure ulcer development highlights the central nature skin assessment plays in the risk assessment process.

RISK ASSESSMENT IN PRACTICE

A review of the evidence suggests that nursing assessment is a dynamic and continuous process involving synthesis of information from a variety of sources including underpinning knowledge, previous experience, specialty-based knowledge, recognition of important indicators and knowledge of the patient. In nursing assessment of potential risk of pressure ulcer development information sources are summarized in Box 6.2. Nursing skill is required in order to select, weight and combine important factors in order to notice, understand and act.

It is recommended, on the basis of the existing research evidence, that nursing assessment of potential risk of pressure ulcer development

---

BOX 6.2   INFORMATION SOURCES IN RISK ASSESSMENT

Underpinning knowledge
◆ Aetiology –
   (a) intensity and duration of pressure
   (b) tolerance of skin
◆ Key prognostic factors
◆ Specialty pressure ulcer risk factors
◆ Specialty – patterns of disease and recovery.

Clinical experience
◆ Patterns of disease and recovery
◆ Expected norms
◆ Local risk factors.

Patient evidence
◆ Mobility – intensity and duration of pressure
◆ Skin response – tolerance of the skin
◆ General condition
◆ Predicted future course.

should consider the following questions simultaneously:

1 Is the patient exposed to prolonged or repetitive pressure (friction and shear)?
2 What is the patient's skin response to pressure?
3 Are there factors present which reduce skin tolerance?

That is, risk assessment requires detailed assessment of mobility, the skin and general risk factors. Assessment of these three aspects of the patient inform judgements about risk and the frequency of monitoring. A decision support tool such as a risk assessment scale may provide a framework for such an assessment but the nurse must incorporate specialty-based knowledge, patient prognosis, previous experience and local knowledge in the assessment of potential risk and anticipation of future care needs. For example, a surgical nurse will recognize preoperatively the likely postoperative needs of a major surgical patient on the basis of prior knowledge and experience of caring for surgical patients, and allocate appropriate resources. Assessment is context-specific, combining knowledge of key risk factors with patient circumstances. Important aspects of mobility, general and skin assessments are discussed next.

Mobility assessment – exposure to pressure, friction and shear

Mobility assessment aims to determine risk resulting from exposure to pressure, friction and shear. Important elements specific to the patient inform the judgement of potential risk. These include:

- knowledge of patient circumstances (e.g. reason for immobility)
- clinical experience of the medical/surgical condition (e.g. expected postoperative period of immobility)
- sensory perception (e.g. stimulus to move)
- motivational and compliance factors (e.g. stimulus to move)
- position required/favoured by patient.

These factors are largely ignored in research, to date, yet impact greatly at an individual level on patient care. For example, a semirecumbent position generates friction and shearing forces which, as previously discussed, exacerbate the pressure effect (Fig. 6.3). Sitting also generates high pressures over the ischial tuberosities, which may be exacerbated if the patient has a tendency to slip forward. Practical problems are also encountered when patients prefer one position and resume their favoured position despite all efforts, or in patients who are haemodynamically unstable and are, as a consequence, too unstable to move.

It is also important to consider immobility and activity factors within the context of the local environment and equipment provision. For example, the type of mattress, chair or other equipment provided within the environment will affect exposure to pressure, friction and shear. Such factors specific to the individual and environment inform the risk assessment process, together with other clinical signs and symptoms relating to the skin response. The variables involved and knowledge required relating to patient factors illustrate that risk assessment is an interactive and dynamic process.

Skin assessment – skin response to pressure

The interpretation of skin assessment in practice relies on practitioner understanding of the clinical manifestations of pathophysiological events and knowledge of the patient, patient-specific risk factors and potential environmental risk factors.

When undertaking clinical assessment of the skin it is useful to relate the pathophysiological events to their visual appearance. This enables informed interpretation of signs and symptoms to support clinical decision making. As described in Chapter 3, if occlusion occurs the release of pressure produces a large and sudden increase in blood flow and the bright red flush so produced is known as reactive hyperaemia. Other skin changes relate directly to the pathology. For example, local oedema, induration, heat, non-blanching hyperaemia, blue/purple/black

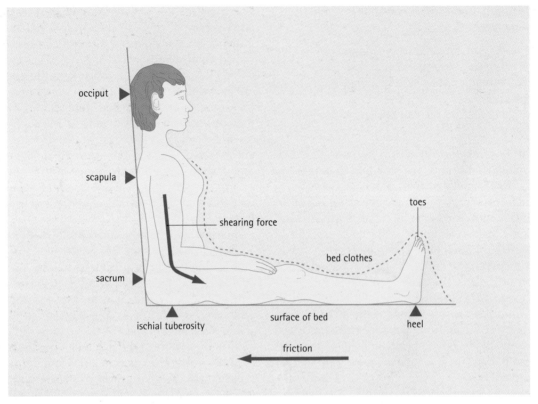

occiput

scapula

shearing force

toes

sacrum

bed clothes

ischial tuberosity

surface of bed

heel

friction

Figure 6.3 Shearing forces, friction and pressure in a semirecumbent position. Reproduced with permission from Morison (1992) A Colour Guide to the Nursing Management of Chronic Wounds, Mosby.

discoloration (Shea 1975, Parish et al 1983, Lowthian 1987, Lyder 1991, Reid & Morison 1994) indicate lymphatic involvement and capillary disruption. Lowthian (1994) emphasizes the importance of detailed skin inspection of non-blanching hyperaemia and describes in detail clinical examination of a pressure area for heat and induration.

Observations of erythema should prompt consideration as to whether the response observed is normal or abnormal and a judgement made regarding the clinical importance of the observation. Such consideration can only be undertaken within the clinical environment and requires consideration of:

1 Circumstances associated with the appearance of the hyperaemic response including:
   (a) nature of pressure assault
        (single/repetitive, duration)

   (b) patient mobility
   (c) patient activity
   (d) prognosis.
2 Nature of the hyperaemic response including:
   (a) intensity of redness
   (b) duration of redness
   (c) presence/absence of blanching under light finger pressure.
   (d) presence/absence of oedema, induration, pain, discoloration.

For example, the observation of a reddened area on a usually mobile patient who has woken from sleep is unlikely to have any clinical importance. However, a reddened area observed when repositioning a spinally injured patient should prompt further observation including signs of blanching and duration of the reactive hyperaemic response.

On the basis of current research evidence best practice can be summarized as follows:

1. Observation of blanching erythema indicates the need for an informed judgement of risk and clinical relevance at individual patient level. It is an indicator of the patient's individual response to pressure and is therefore a key indicator in the evaluation of care interventions.
2. Observation of a non-blanching area indicates that the patient is at high risk of subsequent skin loss and requires active intervention to alleviate pressure.

Although considered clinically important, there is debate regarding the inclusion of these observations within pressure ulcer classification systems (Lyder 1991, Hitch 1995). Debate appears to focus upon the classification of pressure ulcers for research and audit purposes and difficulties in achieving good inter-rater reliability and validity of definition (Lyder 1991, Healey 1996). From a practice perspective, regardless of the classification system used, it is essential that the record of care provides clear descriptions of the skin changes observed and such evidence should direct and support individual patient care (see Key Points).

Tolerance of the skin – other risk factors

Various factors affect the tolerance of the skin to pressure. These include variables which affect the basic structures of the skin and those which affect the nutrient supply. Three themes that emerge from prognostic factor studies serve to underline the need for a comprehensive assessment of the nutritional status of the patient (Ch. 13), an awareness of age and assessment of the various factors affecting tissue perfusion.

Sackett and colleagues warn against blind faith in variables identified as 'predictive': 'Keep in mind that these prognostic factors need not cause the outcome; they need only be associated with its development strongly enough to predict it'. (Sackett et al 1997, p. 90).

KEY POINTS

SKIN ASSESSMENT IN PRACTICE

◆ Skin assessment and interpretation of signs and symptoms is the basis of pressure ulcer prevention and treatment

◆ External force generates a variety of skin changes which are clinically important. These include:
  — reactive hyperaemia – blanching/non-blanching
  — local oedema
  — heat
  — induration
  — blue/purple/black discoloration

◆ It is important at the clinical level to distinguish between a normal and abnormal skin response

◆ Observation of blanching erythema indicates the need for an informed clinical decision regarding the risk of pressure ulcer development

◆ Observation of a non-blanching area indicates that the patient is at high risk of subsequent skin loss and requires active intervention to alleviate pressure

◆ Documentation of skin changes supports clinical decisions.

This is pertinent with respect to factors affecting skin tolerance. The primary risk factor in pressure ulcer development is reduced mobility and it is the interaction between the pressure assault and the tolerance of the skin which leads to tissue damage. The importance attributed to these factors will in part be determined by mobility assessment (that is, if the patient has no mobility deficit these factors are not important) and the skin assessment which provides an indication of the skin's tolerance to pressure.

6

SUMMARY

Patient assessment requires an interactive ongoing approach. It is essential from the outset to identify which patients require baseline skin assessment in order to determine the presence or absence of an existing pressure ulcer. Subsequent assessment of individual patient risk is an ongoing and dynamic process supported by our knowledge of key prognostic factors (in particular mobility), the patient's individual skin response to pressure and prognosis, specialty-based knowledge and clinical experience. It requires the nurse to assimilate information from a variety of sources and make an informed judgement of patient risk and care needs. Risk assessment scales, while limited in construction methodologies and validity, may provide a framework and appropriate prompts for assessment but their use as a single instrument to assess risk is not supported on the basis of current evidence.

 CASE STUDY 6.1

Mrs Rutter is a 79-year-old admitted to hospital for a left hemicolectomy. She has a history of weight loss (2 kg over a 2-month period) but remains obese. She is deaf but has no hearing aids and her understanding of her situation is difficult to determine without loss of privacy and dignity. She is nursed in a six-bedded single-sex ward area.

Mrs Rutter underwent a 3-h surgical procedure during which time no pressure ulcer prevention measures were allocated. She had a general anaesthetic, with a preoperative epidural cannula sited for postoperative pain relief. She was hypotensive for long periods both intra- and postoperatively.

On her first postoperative day Mrs Rutter remained confined to bed and found difficulty in moving because of intravenous cannula, wound drains and epidural. Despite attempts to position Mrs Rutter laterally and explanations for the need to rest on her side she frequently resumed a semirecumbent position. She was nursed on a high-specification foam mattress. Her sacrum and buttock areas were noted as blanching hyperaemia postoperatively by theatre staff and during each shift period in the first 36 h after surgery. A small area on her left buttock was observed to be non-blanching on the morning of her second postoperative day.

1 What are the main aetiological risk factors for pressure ulcer development:
   (a) intraoperatively
   (b) postoperatively

2 What individual management problems exacerbate these risk factors?

3 Using a method of your choice assess the likelihood of Mrs Rutter developing a pressure ulcer.

REFERENCES

Agency for Health Care Policy and Research (AHCPR) 1992 Pressure ulcers in adults: prediction and prevention. AHCPR Publication No. 92–0047. US Department of Health and Human Services, Rockville

Allman R M 1997 Pressure ulcer prevalence, incidence, risk factors and impact. Clinics in Geriatric Medicine 13(3):421–436

Allman R M, Laprade C A, Noel L B et al 1986 Pressure sores among hospitalized patients. Annals of Internal Medicine 105(3):337–342

Allman R M, Goode P S, Patrick M M, Burst N, Bartolucci A A 1995 Pressure ulcer risk factors among hospitalized patients with activity limitation. Journal of the American Medical Association 273(11):865–870

Andersen K E, Jensen O, Kvorning S A, Bach E 1982 Prevention of pressure sores by identifying patients at risk. British Medical Journal 284:1370–1371

Bale S, Finlay I, Harding K G 1995 Pressure sore prevention in a hospice. Journal of Wound Care 4(10):465–468

Barbenel J C, Jordan M M, Nicol S M, Clark M O 1977 Incidence of pressure sores in the Greater Glasgow Health Board Area. Lancet ii:548–550

Barbenel J C, Jordan M M, Nicol S M 1980 Major pressure of sores. Health and Social Service Journal 90(2):1344–1345

Barnes D, Payton R G 1993 Clinical application of the Braden scale in the acute-care setting. Dermatology Nursing 5(5):386–388

Barrois B, Colin D 1995 A survey of pressure sore prevalence in hospitals in the Greater Paris region. Journal of Wound Care 4(5):234–236

Benner P 1984 From novice to expert: excellence and power in clinical nursing practice. Addison-Wesley, Menlo Park

Benner P, Wrubal J 1982 Skilled clinical knowledge: the value of perceptual awareness. Nurse Educator 7:11–17

Bergstrom N, Braden B 1992 A prospective study of pressure sore risk among institutionalized elderly. Journal of the American Geriatrics Society 40(8):747–758

Berlowitz D R, Wilking S V B 1989 Risk factors for pressure sores: A comparison of cross-sectional and cohort-derived data. Journal of the American Geriatrics Society 37(11):1043–1050

Berlowitz D R, Wilking S V B 1990 The short-term outcome of pressure sores. Journal of the American Geriatrics Society 38(7):748–752

Bergstrom N, Braden B J, Laguzza A, Holman V 1987a The Braden scale for predicting pressure sore risk. Nursing Research 36(4):205–210

Bergstrom N, Demuth P J, Braden B J 1987b A clinical trial of the Braden scale for predicting pressure sore risk. Nursing Clinics of North America 22(2):417–428

Bliss M, 1998 Hyperaemia. Journal of Tissue Viability 8(4):4–13

Braden B J, Bergstrom N 1994 Predictive validity of the Braden scale for pressure sore risk in a nursing home population. Research in Nursing and Health 17:459–70

Brandeis G H, Ooi W L, Hossain M, Morris J N, Lipsitz L A 1994 A longitudinal study of risk factors associated with the formation of pressure ulcers in nursing homes. Journal of the American Geriatrics Society 42(4):388–393

Bridel J, 1993 Assessing the risk of pressure sores. Nursing Standard 7(25):32–35

Bridel J, Banks S, Mitton C 1996 The admission prevalence and hospital-acquired incidence of pressure sores within a large teaching hospital during April 1994 to March 1995. In: Cherry G W et al (eds) Proceedings of the 5th European Conference on Advances in Wound Management. Macmillan Magazines, London, pp. 83–85

Capobianco M L, McDonald D D 1996 Factors affecting the predictive validity of the Braden Scale. Advances in Wound Care 9(6):32–6

Clark M, Cullum N 1992 Matching patient need for pressure sore prevention with the supply of pressure redistributing mattresses. Journal of Advanced Nursing 17(3):310–316

Clark M, Watts S 1994 The incidence of pressure sores within a National Health Service Trust Hospital during 1991. Journal of Advanced Nursing 20(3):33–36

Clarke M, Kadhom H M 1988 The nursing prevention of pressure sores in hospital and community patients. Journal of Advanced Nursing 13(3):365–373

Clough N P 1994 The cost of pressure area management in an intensive care unit. Journal of Wound Care 3(1):33–35

Collins J G 1988 Prevalence of selected chronic conditions, United States, 1983–85. Advance Data from Vital and Health Statistics. No. 155. DHHS publication no. (PHS 88–1250). Public Health Service, Hyattsville

Corcoran-Perry S, Graves J 1990 Supplemental-information-seeking behaviour of cardio-vascular nurses. Research in Nursing and Health 13(2):119–127

Crow R A, Chase J, Lamond D 1995 The cognitive component of nursing assessment: an analysis. Journal of Advanced Nursing 22(2):206–212

Cullum N, Nelson E A, Nixon J 1999 Pressure sores. In: Clinical evidence: a compendium of the best available evidence for effective health care. BMJ Publishing Group, London. Issue 1, June 1999, pp. 211–217

David J A, Chapman R G, Chapman E J, Lockett B 1983 An investigation of the current methods used in nursing for the care of patients with established pressure sores. Nursing Research Unit, Northwick Park

Deeks J J 1996 Pressure sore prevention: Using and evaluating risk assessment tools. British Journal of Nursing 5(5):313–320

Edwards M 1995 The levels of reliability and validity of the Waterlow pressure sore risk calculator. Journal of Wound Care 4(8):373–378

Edwards M 1996 Pressure sore risk calculators: Some methodological issues. Journal of Clinical Nursing 5(5):307–312

Effective Health Care 1994 Implementing clinical practice guidelines: Can guidelines be used to improve clinical practice? Effective Health Care Bulletin 1(8):1–11

Effective Health Care 1995 The prevention and treatment of pressure sores: How effective are pressure-relieving interventions and risk assessment for the prevention and treatment of pressure sores? Effective Health Care Bulletin 2(1):1–16

Ek A-C, Unosson M, Larsson J, Von Schenck H, Bjurulf P 1991 The development and healing of pressure sores related to the nutritional state. Clinical Nutrition 10:245–250

Exton-Smith A N, Sherwin R W 1961 The prevention of pressure sores: significance of spontaneous bodily movements. Lancet, ii(7212):1124–1126

Guralnik J M, Harris T B, White L R, Cornoni-Huntley J C 1988 Occurrence and predictors of pressure sores in the National Health and nutrition examination survey follow-up. Journal of the American Geriatrics Society 36(9):807–812

Halfens R J 1997 The reliability and validity of the Braden scale. In: Harding K G, Leaper D J, Turner T D (eds) Proceedings of the 7th European Conference on Advances in Wound Management. Macmillan, London

Healey F 1996 Classification of pressure sores: 2. British Journal of Nursing 5(9):567–574

Hitch S 1995 NHS Executive Nursing Directorate – Strategy for major clinical guidelines – prevention and management of pressure sores: A literature review. Journal of Tissue Viability 5(1):3–24

Hoshowsky V M, Schramm C A 1994 Intraoperative pressure prevention: An analysis of bedding materials. Research in Nursing and Health 17(5):333–339

Jenny J, Logan J 1992 Knowing the patient: one aspect of clinical knowledge. Image: The Journal of Nursing Scholarship 24(4):254–258

Kemp M G, Keithley J K, Smith D W, Morreale B 1990 Factors that contribute to pressure sores in surgical patients. Research in Nursing and Health, 13(5):293–301

Kirshner B, Guyatt G 1985 A methodological framework for assessing health indices. Journal of Chronic Disability 38(1):27–36

Langemo D K, Olson B, Hunter S, Hanson D, Burd C, Catheart-Silberg T 1991 Incidence and prediction of pressure ulcers in five patient care settings Decubitus 4(3):25–36

Larson E 1986 Evaluating validity of screening tests. Nursing Research 35:186–188

Lowthian P 1987 Classification and grading of pressure sores. Care Science and Practice 5(1):5–9

Lowthian P 1989 Identifying and protecting patients who may get pressure sores. Nursing Standard 4(4):26–29

Lowthian P 1994 Pressure sores: A search for definition. Nursing Standard 9(11):30–32

Lyder C H 1991 Conceptualisation of the stage I pressure ulcer. Journal of Enterostomal Nursing 18(5):162–165

MacLeod M L P 1993 On knowing the patient: experiences of nurses undertaking care In: Radley A (ed.) Worlds of illness: biographical and cultural perspectives on health and disease. Routledge, London, pp. 179–197

MacLeod M 1994 'It's the little things that count' the hidden complexity of everyday clinical nursing practice. Journal of Clinical Nursing 3(6):361–368

McGough A J 1999 A systematic review of the effectiveness of risk assessment scales used in the prevention and management of pressure sores. MSc thesis, The University of York, York

Marchette L, Arnell I, Redick E 1991 Skin ulcers of elderly surgical patients in critical care units. Dimensions of Critical Care Nursing 10(6):321–329

Nixon J, McElvenny D, Mason S, Brown J, Bond S 1998 A sequential randomised controlled trial comparing a dry visco-elastic polymer pad and standard operating table mattress in the prevention of post-operative pressure sores. International Journal of Nursing Studies 35(4):193–203

Nixon J, Smye S, Scott J, Bond S 1999 The diagnosis of early pressure sores: Report of the pilot study. Journal of Tissue Viability 9(2):62–66

Nixon J, McElvenny D, Mason S, Brown J, Bond S 2000 Prognostic factors associated with pressure sore development in the immediate post-operative period. International Journal of Nursing Studies, 37(4): 279–289

Norton D, McLaren R, Exton-Smith A N 1962 An investigation of geriatric nursing problems in hospital. Churchill Livingstone, Edinburgh

Parish L C, Witkowski J A, Chrissey J T 1983 The decubitus ulcer. Masson, New York

Parkinson H, Coleman S, Nixon J, Scott J 1999 Peri-operative pressure area care implementation of a research based assessment and management flow chart. Poster Presentation, National Association of Theatre Nurses 35rd Congress and Exhibition, Harrogate

Prescott P A, Soeken K L, Ryan J W 1989 Measuring patient intensity: a reliability study. Evaluation and The Health Professions 12(3):255–269

Pyles S H, Stern P N 1983 Discovery of nursing gestalt in critical care nursing: the importance of the gray gorilla syndrome. Image: The Journal of Nursing Scholarship 15(2):51–57

Ramundo J M 1995 Reliability and validity of the Braden scale in the home care setting. Journal of Wound Ostomy and Continence Nursing 22(3):128–34

Reid J, Morison M 1994 Towards a consensus: Classification of pressure sores. Journal of Wound Care 3(3):157–160

Richardson R R, Meyer P R 1981 Prevalence and incidence of pressure sores in acute spinal cord injuries. Paraplegia 19:235–247

Robnett M K 1986 The incidence of skin breakdown in a surgical intensive care unit. Journal Nursing Quality Assurance 1(1):77–81

Sackett D L, Richardson W A, Rosenberg W, Haynes R B 1997 Evidence-based medicine how to practice and teach EBM. Churchill Livingstone, Edinburgh

Salzberg C A, Byrne D W, Cayten C G et al 1996 A new pressure ulcer risk assessment scale for individuals with spinal cord injury. American Journal of Physical Medicine & Rehabilitation 75(2):96–104

Shea J D 1975 Pressure sores. Classification and management. Clinical Orthopaedics 112:89–100

Simon R, Altman D G 1994 Statistical aspects of prognostic factor studies in oncology. British Journal of Cancer 69:979–985

Stotts N A, Paul S M 1988 Pressure ulcer development in surgical patients. Decubitus 1(3):24–30

Tanner C A, Benner P, Chesla C, Gordon D R 1993 The phenomenology of knowing the patient. Image: The Journal of Nursing Scholarship 25(4):273–280

Thomas D R, Goode P S, Tarquine P H, Allman R M 1996 Hospital-acquired pressure ulcers and risk of death. Journal of the American Geriatrics Society 44(12):1435–1440

Towey A P, Erland S M 1988 Validity and reliability of an assessment tool for pressure ulcer risk. Decubitus 1(2):40–48

Versluysen M 1986 How elderly patients with femoral fracture develop pressure sores in hospital. British Medical Journal 292:1311–1313

Wai-Han C, Kit-Wai C, French P, Yim-Sheung L, Lai-Kwan T 1997 Which pressure sore risk calculator? A study of the effectiveness of the Norton scale in Hong Kong. International Journal of Nursing Studies 34(2):165–169

Waterlow J 1988 The Waterlow card for the prevention and management of pressure sores: Towards a pocket policy. Care Science and Practice 6(1):8–12

Watts S, Clark M 1993 Pressure sore prevention: a review of policy documents. Nursing Practice Research Unit, University of Surrey

Yates J F 1990 Judgements and decision making. Prentice-Hall, London

7 *Michael Clark*

Pressure ulcer prevention

INTRODUCTION

Current attitudes towards pressure area care aptly reflect the old proverb 'an ounce of prevention is worth a pound of cure'. The present emphasis upon pressure ulcer prevention primarily derives from three key beliefs.

1 Preventing pressure ulcers prevents needless pain, distress and even death.
2 Preventing pressure ulcers costs less money than does their treatment.
3 The majority of pressure ulcers are preventable.

Few would disagree that avoiding the development of a pressure ulcer is likely to benefit patients. Pressure ulcers are likely to reduce one's health-related quality of life (see Ch. 4). The person with a pressure ulcer may experience pain, embarrassment and may feel barred from participation in everyday activities among other deleterious effects. Most pressure ulcers involving skin breaks are painful (Szor & Bourguignon 1997): 28 out of 32 (87.5%) subjects reported pain, of whom five described the pain as being either horrible or excruciating). Interestingly Szor & Bourguignon reported that the description of the pain caused by partial- and full-thickness ulcers did not differ. While they may be painful, pressure ulcers are rarely a primary reason for admission to hospital. Of the 961 patients with established pressure ulcers reported by David et al (1983), only 5.7% had been admitted as a consequence of having developed a pressure ulcer. The presence of a pressure ulcer does not necessarily delay discharge from hospital. So while the majority of pressure ulcers (where the skin is broken) may be painful, typically these wounds do not present as life-threatening clinical problems. However, while full-thickness (severe) pressure ulcers may be relatively rare, affecting perhaps 1 in every 500 hospital in-patient admissions in the UK (Clark & Watts 1994), their impact can be devastating, and such wounds may result in death. In 1986, 171 people died in the UK as a direct consequence of having developed pressure ulcers, with these being noted on the death certificates of a further 1929 people (Davies et al 1991).

Patients clearly benefit from avoiding pressure ulcers, but does aggressive pressure ulcer prevention save money? At an individual patient level, pressure ulcer prevention may be less expensive; Clark (1994a) reported the daily cost of prevention in a UK hospital to be £1.83 per patient, while the daily cost of treatment (primarily of partial-thickness pressure ulcers) was £3.91. However, if the perspective of the analysis is changed from the individual patient to the overall hospital, then prevention may cost more than treatment. Clark (1994a) calculated the annual costs of treatment within a District General Hospital to be £78 228.93, while the annual costs of prevention were higher (£90 118.35) due to the greater numbers of patients requiring preventive care. Touche Ross (1993) also discussed the potential higher costs of prevention.

The third, and perhaps most important, belief supporting pressure ulcer prevention is that most established pressure ulcers could have been avoided. In a widely quoted comment, Hibbs (1988) suggested that 95% of all established ulcers could have been prevented, with only 5% being inevitable despite preventive care. While such statements focus attention upon the potential benefits of prevention, they may have little or no basis in fact. If pressure ulcers are indeed preventable, this infers that the natural history of the developing pressure ulcer can be altered through actions taken by either health care professionals or by the patient. Knowledge of the natural history of pressure ulcers is still incomplete and without a precise definition of 'risk' it is impossible to ascertain when this risk has been averted, and a pressure ulcer prevented.

Measuring the success of preventive care?

To date, there is no universally recognized marker of the success of preventive care. Typically 'successful' pressure ulcer prevention has been inferred through apparent reductions in either the prevalence or incidence of the ulcers. Viewed uncritically, such an approach appears to offer strong evidence of improvements in practice. However, the reasons why longitudinal surveys may show reduced, or increased, rates of pressure ulcer occurrence may be complex. Has the introduction of preventive care affected patient outcomes, or has the patient population along with the organization and delivery of care changed between the time of successive surveys? Such confounders of pressure ulcer occurrence rates can be controlled through the adjustment of raw prevalence or incidence data using both structural and process variables. Case-mix adjustment of pressure ulcer prevalence and incidence rates has begun to be reported in both North America and the UK. In the UK, Williams et al (1997) reported the adjustment of incidence data to control for both differences in patients' vulnerability to developing ulcers, as measured using the Waterlow Scale, and their length of stay in hospital. Comparing the incidence of ulcers upon two medical wards drawn from different hospitals, case-mix adjustment reduced the crude incidence by 0.2%, from 9.9% to 9.7% in one ward, with an increased incidence calculated upon the second ward following case-mix adjustment, from 6.1% to 6.3%. While these

changes following case-mix adjustment may be relatively small they had the overall effect of reducing the apparent difference between wards, as inferred by the crude incidence rates. Other authors have used more complex approaches towards case-mix adjustment. Mukamel (1997), using 14 patient characteristics, modelled the likelihood of a pressure ulcer deteriorating between successive assessments, while Berlowitz et al (1996) constructed a model based upon 11 factors to adjust the incidence rates measured across 143 long-term care facilities in the USA. While case-mix adjustment should be performed if the rate of pressure ulcer occurrence across different sites is to be compared, or a single site is to be compared over time, several issues remain unresolved. Beyond important practical issues regarding how health care providers are to collect and adjust pressure ulcer incidence data, two fundamental questions remain – which factors should be controlled (for example, should age be controlled, or mobility or nutritional status?) and are these factors constant in different care settings?

'Conversion rates': how many vulnerable patients develop pressure ulcers?

Regardless of the lack of a universal case-mix adjustment factor, what proportion of patients vulnerable to developing pressure ulcers actually experience these wounds, or what is the 'conversion rate' between risk and pressure ulcers? It could be assumed that if risk was precisely defined, and no preventive care delivered, then all vulnerable patients would develop pressure ulcers – a conversion rate of 100%. Published data upon the occurrence of pressure ulcers in the absence of preventive care are rare. Xakellis et al (1998) reported the incidence of pressure ulcers within a long-term care facility in the USA before and following the introduction of preventive care. Prior to any preventive care being delivered, 34 patients were considered to have been vulnerable to developing pressure ulcers from a retrospective calculation of their Braden scores; of this group, 13 developed pressure ulcers, giving a 'conversion rate' of 38.2%. Following the introduction of a range of preventive care (including a new guideline, staff training, patient repositioning, the use of mattress overlays and employment of additional nursing staff), the conversion rate fell to 11.5% (three developed pressure ulcers among 26 vulnerable patients). While these rates (38.2% and 11.5%) are not case-adjusted, they do suggest that the introduction of preventive care may reduce the number of vulnerable patients who subsequently develop pressure ulcers. It is interesting to note that the pre-prevention conversion rate (38.2%) falls below the theoretical 100% conversion that could be predicted in the absence of pressure ulcer preventive care. This could be explained either by the informal performance of preventive care in Xakellis et al's pre-intervention stage, or that the denominator is incorrect, reflecting the presence of false positives when predicting risk using assessment tools such as the Braden or Waterlow scales. As long as prediction of risk is based upon an incomplete understanding of pressure ulcer aetiology, the 'conversion rate' is likely to be artificially low because of the reduced sensitivity of the tools used to predict risk.

KEY POINTS

◆ There is no single recognized marker of successful pressure ulcer prevention

◆ Observed incidence and prevalence rates may be misleading if not adjusted to reflect patient and organizational characteristics

◆ Little knowledge is available regarding 'conversion rates' or the number of vulnerable patients who develop pressure ulcers in the absence of preventive care.

THE AIM OF PRESSURE ULCER PREVENTION

Successful prevention of pressure ulcers results from reducing or removing the causes of these wounds. Unfortunately, our knowledge of pressure ulcer aetiology is incomplete. Given such uncertainty, the focus of pressure ulcer prevention remains the mitigation of the effects of patient immobility. Immobility prolongs weight bearing over bony prominences of the body. Therefore, preventive care either reduces the period of time prominences are loaded (through patient repositioning and the use of alternating-pressure air mattresses, APAMs), or minimizes the magnitude of the forces applied during tissue loading (through the use of static or soft patient support surfaces); rarely have attempts been reported where the integral 'tolerance' of soft tissues to loading has been manipulated. The prevention of pressure ulcers is helped through the use of skin dressings and lotions to protect against abrasion, through the implementation of local and national guidelines promoting best practice and through providing knowledge to both practitioners and their patients. The various actions that, in combination, may lead to successful pressure ulcer prevention are illustrated in Figure 7.1.

PREVENTING PRESSURE ULCERS THROUGH MOVING OR POSITIONING THE PATIENT (Fig. 7.2)

Clark (1998) reviewed the evolution and impact of regular patient positioning upon the development of pressure ulcers. Seven fundamental questions regarding repositioning remain unanswered. These are discussed below.

Why do so few local guidelines include specific reference to the repositioning of patients?

Although evidence-based national guidelines strongly support repositioning of patients, specific guidance upon repositioning was given in only 5.8% (5/86) of local policies and guidelines in the UK (Watts & Clark 1993).

Why should some vulnerable patients be repositioned, but others not?

Failure to reposition all vulnerable patients was reported by Bergstrom et al (1996), where 48.9% of subjects at moderate to high risk (based upon their Braden Scores) were not repositioned.

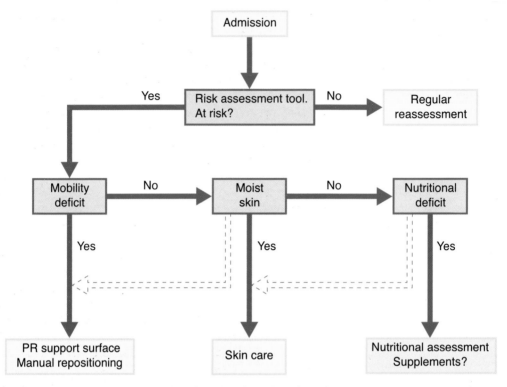

Figure 7.1   Pressure ulcer prevention algorithm. (Based on algorithm constructed by the Panel for the Prediction and Prevention of Pressure Ulcers in Adults, 1992).

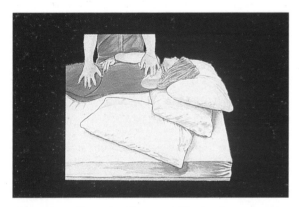

Figure 7.2   Manual patient repositioning (reproduced with permission from Medical Support Systems Ltd).

How often should patients be repositioned?

Traditionally, repositioning is considered to be most effective when performed at 2-h intervals.

This has been reinforced within national guidelines; for example repositioning should be performed 'at least every 2 hours' (Panel for the Prediction and Prevention of Pressure Ulcers in Adults 1992). Practitioners also accept 2-hourly changes in position as being the most effective; for example Buss & Halfens (1995) reported how over half (55%) of participants in a Dutch pressure ulcer symposium considered 2-hourly turns to be the most effective interval for repositioning patients. When asked, fewer participants (8%) considered repositioning at hourly intervals to be the optimum frequency.

Does turning always reduce the incidence of pressure ulcers?

In a report by Bergstrom et al (1996), patients who were repositioned (position changes at unspecified intervals) developed more pressure ulcers, with all the ulcers considered to be superficial. Among those at minimal risk, this difference was striking: 28% of those repositioned developed pressure ulcers compared with an incidence of only 7% among those who were not repositioned. As vulnerability to pressure ulcers increased, the difference between incidence among those repositioned or not decreased; 42% moderate to high risk patients who were repositioned developed pressure ulcers, while 39.5% of non-repositioned patients also developed pressure ulcers. Perhaps such differences relate to the techniques used to reposition patients? If subjects were in part 'dragged' across the bed surface then the apparent discrepancy between the allocation of turning and the incidence of pressure ulcers may simply indicate skin abrasion as a result of inappropriate repositioning (Clark 1996a).

Why are patients repositioned 2-hourly?

Clark (1998) highlighted the anecdotes that have arisen regarding the origins of 2-hourly turning. This interval between changing a patient's position has been attributed to the ward regimens instituted by Florence Nightingale and to the classic aetiology study reported by Kosiak in 1961. However, it would appear that 2-hourly turning stems from observations made during attempts to prevent the development of pressure ulcers among paraplegic patients.

Is '2-hourly turning' effective?

The investigations reported by Norton et al (1962) are considered to provide strong support for the efficacy of 2-hourly turning. Norton and colleagues have been described as having 'manipulated the repositioning schedule and measured the effect on the incidence of pressure ulcers in at-risk elderly individuals' (Panel for the Prediction and Prevention of Pressure Ulcers in Adults 1992). This description of Norton et al (1962) is incorrect. Norton et al (1962) reported the fate of 100 elderly in-patients, without established pressure ulcers, all newly admitted to a 'Care of the Elderly' ward. This group could be divided into

two cohorts: the first ($n = 68$) were considered to be mobile; the remainder ($n = 32$) were deemed to be immobile while in bed. Among the mobile subjects, 27 were repositioned every 4 h, with the majority ($n = 41$) rarely repositioned (reported interval between nurse-initiated changes of position was between 6- and 12-hourly). Few of these mobile patients developed pressure ulcers ($n = 3$, all developed superficial ulcers). Among the immobile patients, 18.7% ($n = 6$) developed ulcers, all superficial. At no time did Norton and colleagues 'manipulate the repositioning schedule'. As such, this classic study simply informs us that patients who are immobile are prone to developing pressure ulcers, often despite regular repositioning. All the superficial pressure ulcers that developed resolved within 5 weeks when patients were repositioned at strict 2-h intervals. As Clark (1998) noted, 'this uncontrolled observation of a cohort of patients tells us little about the optimal frequency of regular repositioning'. Little attention has been paid to the optimum frequency of repositioning since the work of Norton et al (1962). In 1994, Knox and colleagues described the consequences of resting in one position for 1, 1.5 and 2 h upon four outcomes: skin temperature, contact (interface) pressure, pain and skin colour changes. Elderly volunteers ($n = 16$, mean age 70.5 years, range 61–78) lay upon plastic-coated mattresses in either a supine or 90° lateral position, with measurements made at the sacrum and greater trochanters, respectively. Unsurprisingly, contact pressures did not show any marked change while subjects rested in one position, although skin temperature increased significantly, particularly over the greater trochanters after 2 h of immobility. The majority of subjects presented with moderate to severe redness over the greater trochanter or sacrum regardless of the duration of immobility; after 1 h immobile 10 subjects had red areas, with eight showing similar skin changes after 2 h in a constant position. From this data, Knox et al (1994) suggested that patients should perhaps be repositioned after 1.5 h, rather than 2-hourly, with the frequency reducing to hourly changes if the skin colour changes within 90 min of immobility. Another interpretation of their data is possible:

the majority of subjects showed evidence of skin changes after only 1 h in a constant position. This may suggest that even hourly turns may not be sufficient to protect all vulnerable patients from developing pressure ulcers. While 'two-hourly turns' may appear to be a strong foundation for successful pressure ulcer prevention, there remains great uncertainty regarding the optimal frequency of repositioning, largely because 'the effectiveness of different schedules of manual repositioning has not been adequately studied' (Cullum et al 1995).

Can any turning schedule guarantee to prevent pressure ulcers?

Perhaps turning schedules cannot provide adequate protection for all patients. Salisbury (1985) measured the availability of oxygen at the greater trochanters while both volunteers and burns patients rested upon different support surfaces. Transcutaneous oxygen levels fell rapidly within the first few minutes after adopting a constant position upon a standard hospital mattress; similar changes were recorded when the mattress was covered with a sheepskin fleece. He commented that following the onset of immobility 'the rapid drop of recorded cutaneous PO_2 was alarming. Thus, in patients at high risk for pressure ulcer development, the accepted regimen of position changes every 2 h would not be adequate. It is now obvious that even if nursing personnel were following this regimen completely, the patient would still be at risk'.

Positioning patients: the 30° tilt (Fig. 7.3) Shea (1975) commented that 'position can be changed every two to three hours with minimal physical and professional effort if one does not attempt to turn the patient a full 180 degrees each time but merely rolls him 20 to 30 degrees to a slightly tilted position supported by pillows'. Perhaps a greater emphasis upon the positioning of patients may generate greater benefits, in terms of fewer pressure ulcers, than a continued search for a, perhaps unrealistic, optimum interval between repositioning? The 30° tilt, as suggested by Shea (1975), has been investigated in the lab-

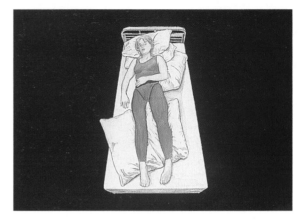

Figure 7.3 The 30° tilt (reproduced with permission from Medical Support Systems Ltd).

oratory with encouraging results. Adoption of this posture appears to reduce pressures compared with the conventional supine position, while also maintaining the supply of oxygen to vulnerable anatomical locations. However, there are no patient outcome studies that question whether fewer pressure ulcers develop when patients are positioned at a 30° tilt. Until such time that well-executed comparative outcome studies are available, the 30° tilt must remain an interesting, yet unproven, method for preventing pressure ulcers.

SURFACES TO PREVENT PRESSURE ULCERS

Support surfaces, be they beds, mattresses or chair cushions, have been used for many years to assist the prevention of pressure ulcers. The value of support surfaces in pressure ulcer management has been recognized from at least 1569. In the sixteenth century, Paré advised upon the treatment of a large pressure ulcer on the buttock. According to Levine (1992), Paré requested that 'we should put him in another bed, very soft' and also that 'we should make him a little pillow of down to keep his buttock in the air, without his being supported on it'. Although the potential value of support surfaces has clearly been long recognized, their common use within health care systems is relatively recent, while their efficacy remains largely unknown.

Definitions of support surfaces

All patient support surfaces can be placed into one of three groups based upon their mode of operation. *Static* (also known as constant low pressure, CLP) support surfaces seek to maximize the area of the patient's body in contact with the mattress surface, so reducing the magnitude of the interface (or contact) pressure at any given anatomical location. The second category of support surface is the *dynamic* group, which includes alternating-pressure air mattresses. These devices aim systematically to vary the anatomical locations of the body that bear weight, usually through the cyclical inflation and deflation of different sections of the support surface. The final category, *turning* or *tilting* support surfaces systematically vary the body's centre of gravity, and hence alter the loading upon specific anatomical points, through raising and lowering (tilting) the support surface along its longitudinal axis. This final support surface group is rarely encountered when used primarily to prevent pressure ulcers and, as such, is not discussed further within this chapter.

During the early 1990s, further definitions of the actions of different support surfaces emerged. Supports, whether they are static or dynamic, are said to be either pressure reducing or pressure relieving. These definitions relate to a support surface's ability to reduce contact pressures to below 32 mmHg, the assumed 'safe' loading that will not compromise flow in the microcirculation. Pressure-reducing surfaces apply lower pressures than standard hospital mattresses, but do not always reduce these pressures to below 32 mmHg across all vulnerable bony prominences, while pressure-relieving surfaces do reduce contact pressure to below 32 mmHg at all vulnerable body sites. While the validity of accepting 32 mmHg as the critical load initiating pressure damage is not discussed here, the definition of 'pressure relief' would appear to exclude all support surfaces! Contact pressures under the heels are typically much

higher than 32 mmHg with high heel-contact pressures reported upon air-fluidized beds which are usually described as 'pressure relieving' (Allen et al 1993). Defining support surfaces using criteria that no support surface may achieve would appear to be without value and offers no assistance to clinical decision-makers. Support surfaces have also been defined as being pressure redistributing (PR). This definition highlights that when load is reduced upon one bony prominence, other parts of the body must be under increased load given that the force applied to the support surface (body weight) remains unchanged. Support surfaces will be described as being pressure redistributing, abbreviated to PR, within this chapter.

When are support surfaces used?

The initial local pressure ulcer prevention policy in the UK (Hibbs 1988) simply listed the number and type of PR support surfaces that may be required by a hospital of a particular size. No specific guidance was offered upon the most effective methods for allocating these support surfaces to the patients at greatest risk of developing pressure ulcers. It is not unreasonable to think that the rapid spread of the Waterlow Scale, currently the most commonly encountered risk assessment tool in the UK, may be due to its explicit linking of risk assessment and equipment allocation. However, in the wake of its increased use, the Waterlow Scale has been criticized in that it is believed to vastly overpredict the need for PR support surfaces. Such criticism is unfounded; a risk assessment tool's tendency to overpredict risk can be determined from its sensitivity, a measure derived from the number of patients identified as being at risk and who subsequently develop pressure ulcers divided by the total number of vulnerable subjects. Clark & Farrar (1991) reported that, when used correctly, there were no significant differences between the sensitivities of the Waterlow Scale and five alternative tools.

Accepting that overprediction of risk will be an inevitable consequence of the use of imprecise measures of patients' risk of developing pressure ulcers, the allocation of PR equipment based upon a risk score deserves comment. Based upon the Waterlow Scale, an elderly female patient, who is totally mobile, but is overweight, incontinent and a diabetic, may present with a Waterlow Score of at least 16; if PR equipment was to be allocated solely upon risk scores, this mobile patient would be likely to be allocated a PR support surface. Obviously, PR support surfaces cannot correct all the reasons why an individual may be at risk of developing pressure ulcers; at best they may enable an immobile patient to remain in one position for a longer period without experiencing skin damage. It would therefore appear sensible to refine the allocation of PR support surfaces to better reflect the immobility of patients.

Has the focus upon PR support surfaces improved patient outcomes?

Regardless of how we allocate support surfaces, there is a lack of evidence that the increased number of PR support surfaces available in the UK since 1988 has improved patient outcomes. Clark & Cullum (1992) reported how the prevalence of pressure ulcers within four hospitals increased from 6.7% to 14.2%, despite a concurrent increase in the number of available PR support surfaces from 69 to 187. While data are scant, support surfaces became commonly available across the UK Health Service following the publication of the first local pressure ulcer management guidelines. Despite this, pressure ulcers appear to be more common. For example, in 1983, David and colleagues reported upon the treatment of pressure ulcers within hospitals in England and Wales. This survey covered 132 hospitals drawn from a random, stratified sample of four Regional Health Authorities and 20 District Health Authorities. Within the 737 wards recruited to the investigation, 961 out of 14 448 (6.65%) patients had established pressure ulcers. While this survey has not been replicated, other large prevalence surveys have been conducted across acute care providers in the UK. O'Dea (1995) reported prevalence surveys conducted in hospitals across four European countries; within

the UK, a total of 8123 hospital patients were surveyed between May 1993 and May 1994, and of these, 18.6% (n = 1511) were reported to have pressure ulcers. While methodologies are dissimilar, and no account has been taken of possible changes in patient populations, these two surveys superficially suggest that pressure ulcers could be up to three times more common, despite changes in the structure and processes of care.

While absolute numbers of pressure ulcers may not reflect the impact of introducing PR support surfaces, there is perhaps a general perception that severe pressure ulcers are rarer at the end of the 1990s. However, there is insufficient data to support this perceived effect of the use of PR support surfaces and it would appear that the incidence of severe pressure ulcers dropped prior to the widespread diffusion of PR support surfaces within the UK. In 1962, Norton et al reported a pressure ulcer incidence rate of 23.6% among elderly hospital patients, with the incidence of severe pressure ulcers being 18.9% among patients with a Norton Score of 14 or less. Ten years later, Green et al (1974) reported an incidence rate of severe pressure sores of 6.6% within a similar patient population. Unfortunately, comparable data is not available since PR support surfaces became widely available across the UK.

The effectiveness of PR support surfaces

Pressure redistributing support surfaces are now widely used throughout advanced health care systems and are commonly encountered in all health care settings. This diffusion has not been inexpensive; the UK National Health Service (NHS) currently spends approximately £40 million annually upon the acquisition and maintenance of PR support surfaces. In other health systems expenditure upon PR support surfaces may be higher; for example Moody et al (1988) reported the annual cost of special beds within a single 350-bed hospital in the USA to be over $162 000 (1988 prices). While these costs are high, support surface use typically represents 7–8% of the total cost of pressure ulcer prevention and treatment (Haalboom 1991, Clark et al 1993).

Given their wide use and the high associated costs, it is unsurprising that a major theme in pressure ulcer research has been establishing that PR support surfaces 'work'. In 1975, the first major UK meeting on pressure ulcers was held in Glasgow (Kenedi et al 1976). Of the 41 papers presented during this meeting, 14 (34.1%) considered the effectiveness of PR support surfaces. This focus upon the action of PR support surfaces remains today: the electronic database MEDLINE returns 206 references from 1998 when searched using the term 'pressure sore'; of these references 33 (16%) are specifically focused upon the effectiveness of PR support surfaces. While the assessment of PR support surfaces has been a common theme in pressure ulcer research, several approaches to support surface evaluation have been reported. Predominantly, PR support surfaces have been investigated using a range of intermediate outcome measures accessible in the laboratory.

Laboratory measures of effectiveness

Clark (1994b, 1997) reviewed the use of intermediate outcome measures to compare the likely effectiveness of PR support surfaces. Seven key areas of measurement activity can be identified from past literature (Box 7.1). With one exception, there has been limited investigation of these aspects of the likely effectiveness of PR support surfaces (since 1990 the number of references offering primary data and retrievable using MEDLINE ranges from 2 (humidity) to 13 (both LDF and skin temperature)). However, over the same period, 71 references are available within MEDLINE that report contact (or interface) pressure.

While measurement of the pressures exerted between anatomical 'landmarks', such as the sacrum, and various mattresses and cushions may be commonly reported, the value of such data is questionable. Comparisons of PR surfaces may be influenced by the choice of study protocol (Clark 1996b). In this investigation, Clark compared the pressure redistribution achieved using four PR support surfaces: two intended to be used on top of the standard mattress and two to replace the standard mattress. The replace-

---

BOX 7.1 PHYSICAL AND PHYSIOLOGICAL PARAMETERS MEASURED IN THE LABORATORY TO COMPARE THE LIKELY EFFECTIVENESS OF PRESSURE-REDISTRIBUTING (PR) SUPPORT SURFACES

- Contact (interface) pressure
- Blood flow, either directly (typically using laser Doppler flowmetry, LDF) or indirectly using transcutaneous gas measurements
- Shear
- Temperature at the interface between subjects and PR support surfaces
- Humidity at the interface between subjects and PR support surfaces
- Abrasiveness (including measurements of coefficients of friction)
- Comfort.

---

ment mattresses were a foam mattress with a vapour-permeable cover (Mattress A) and an alternating-pressure air mattress (Mattress D). The overlay mattresses were a fibre-filled static overlay (Mattress B) and a different type of alternating-pressure air mattress (Mattress C).

This study showed that the anatomical site at which contact pressure is measured could affect the results. At the sacrum, for example, the four mattresses applied similar pressure impulses (defined as the amount of pressure applied during 1 h of resting upon the mattress) and could therefore be predicted to have a similar effect on tissue viability. However, at the heel, the lowest pressure impulse was applied by Mattress B, while at the trochanter the measured pressure impulses supported the use of Mattress D, the replacement alternating-pressure air mattress. Changing the site at which contact pressures were measured produced three separate impressions of mattress effectiveness: one favoured a static product, one provided 'evidence' for selecting a dynamic product while the final ranking suggested that the four mattresses were of similar effectiveness. Such sensitivity to changes in study protocol seriously devalues the use of contact pressure measurements to compare PR support surfaces.

The validity of contact pressure measurements as predictors of clinical outcome is also unclear. Clark (1996a) reported the fate of 90 elderly hospital patients who were free from pressure ulcers when admitted to hospital. Eleven patients developed ulcers; six of these were superficial pressure ulcers over the sacrum – superficial ulcers being defined as either grade I (non-reactive erythema) or grade II (superficial break in the skin). Three factors appeared to predict the development of superficial sacral pressure ulcers;

- increased relative humidity between the sacrum and mattress
- the presence of chronic diseases of the central and peripheral circulation
- the amount of oxygen available at the sacrum following loading (surprisingly this was higher among subjects who subsequently developed ulcers).

No significant differences were found between patients who developed superficial sacral ulcers and those that did not with regard to many of the factors that could prolong or increase tissue compression at the sacrum (for example, immobility and contact pressures). Given these challenges to both the reliability and validity of support surface comparisons based solely upon contact pressure measurements, it is unsurprising that a recent Effective Health Care Bulletin commented that 'interface pressure is an intermediate or surrogate outcome measure which has serious limitations as a proxy for clinical outcome' (Cullum et al 1995).

Leaving the laboratory: why are case studies considered to be weak evidence?

The case study remains a favoured design for highlighting the apparent effect of a PR support surface. Many reports exist where either a single subject or a series of case histories are presented, usually to illustrate the healing of established pressure ulcers. Reliance upon this form of evidence is inappropriate because it fails to take

account of the likely heightened interest of the staff caring for that patient or the quality of the care delivered. In a classic study, Fernie & Dornan (1976) introduced a new intervention to two hospitals in Canada. This was a device emitting electromagnetic radiation at three intensities – low, medium and high power. This device was aimed at the previously non-healing pressure ulcers of five patients (site and severity of the ulcers unreported), with each ulcer exposed to the device for 30 min in each 2 h throughout the day and night. All pressure ulcers responded to this intervention, with rapid reductions in the surface area of each ulcer (one pressure ulcer healed within 14 days of commencing this new treatment). Fernie & Dornan noted that 'the staff involved in the study became convinced of the efficacy of the machine'. However the device was a placebo, with no emission of any electromagnetic radiation. Fernie & Dornan concluded that any comparative study of pressure ulcer interventions should include a placebo arm to measure the likely impact of the nursing practice delivered during the study. In many examples, the data presented within case series may simply reflect the delivery of high-quality nursing and so prevent detection of an ineffective support surface.

Strong research designs highlighting efficacy

The randomized controlled trial (RCT) is typically considered to be the research design that can provide the best evidence of efficacy. Often considered to be the gold standard, the implementation of a well-designed RCT imparts high internal validity to a study, defined by Moher et al (1996) as 'the confidence that the trial design, conduct, analysis and presentation has minimised or avoided biases in its intervention comparisons'. Through minimizing any bias (on the part of the researchers, clinicians and patients), RCTs can provide objective information comparing the efficacy of different PR support surfaces. By the beginning of 1998, 33 RCTs of PR support surfaces (beds, mattresses and seat cushions) had been reported worldwide, but these have been considered to be largely 'of poor quality and are often too small to be informative' (Cullum et al 1995, Clark 1999).

While the available RCT data do not allow the identification of the PR support surface that is likely to be the 'best' in terms of preventing and treating pressure ulcers, several trends can be identified from the limited pool of support surface RCTs.

Replacing the standard mattress   Patients nursed upon standard hospital mattresses are more likely to develop pressure ulcers than are those nursed upon alternative low-pressure foam mattresses (Fig. 7.4). Three RCTs have compared the incidence of pressure ulcers upon standard and alternative foam mattresses. Hofman et al (1994) compared the Dutch standard hospital mattress with a modular foam replacement mattress. All newly admitted patients, considered to be at risk of developing ulcers, and with a femoral-neck fracture, were eligible for recruitment into this unblinded study. A total of 46 subjects were recruited, with equal numbers being allocated to the two mattresses. Two of the subjects allocated to the low-pressure foam mattress were excluded through incorrect application of the randomization process and no data are provided on their skin condition. Subjects were eligible for recruitment if they showed non-reactive erythema over pressure areas, and three subjects (two on standard mattress) were recruited upon this basis.

Eight subjects were 'lost' to the study within the 2 weeks after mattress allocation – five were discharged and three died. The condition of the pressure areas of these subjects at the time of their leaving the study was not reported. At 2 weeks' use of the mattresses, 20 subjects showed evidence of pressure damage: six on the alternative mattress, and 14 on the standard. Of these pressure ulcers, three (two on alternative mattresses) presented as non-reactive erythema and were considered by the researchers to be clinically irrelevant. The remaining pressure ulcers were classed as blisters ($n = 6$, five on standard mattresses), superficial ulcers ($n = 8$, five on standard mattresses), while three presented as severe full-thickness pressure ulcers (all on standard mattresses). Hofman et al (1994) concluded that the distribution of ulcers after 2 weeks' use of the mattress was such that there was a statistically significant difference in favour of the alternative foam mattress.

Do alternating-pressure air mattresses provide better clinical outcomes than constant low-pressure devices?   While RCT data have not yet answered questions regarding the relative efficacy of different alternating-pressure air mattresses (Fig. 7.5), 12 studies have compared alternating devices with static pressure support surfaces. Excluding comparisons against various standard hospital mattresses, only two studies,

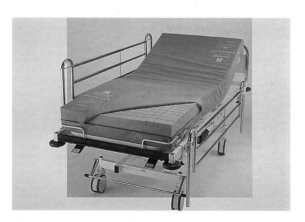

Figure 7.4   Low-pressure foam mattress (reproduced with permission from Huntleigh Technology Plc).

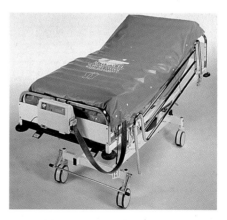

Figure 7.5   Alternating-pressure air mattress (reproduced with permission from Huntleigh Technology Plc).

both from the same research group, have shown a significant reduction in the incidence of pressure ulcers when patients were nursed upon alternating-pressure air mattresses. Gebhardt et al (1996) recruited 52 subjects within an intensive care unit (ICU); of these nine were not included in the analysis (four served as an informal pilot for the study, while five either died or were discharged from the ICU prior to the second skin assessment). All subjects were initially free from pressure ulcers and were considered to be vulnerable to their development (Norton Score under 13). A total of 23 subjects were allocated alternating-pressure air mattresses, while 20 received static pressure devices. Subjects were followed until they left the ICU; only one subject in the alternating-pressure air mattress group exhibited pressure damage (non-reactive erythema) while 11 subjects nursed on static pressure devices developed skin damage (three developed non-reactive erythema, while eight subjects developed open pressure ulcers, and four of these developed full-thickness wounds). In all other comparisons ($n = 8$) no significant differences were found between the incidence of new pressure ulcers and/or the appearance of the skin of patients nursed on alternating or static pressure support surfaces. However, these studies were generally small, with the numbers recruited to the alternating device in six of the seven investigations ranging from 14 to 72. In the final study, Andersen et al (1982) recruited 321 newly admitted hospital patients and randomly allocated these to an alternating-pressure air mattress overlay ($n = 166$) and a water mattress ($n = 155$), respectively. All subjects were assessed to be at risk of developing pressure ulcers but were free from these at the time of mattress allocation. Within 10 days of mattress use, seven subjects developed pressure ulcers (severity unreported) within each group. This study, albeit unblinded and not analysed upon an intention-to-treat basis, 'does not support any choice between air- vs. water-mattresses'. These studies highlight that the available RCT data have not yet satisfactorily answered fundamental questions regarding the relative effects of alternating and static support surfaces.

What about special beds? Excluding comparisons against standard mattresses, there have been no randomized controlled trials comparing the incidence of new pressure ulcers upon air-fluidized or low-air-loss beds and other PR surfaces.

What about seat cushions? Of the 33 RCTs, only one has compared different seat cushions used to prevent pressure ulcers (Fig. 7.6). Lim et al (1988) compared the incidence of new pressure ulcers among elderly subjects. At the beginning of the study, all eligible subjects were considered to be vulnerable to developing pressure ulcers, based upon their Norton Score and all were free from these (including non-reactive erythema). Sixty-two subjects were recruited, all sat upon either a standard foam cushion or a contoured foam cushion for at least 3 h each day for 5 months. The study appeared to be single-blinded (in that the skin assessor did not know the allocation of subjects to the two cushions), with no intention to treat analysis and also too small (only 52 subjects completed the 5-month study period). Over a 5-month period, the majority of subjects developed pressure ulcers (69% on contoured cushions and 73% on standard cushions), the majority of these pressure ulcers were areas of non-reactive erythema (44 out of 72 ulcers reported, 61%). No full-thickness pressure ulcers developed in either group. This study indicated

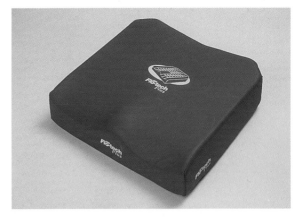

Figure 7.6 Low-pressure seat cushion (reproduced with permission from Medical Support Systems Ltd).

that the incidence of ulcers upon both cushions was high albeit that the ulcers were relatively superficial.

Reducing pressure ulcer incidence in the operating theatre   Since the work of Versluysen (1986), the combination of lengthy surgical procedures and firm operating theatre tables has been assumed to be the cause of many nosocomial pressure ulcers. Alternative theatre tables have been compared with 'standard' surfaces in four controlled studies. In each investigation, the numbers of subjects developing pressure damage, other than areas of non-reactive erythema are relatively small. Nixon et al (1998) reported an incidence of skin breaks of 1.3% (6/446) by the eighth day following prolonged surgery (over 90 min duration, but restricted to elective major general, gynaecological or vascular procedures). None of these pressure ulcers presented as full-thickness wounds. Including areas of both reactive and non-reactive erythema as negative outcomes, Nixon et al (1998) noted that the incidence of pressure damage was reduced following use of a dry visco-elastic polymer pad compared with standard theatre tables. Vacuum-moulded mattresses when used in casualty, ward and then theatre environments appeared to reduce the incidence of pressure ulcers compared with the use of standard patient support surfaces among patients who had experienced a femoral fracture (Goldstone et al 1982). In this small study with alternate unblinded allocation of patients to either vacuum-moulded support or standard care, five subjects (15.6% incidence) developed pressure ulcers within the vacuum-moulded group, and 21 out of 43 (48.8% incidence) developed pressure damage in the control group. The severity of these pressure ulcers was unreported. This study essentially compares two systems for providing pressure redistribution, and in itself does not lend weight to the use of vacuum-moulded supports in theatre alone. While pressure ulcers are commonly believed to begin during surgical procedures, the controlled trial data, perhaps as a consequence of the types of surgical procedure considered, reveal low incidences of skin breaks, which may be further reduced through the use of dry visco-elastic polymer overlays.

Efficacy or effectiveness?

The difference between efficacy and effectiveness is subtle but may have profound consequences when interpreting the results of a formal evaluation of an intervention. Efficacy refers to the ability of an intervention to achieve a desired result under ideal circumstances (for example, within the rigid design of an RCT), while effectiveness defines the intervention's ability to achieve the same outcome under normal or typical clinical circumstances. Many authors have stressed the need for studies to highlight the effectiveness of PR support surfaces, although such investigations remain rare. The preceding review of the limited RCT data concentrated upon the efficacy of support surfaces, but what about their effectiveness? Conine & Hershler (1991) defined several parameters of 'effectiveness' including cost, user-friendliness and compliance with local standards. 'User-friendliness' has typically been reported as the perceived comfort of subjects sleeping upon the support surface. However, there is no single accepted method for recording comfort, which reduces the comparability of studies. Despite this lack of standard measurement, it would appear, at least to volunteers and to patients unlikely to develop pressure ulcers, that alternating pressure systems that apply low minimum contact pressures when cells are deflated and high maximum contact pressures when inflated are perceived to be uncomfortable. The cost of support surfaces is complex and, for purchased devices, is dependent upon the period of time the device can be reliably used (the 'useful life' of the product) and the need for maintenance and repair during that lifetime (Table 7.1).

Support surfaces are now in common use, although their efficacy and effectiveness are largely unknown. Fundamental questions remain unanswered; for example, do alternating-pressure air mattresses really convey benefits beyond the use of simple static devices? Answering such questions will clearly have a

Table 7.1 How much does that mattress cost?* An example of how to derive the costs of purchased PR support surfaces

Cost	Low-pressure foam mattress	Alternating-pressure air mattress
Purchase price (£)	150	4000
'Useful life' in years	3	7
Annual depreciated cost (£)	50 (150/3)	571.43 (4000/7)
Annual maintenance and operation	25 (Laundering of cover)	400 (Service charge)
Overall annual cost of use	75 (Annual cost + maintenance)	971.43
Cost per day of use	0.20 (75/365 days)	2.66

* This costing model assumes straight-line depreciation of purchase costs, and constant mattress use.

large impact upon the pattern of health care delivery, but how best should such questions be tackled? Laboratory measures currently leave doubts regarding the validity of the measures adopted; one solution for this would be for studies to identify which subset of physiological parameters best reflects the efficacy of support surfaces, as shown through RCTs. RCT design is worthy of comment; such designs do minimize bias if correctly applied and for this reason sound RCTs are probably the best solution to understanding support surface efficacy. However, many of the available RCTs presented have severe methodological flaws; many are unblinded, in that the researchers, clinicians and patients were all aware of which mattress had been allocated to any particular subject. Clinicians who knew which mattress the subject had been allocated assessed the presence and severity of the pressure ulcers. The lack of blinding, particularly during the recording of skin outcomes, potentially introduces a strong bias in favour of the intervention. Other weaknesses in RCT design and implementation are highlighted in Box 7.2. Such design constraints may require further theoretical consideration. Can an

BOX 7.2 WEAKNESSES IN THE DESIGN OF RANDOMIZED CONTROLLED TRIALS OF PRESSURE-REDISTRIBUTING SUPPORT SURFACES

◆ Lack of blinding to treatment allocation

◆ Non-random allocation of interventions

◆ Failure to analyse data upon an 'intention-to-treat' basis

◆ Short periods of follow up of subjects, typically days rather than months

◆ Inadequate sample sizes

◆ No a priori calculation of the sample size required

◆ Project timescale is longer than product lifespan! Data are not available in a timely fashion to guide equipment selection.

KEY POINTS

◆ The effectiveness of support surfaces should not be judged solely on the basis of interface (contact) pressure measurements

◆ The positive results cited in case studies may reflect high-quality nursing care and not the effect of any support surface

◆ Randomized controlled trials comparing support surfaces are rare and often badly designed

◆ Low-pressure foam mattresses appear to reduce the incidence of pressure ulcers compared with standard hospital mattresses

◆ There is inconsistent evidence regarding the relative merits of static and dynamic support surfaces.

amended design be considered which can provide robust impressions of efficacy with smaller sample sizes? Addressing questions of effectiveness may require designs other than the RCT, perhaps naturalistic experiments following patient outcomes and support surface performance criteria may be one potential alternative approach, although bias would not be minimized through such observational studies.

THE USE OF WOUND DRESSINGS AND TOPICAL LOTIONS TO PREVENT THE DEVELOPMENT OF PRESSURE ULCERS

A wide variety of local skin preparations have been used in support of pressure ulcer prevention; for example, Norton et al (1962) commented how 14 different materials were applied to intact skin. Following a cohort of 205 elderly patients, 25% developed pressure ulcers despite the use of a variety of local skin applications. The percentage developing pressure ulcers ranged from 15% (zinc cream preparation) to 39% (soap and witch hazel), although little guidance regarding the effect of skin preparations can be extrapolated from this uncontrolled series of observations. Few controlled studies ($n = 3$) have examined the use of skin preparations in the prevention of pressure ulcers. These have compared the application of essential fatty acids to the skin of patients nursed in an intensive care unit (Declair 1997), while other studies reported the use of a hexachlorophane-containing skin cream (Green et al 1974, van der Cammen et al 1987). The three studies mentioned reported double-blinded investigations in which the active intervention was compared with an inactive carrier (Green et al 1974, Declair 1997) or with a second skin preparation (van der Cammen et al 1987). The incidence of pressure ulcers was lower within the active treatment groups, with no significant difference recorded when two active compounds were compared (although the possibility of a type II error is high given the small sample size, 54 and 50, within the two comparison groups). These studies, albeit limited in number, appear to suggest that some skin preparations may delay

the onset of pressure damage, and this potential should be explored in further clinical trials.

Drug-based prevention of pressure ulcers has been reported on one occasion. Barton & Barton (1976) described the incidence of pressure ulcers following either elective hip replacement or emergency repair of a fractured femur. In this double-blind study, subjects were given an intramuscular application of either adrenocorticotrophic hormone (ACTH) in a gelatin solvent or the gelatin solvent alone. Each application was given 4 h prior to surgery. No subject who received ACTH developed ulcers after their hip replacement, with five (26%) experiencing pressure ulcers following their fracture femur repair. However, in the control group, 31% (5/16) and 26% (7/27) developed pressure ulcers after their hip replacement or repair of their fractured femur, respectively. Unfortunately, no details were provided regarding the severity of the ulcers that developed. This interesting study suggests that pharmaceutical interventions may help to reduce the incidence of pressure ulcers, although such benefits may only be achievable where the drug can be delivered at a specified time prior to the likely cause of the ulcer. In this example, Barton & Barton (1976) suggest that the ACTH must be applied in time to allow maximum cortisol levels to be reached prior to endothelial damage occurring as a consequence of applied pressure. The importance of the timing of drug interventions could be seen in the case of the fractured femur patients in whom endothelial cell separation may have occurred prior to their arrival in hospital, as a result of experiencing variable periods of immobility following the fracture.

Prophylactic use of wound dressings to protect intact skin has been reported anecdotally for many years, but controlled studies are rare. Hall (1983) reported the use of a film dressing to prevent ulcer development. In this study, elderly orthopaedic patients admitted to one ward with a femoral fracture or requiring a knee or hip arthoplasty were allocated the film dressing. Patients with similar medical problems nursed in a second ward were recruited as a comparison group and were not allocated the film dressing.

Eighteen patients received film dressings applied to 'all pressure points' and of these one developed a pressure ulcer (severity and location were unreported), giving an incidence of 5.5%. Within the comparison group ($n = 16$), seven developed pressure ulcers (an incidence of 43.7%), with four of these being described as severe. Such results must, however, be treated with some caution; the organization and quality of care delivered may have differed between wards, this study did not randomly allocate patients to the treatment and control groups, and other forms of preventive care differed between wards. This final point deserves comment; on the ward where the film dressing was used, patients were repositioned every 2 h during the day, and 4-hourly at night. On the comparison ward, patients were repositioned 2-hourly day and night, with patients' skin being massaged with soap and water at unspecified intervals. These differences between the interventions received may have made a significant contribution towards the variations in incidence reported in the two wards.

Several authors have reported the consequences of using dressings to prevent pressure ulcers upon the costs of pressure area care. These reports have highlighted the relatively high cost of hydrocolloid and other advanced dressings when used to prevent pressure ulcers. Frantz et al (1991) noted that the mean cost of treating grade I ulcers per day within a single US long-term care provider was $7.22. The same provider spent less when treating more severe ulcers, where the mean daily cost of treating grade IV ulcers was $4.79; this difference arose through the common application of advanced dressing materials upon early stages of pressure ulcers. There is little evidence to suggest that advanced dressing materials are required to protect skin from abrasion. Callaghan & Trapp (1998) compared the use of a hydrocolloid dressing, a gel pad and no dressing, upon the incidence of skin damage at the nasal bridge following nasal intermittent positive pressure ventilation using face masks. This non-randomized evaluation recruited 10 patients to each intervention group. Of these, 90% showed skin deterioration where no dressing was used to protect the nasal bridge after 2 days' use of the face mask; 70% deteriorated in the same period using the gel pad, with 30% deterioration where the hydrocolloid dressing was used. Were similar results to be obtained with random allocation to intervention groups then the use of advanced dressing material to protect skin may be cost effective regardless of the higher unit costs of these dressing materials.

Improving tissue tolerance to loading

The preceding sections have considered the use of external devices to minimize the deleterious effects of prolonged tissue loading. However, similar results (in terms of reductions in pressure ulcer incidence) could theoretically be achieved if the tissues themselves could be strengthened. Such a hypothesis would appear to underpin the emphasis upon impaired nutrition in pressure ulcer prevention. If nutritional deficits and frank weight losses could be reversed, then tissues may be able to better withstand prolonged compression. Such a view is attractive, but has very rarely been supported by well-designed studies. Generally, studies associating pressure ulcers and malnutrition have demonstrated how patients with pressure ulcers, and even those vulnerable to developing these wounds, have altered nutritional intakes and may have lowered serum protein concentrations (see, for example, Cullum & Clark 1992, Green et al 1999). Of the 36 studies identified in MEDLINE using the terms 'pressure sore' and 'nutritional deficiency' only one described a study designed to explore the relationship between reducing pressure ulcer incidence through improving nutrition (Hartgrink et al 1998). Hartgrink and colleagues investigated the effect of supplemental nasogastric tube feeding upon the incidence of pressure ulcers among patients with hip fractures within a prospective randomized controlled trial. Initially, 62 subjects were allocated to receive supplemental feeding, with 67 in the control arm; however, few subjects could tolerate the experimental regimen, with only 25 remaining in the tube-fed group after 7 days and 16 after 2 weeks. There were no significant differences between either the incidence or severity of pressure ulcers within the experimental and control groups, suggesting either that nutritional supplementation may not improve tissue 'tolerance' to prolonged loading or that the poor compliance with the tube-feeding obscured a real difference between groups. It would appear that the link between improving nutrition and reducing the occurrence of pressure ulcers remains unproven and further well-designed studies should now be initiated to resolve this question.

Mawson et al (1993) reported an alternative approach to improving tissue tolerance to prolonged loading. They postulated that electrical stimulation, and in particular high-voltage pulsed galvanic stimulation (HVPGS) could increase blood flow and raise tissue oxygen levels among spinal-cord injured subjects into the range observed in uninjured subjects. However, while significant but perhaps transient, increases in tissue oxygen could be demonstrated in the laboratory using HVPGS, this method has yet to be compared in an RCT with an appropriate control intervention. As with so many aspects of pressure ulcer prevention and treatment, the use of interventions to improve the resistance of soft tissues to prolonged compression remains largely untested and no firm conclusion can yet be drawn as to the value of such interventions.

To massage or not to massage?

'Gentle' massage of pressure areas has been a traditional method for preventing the development of pressure ulcers. Such practice remains commonly applied in parts of mainland Europe; for example, Buss & Halfens (1995) reported the views of 339 Dutch participants within a national pressure ulcer symposium. Most (67%) considered that massage was harmless, with almost one-quarter (24%) considering that skin massage at 4-hourly intervals was a useful preventive intervention. However both the Panel for the Prediction and Prevention of Pressure Ulcers in Adults (1992) and European Pressure Ulcer Advisory Panel (1998) recommend that massage may be harmful. This discrepancy between the exponents of national guidelines and the views of practitioners (at least in The Netherlands) may hinge upon the definition of 'gentle' massage. Vigorous skin rubbing may increase pressure

damage, as suggested by the work of Dyson (1978). This frequently cited study reports a 38% higher incidence of pressure ulcers among wards where patients' skin was rubbed, compared with wards where no massage was performed. The effect of rubbing upon subcutaneous tissues over the sacrum was examined through post-mortem observations; where rubbing had been performed then the tissues were macerated 'and very degenerated'. However the data are difficult to interpret since no data are provided upon the numbers of ulcers that developed, their severity or even the numbers of patients included in the study. No indication is given of the number of post-mortems performed and there is no quantitative index of tissue 'degeneration' provided. Skin blood flow has been measured following massage (Ek et al 1985) with marked inter- and intra-subject variability in response to massage reported. Where massage was applied to areas of discoloured skin (grade I pressure ulcers), blood flow in the affected area tended to decrease in 10 out of 15 subjects. Olson (1989) noted how extended massage (60 s duration) reduced sacral skin temperature compared with shorter duration manipulation (30 s). This reduced temperature was suggested to represent ischaemic tissue, with prolonged massage causing an 'impaired circulation to the pressure area'. If one excludes the unquantified observations of Dyson, then massage may have variable results upon skin blood flow, with prolonged massage likely to have a greater deleterious effect. We have yet to be able to standardize what is meant by 'massage' – what duration and force should be applied, and how is this force to be applied? – and this imprecision in the definition of massage precludes a definitive answer to its biological effects.

EFFECT OF PRESSURE ULCER PREVENTION GUIDELINES UPON THE PREVENTION OF PRESSURE ULCERS

The earliest pressure ulcer prevention guideline was derived, through a consensus process in The Netherlands in 1985. Over 15 years later, the extent of implementation of the guideline recommendations in The Netherlands remains variable, with little knowledge of any changes in the incidence of pressure ulcers. Unfortunately, such a scenario is common, as the development of guidelines within the USA (Panel for the Prediction and Prevention of Pressure Ulcers in Adults 1992) and various European countries (European Pressure Ulcer Advisory Panel 1998; Fig. 7.7) has not yet been associated with either consistent changes in practice, reduced costs of care or in improved patient outcomes. Of the available national guidelines, the United States Agency for Health Care Policy and Research (AHCPR) pressure ulcer prevention guidelines (1992) have been subjected to the greatest formal

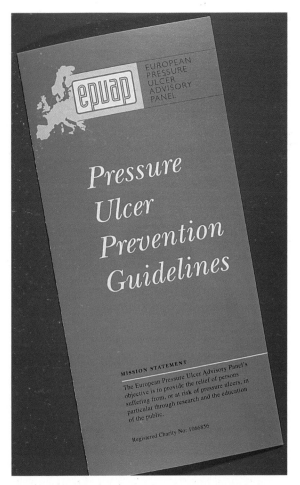

Figure 7.7 European Pressure Ulcer Prevention Guidelines (reproduced with permission from the European Pressure Ulcer Advisory Panel).

evaluation. Impressive reductions in the occurrence of pressure ulcers have been reported following implementation of the AHCPR guidelines, with Xakellis et al (1998) reporting that the incidence of ulcers fell from 23.2% to 4.7% following AHCPR guideline implementation. However, these claims are confounded by concurrent changes in organizational structure within the provider units studied. Xakellis et al (1998) introduced the AHCPR guidelines within a single 77-bedded long-term care facility; concurrent with the introduction of the guidelines the facility altered its organization of nursing care, resulting in an increased number of nurses per shift, with a higher proportion of registered nurses. This organizational change was complemented by training on pressure ulcer prevention during the orientation of the new nursing staff. It would appear that the facility studied by Xakellis and colleagues did achieve reductions in the incidence of pressure ulcers; however, it is not possible to isolate the effects of the AHCPR guidelines from the other changes. Process changes following introduction of the AHCPR guidelines have been reported; in particular the use of consistent risk assessment and pressure ulcer grading tools. The adoption of a common vocabulary both within and between health care providers could be expected to reduce the likelihood of the quality of patient care deteriorating as a consequence of disjointed professional communication regarding pressure ulcers and their prevention. The cost of care has remained similar regardless of the implementation of the AHCPR guidelines (Hu et al 1993, Xakellis et al 1998). Hu et al (1993) recorded the variable costs associated with the preventive care received by 27 vulnerable patients nursed either in hospital ($n = 19$) or in a nursing home ($n = 8$). The sample was divided into four groups: those with a hip fracture, patients in intensive care, paraplegics and those in a nursing home. Prior to guideline implementation the daily costs of prevention ranged from $12.20 (nursing home) to $45.07 (paraplegics). Following the introduction of the AHCPR guidelines, daily costs were predicted to rise in intensive care and in nursing homes by 21.2% and 24.0%, respectively. Cost reductions were predicted post-guideline implementation in the case of paraplegic care and for hip fractures, by 18.7% and 4%, respectively. Overall, Hu and colleagues (1993) considered that the implementation of the AHCPR guidelines may be no more costly than pre-guideline practice. Xakellis et al (1998) reported similar conclusions regarding the likely costs of implementing the AHCPR guidelines; before guideline implementation, no costs were incurred through prevention, with the mean cost of treatment per patient being $113 ± $345. Following guideline implementation, the overall average cost of prevention and treatment per patient was $100 ± $157 (a non-significant difference). It would appear that three general conclusions may be advanced when considering the impact of guidelines upon pressure ulcer prevention:

1. Process changes may be achieved, leading to improved communication between health professionals.
2. These process changes may be achieved without significantly increased expenditure on pressure area care.
3. Improvement in patient outcomes may be harder to identify given the confounding role of concurrent organizational changes.

CAN EDUCATION IMPROVE PATIENT OUTCOMES?

The AHCPR pressure ulcer prevention guidelines contained 27 specific recommendations; of these, only six were supported by 'good' ($n = 2$) and 'fair' ($n = 4$) evidence from appropriate research. Two of the six 'research supported' recommendations concerned the value of educational programmes as a means of reducing the incidence of pressure ulcers. The belief that providing staff education, on its own, can bring about reductions in the occurrence of pressure ulcers largely rests upon the work of Moody et al (1988). In this seminal study, Moody and colleagues measured the incidence of new pressure ulcers among patients in medical, surgical and orthopaedic wards within a 350-bed teaching hospital, excluding those patients with an expected length-of-stay of less than 3 days.

Incidence data were gathered from medical and nursing record review, while the research team validated the record content by reviewing each patient's notes within 24 h of admission to hospital, supported with inspection visits to wards to check the record content against patients' actual skin condition. Over a 2-month period (December 1985–January 1986), 157 patients were recruited, and of these 123 had no pressure ulcers on admission. Upon discharge, 18 of the 123 patients (14.6%) had developed some stage of pressure ulcer, although the severity of these wounds is unreported. Following this stage, Moody et al instituted training programmes for both doctors and nurses. These courses included information on the aetiology, prevention and treatment of ulcers, including the cost implications of the treatment of more serious pressure ulcers. Weekly teaching sessions were organized for medical staff, and videotapes aimed at nursing staff were also available. Concurrently, Moody et al implemented guidelines on pressure ulcer prevention and treatment. The impact of such an intensive teaching programme was reviewed during the early summer of 1996 (May–June), 4 months after the introduction of the educational programme. Following a similar methodology to the pre-education phase, Moody and colleagues reviewed the outcome of 111 patients admitted without pressure ulcers; of these six (5.4%) developed ulcers, with their severity again unreported. The apparent reduction in incidence from 14.6% to 5.4% is held as a strong indicator that educational programmes, perhaps simply through their effect upon raising general awareness of pressure ulcers, can lead to significant reductions in the scale of the problem. However, some caution must be exercised when interpreting this apparent success of education. It remains possible that the reduced incidence simply marked a natural seasonal variation in the incidence of pressure ulcers between the winter and summer months. Once again, the use of non-case-mix adjusted incidence data may have led to inappropriate study conclusions because of the failure to control the impact of changes in the characteristics and medical problems of patients admitted at different times of the year. Similar problems with the interpretation of pressure ulcer incidence data when used to mark the effect of educational programmes can be seen in the work of Danchaivijitr et al (1995). Prior to the introduction of education on pressure ulcer prevention, the mean incidence across 33 hospitals in Thailand was 8.7% (data collected from medical, surgical and private wards, along with intensive care units). Following the introduction of educational programmes, the incidence apparently fell to 6.5%, with significant reductions in both general medical and surgical wards (medical, from 7.8% to 5.8%; surgical, from 7.9% to 5.0%). However, the total number of patients recruited in the post-education phase was 2893, a 27.5% reduction upon the numbers recruited prior to the educational programmes. This reduced recruitment was explained by the fact that the post-education data collection coincided with the Thai New Year. It is not inconceivable that hospital admission practices varied over the holiday period, so preventing any direct comparison between the pre- and post-education phases of this study. It would appear that the contribution of educational programmes towards reducing the incidence of pressure ulcers remains 'not proven' with further investigation required in which extraneous effects upon incidence rates are controlled.

THE WAY FORWARD

Perhaps Alterescu (1989) provided the most appropriate and elegant summary of our current understanding of pressure area care. Although commenting specifically upon pressure ulcer costing studies, his opinion that '"Estimates" get converted to "studies" and "guesses" become "calculations" while the misinformation in this area gets compounded' well illustrates the myriad aspects of pressure ulcer prevention. If we are to move forward and define effective and efficient systems of prevention then 'studies' and 'calculations' will be required. Fundamentally, we need to determine how to measure the success of any preventive intervention, and to separate this from the impact of the many other structural and process variations present in health care systems. Case-mix adjustment of incidence rates may provide the essential tool, allowing appropriate and meaningful comparisons between provider units and over time.

The efficacy and effectiveness of all interventions offered to assist pressure ulcer prevention should be known. Without this knowledge, gleaned from RCTs, naturalistic experiments and appropriate laboratory measurements, we will continue to gamble upon which guideline, what educational programme and which support surface can provide greatest benefits to patients likely to develop pressure ulcers.

Finally, we need to decide when all reasonable steps have been taken to prevent pressure ulcer development. If we accept the belief that the majority of pressure ulcers can be prevented, this assumes that we also accept that some ulcers are beyond our current ability to prevent. If we accept that pressure ulcers will continue to occur, albeit in much smaller numbers, following the implementation of effective and efficient prevention programmes, then we should consider what level of incidence is acceptable within different health care systems and settings. Just as insuffi-

KEY POINTS

♦ Implementing evidence-based guidelines does not appear to increase the cost of preventive care

♦ The impact of guidelines upon pressure ulcer incidence is hard to determine given concurrent changes in both the structures and processes of health care

♦ Similarly, the effects of providing education upon pressure ulcer prevention is difficult to interpret

♦ What incidence rate marks 'optimal' prevention? Considerable incremental investment may be required to reduce, for example, a 2% rate to 1%. Could such investment be better used within other areas of health care?

cient preventive care may be wasteful of scarce resources, over-investment in prevention may be an equally profligate use of resources. We need to search for the correct balance between under- and over-investment in prevention; however, this balance will be hard to define in the absence of measures of success in prevention and the current ignorance regarding the value of the majority of interventions we use in everyday clinical practice.

In conclusion, while prevention is 'better' than cure, we remain unsure of what constitutes successful preventive care: do we really need expensive support surfaces, national or local guidelines and intensive education to prevent the development of pressure ulcers? These questions must be answered if we are really to achieve major improvements in reducing the morbidity and mortality associated with this common clinical complication, the pressure ulcer.

ACKNOWLEDGEMENTS

Sections of this chapter have been based, with permission, upon articles first published in the following titles; *Nursing Standard*, *Journal of Tissue Viability* and *Journal of Wound Care*. I would like to thank the editorial teams of each title for allowing me to revisit ideas first raised within their publications. Thanks are also due to the commercial organizations that provided illustrations of pressure-redistributing devices. However, the illustrations do not constitute an endorsement of these particular products.

 SELF-ASSESSMENT QUESTIONS

1   Can you list three reasons why increasing the numbers of PR support surfaces may not reduce the number of patients with pressure ulcers?

    Points to consider
    Reasons why increasing the availability of mattresses may fail to reduce the number of patients with sores include:
    ◆ The support surfaces may be ineffective.
    ◆ They may be allocated to the 'wrong' patients, where 'vulnerability' has been incorrectly assessed.
    ◆ They may be used incorrectly.
    ◆ The use of the PR support surfaces may displace other forms of nursing care.
    ◆ The number of patients admitted with ulcers may be high. This would maintain a high prevalence rate in spite of the investment in resources.

2   One hospital has a pressure ulcer prevalence rate of 33%, its neighbouring hospital only 5%. For what reasons may these prevalence rates mislead if directly compared?

    Points to consider
    There are several factors that may distort the apparent relationship between the two organizations. These include:
    ◆ Do the two hospitals record pressure ulcers in the same manner? Does one site include areas of blanching erythema as an ulcer while the other does not?
    ◆ Has the data been collected in similar medical specialities? For example, did the second hospital survey areas where pressure ulcers may be rarely encountered, such as maternity units? Inclusion of specialities with high numbers of patients at low risk of developing ulcers is likely to reduce prevalence rates.
    ◆ Did the hospital with the high prevalence have a patient population all at high risk of developing ulcers? Did the second hospital have few vulnerable

patients? Failing to take account of differences between the populations served by different health care providers may also distort prevalence rates. For this reason, comparison of such data should be based upon 'case-mix adjusted' rates rather than observed rates of pressure ulcers.

3   'Wondermattress' applies only 23 mmHg pressure to the sacrum and for this reason the pressure ulcers of six patients healed rapidly. Would this claim for the device's effectiveness impress you? If not, why? (give five reasons).

Points to consider

'Wondermattress' may not be effective despite the superficially impressive claim. Several questions remain unanswered that would reduce one's confidence in the effectiveness of the device; these include:

◆ Was 23 mmHg the lowest, or the average or the highest pressure this mattress applied to the sacrum?

◆ Whose sacrum? Does the data reflect pressures measured under young healthy subjects? Or under patients? Contact pressures tend to be higher among patient populations compared with the results obtained from young, healthy volunteers.

◆ How did this pressure compare with those applied by alternatives to 'Wondermattress'? Contact pressure data should be comparative, showing differences between devices and not reported as absolute measures.

◆ Did all subjects experience 23 mmHg when lying on the mattress? What is the range of pressures measured upon this device, preferably described using either the standard deviation or the 95% confidence interval about the mean applied pressure?

◆ What about the six patients? Where were their pressure ulcers located? How severe were these wounds? How long did they take to heal?

◆ Would similar results have been obtained using a different mattress?

◆ What other care did these six patients receive? Perhaps the impressive healing upon 'Wondermattress' reflected high-quality nursing care not the effect of the device?

REFERENCES

Allen V, Ryan D W, Murray A 1993 Air-fluidized beds and their ability to distribute interface pressures generat_d between the subject and the bed surface. Physiological Measurement 14:359–364

Alterscu V 1989 The financial costs of inpatient pressure ulcers to an acute care pacility. Decubitus 2(3):14–23

Andersen K E, Jensen O, Kvorning S A, Bach E 1982 Decubitus prophylaxis: a prospective trial on the efficiency of alternating-pressure air-mattresses and water-mattresses. Acta Dermatovener (Stockholm) 63:227–230

Barton A A, Barton M 1976 Drug-based prevention of pressure sores. Lancet ii:443–444

Bergstrom N, Braden B, Kemp M, Champagne M, Ruby E 1996 Multi-site study of pressure ulcers and the relationship between risk level, demographic characteristics, diagnoses and prescription of preventive interventions. Journal of the American Geriatrics Society 44:22–30

Berlowitz D R, Ash A S, Brandeis G H, Brand H K, Halpern J L, Moskowitz M A. 1996 Rating long-term care facilities on pressure ulcer development: importance of case-mix adjustment. Annals of Internal Medicine 124(6):557–563

Buss I C, Halfens R J G 1995 The expectations of experts on the usefulness of position changes and massage in preventing pressure sores. In: Cherry G W, Gottrup F, Lawrence J C, Moffatt C J, Turner T D (eds) Proceedings of the 5th European Conference on Advances in Wound Management, Harrogate. Macmillan Magazines, London, pp. 87–89

Callaghan S, Trapp M 1998 Evaluating two dressings for the prevention of nasal bridge pressure sores. Professional Nurse 13(6):361–364

Clark M 1994a The financial cost of pressure sores to the UK National Health Service. In: Cherry G W, Leaper D J, Lawrence J C, Milward P (eds) Proceedings of the 4th European Conference on Advances in Wound Management, Copenhagen. Macmillan Magazines, London, pp. 48–50

Clark M 1994b Problems associated with the measurement of interface (or contact) pressure. Journal of Tissue Viability 4(2):37–43

Clark M 1996a The aetiology of superficial sacral pressure sores. In: Leaper D L, Cherry G W, Dealey C (eds) Proceedings of the 6th European Conference on Advances in Wound Management, Amsterdam. Macmillan Press, London, pp. 167–169

Clark M 1996b Are contact pressure measurements useful when selecting pressure-redistributing support surfaces? In: Leaper D L, Cherry G W, Dealey C (eds) Proceedings of the 6th European Conference on Advances in Wound Management, Amsterdam. Macmillan Press, London pp. 44–45

Clark M 1997 Evidence of effectiveness. Journal of Wound Care 6(8):400–401

Clark M 1998 Repositioning to prevent pressure sores – what is the evidence? Nursing Standard 13(3):58–64

Clark, M 1999 Beds and mattresses (Editorial). Journal of Wound Care 8(7):323

Clark M, Cullum N 1992 Matching patient need for pressure sore prevention with the supply of pressure-redistributing mattresses. Journal of Advanced Nursing 17:310–316

Clark M, Farrar S 1991 Comparison of pressure sore risk calculators. In: Harding K G, Leaper D L, Turner T D (eds) Proceedings of the 1st European conference on advances in wound management, Cardiff. Macmillan Press, London, 158–161

Clark M, Watts S 1994 The incidence of pressure sores within a National Health Service Trust hospital during 1991. Journal of Advanced Nursing 20:33–36

Clark M, Watts S, Chapman R G, Field K, Carey G 1993 The financial costs of pressure sores to the National Health Service: a case study. Final report to the Department of Health. University of Surrey, Guildford

Conine T A, Hershler C 1991 Effectiveness: a neglected dimension in the assessment of rehabilitation devices and equipment. International Journal of Rehabilitation Research 14:117–122

Cullum N, Clark M 1992 Intrinsic factors associated with pressure sores in elderly people. Journal of Advanced Nursing 17(4):427–31

Cullum N, Deeks J, Fletcher A, et al. 1995 The prevention and treatment of pressure sores. Effective Health Care 2(1):1–16

Danchaivijitr S, Suthisanon L, Jitreecheue L, Tantiwatanapaibool Y 1995 Effects of education on the prevention of pressure sores. Journal of the Medical Association of Thailand 78, Supplement 1:1–6

David J A, Chapman R G, Chapman E J, Lockett B 1983 An investigation of the current methods used in nursing for the care of patients with established pressure sores. Final report to the Department of Health. Nursing Practice Research Unit, Northwick Park

Davies K, Strickland J, Lawrence V, Duncan A, Rowe J 1991 The hidden mortality from pressure sores. Journal of Tissue Viability 1(1):18

Declair V 1997 The usefulness of topical application of essential fatty acids (EFA) to prevent pressure ulcers. Ostomy and Wound Management 43(5):48–54

Dyson R 1978 Bed sores – the injuries hospital staff inflict on patients. Nursing Mirror 146(24):30–32

Ek A-C, Gustavsson G, Lewis D H 1985 The local skin blood flow in areas at risk for pressure sores treated with massage. Scandinavian Journal of Rehabilitiation Medicine 17(2):81–86

European Pressure Ulcer Advisory Panel (EPUAP) 1998 Pressure Ulcer Prevention Guidelines. EPUAP, London

Fernie G R, Dornan J 1976 The Problems of clinical trials with new systems for preventing or healing decubiti. In: Kenedi R M, Cowden J M, Scales J T (eds) Bed sore biomechanics. Macmillan Press, London pp. 315–320

Frantz R A, Gardner S, Harvey P, Specht J 1991 The cost of treating pressure ulcers in a long-term care facility. Decubitus 4(3):37–45

Gebhardt K S, Bliss M R, Winwright P L, Thomas J 1996 Pressure-relieving supports in an ICU. Journal of Wound Care 5(3):116–121

Goldstone L A, Norris M, O'Reilly M, White J 1982 A clinical trial of a bead bed system for the prevention of pressure sores in elderly orthopaedic patients. Journal of Advanced Nursing 7:545–548

Green M F, Exton-Smith A N, Helps E P W, Kataria M S, Wedgwood J, Williams T C P 1974 Prophylaxis of pressure sores using a new lotion. Modern Geriatrics 4(9):376–384

Green S M, Winterberg H, Franks P J et al 1999 Nutritional intake in community patients with pressure ulcers. Journal of Wound Care 8(7):325–332

Haalboom J R 1991 De kosten van decubitus. Ned Tijdschr Geneeskd 135(14):606–610

Hall P 1983 Prophylactic use of Op-Site on pressure areas. Nursing Focus Jan/Feb:148

Hartgrink H H, Wille J, Konig P et al 1998 Pressure sores and tube feeding in patients with a fracture of the hip: a randomized clinical trial. Clinical Nutrition 17(6):287–292

Hibbs P J 1988 Pressure area care for the City and Hackney Health Authority. City and Hackney Health Authority, London

Hofman A, Geelkerken R H, Wille J, Hamming J J, Hermans J, Breslau P J 1994 Pressure sores and pressure-decreasing mattresses: controlled clinical trial. Lancet 343:568–571

Hu T-W, Stotts N A, Fogarty T E, Bergstrom N 1993 Cost analysis for guideline implementation in prevention and early treatment of pressure ulcers. Decubitus 6(2):42–46

Kenedi R M, Cowden J M, Scales J T, eds 1976 Bedsore biomechanics. Macmillan Press, London

Knox D M, Anderson T M, Anderson P S 1994 Effects of different turn intervals on skin of healthy older adults. Advances in Wound Care 7(1):48–52

Kosiak M 1961 Etiology of decubitus ulcers. Archives of Physical Medicine and Rehabilitation 42:19–29

Levine J M 1992 Historical notes on pressure ulcers: The cure of Ambrose Paré. Decubitus 5(2):23–27

Lim R, Sirett R, Conine T A, Daechsel D 1988 Clinical trial of foam cushions in the prevention of decubitis ulcers in elderly patients. Journal of Rehabilitation Research and Development 25(2):19–26

Mawson A R, Siddiqui F H, Biundo J J 1993 Enhancing host resistance to pressure ulcers: a new approach to prevention. Preventive Medicine 22:433–450

Moher D, Jadad A R, Tugwell P 1996 Assessing the quality of randomized controlled trials: current issues and future directions. International Journal of Technology Assessment in Health Care 12(2):195–208

Moody B L, Fanale J E, Thompson M, Vaillancourt D, Symonds G, Bonasoro C 1988 Impact of staff education on pressure sore development in elderly hospitalized patients. Archives of Internal Medicine 148:2241–2243

Mukamel D B 1997 Outcome measures and quality of care in nursing homes. Medical Care 35(4):367–385

Nixon J, McElvenny D, Mason S, Brown J, Bond S 1998 A sequential randomized controlled trial comparing a dry visco-elastic polymer pad and standard operating table mattress in the prevention of post-operative pressure sores. International Journal of Nursing Studies 35:193–203

Norton D, McLaren R, Exton-Smith A N 1962 An investigation of geriatric nursing problems in hospital. Churchill Livingstone, London (Reprinted 1975)

O'Dea K 1995 The prevalence of pressure sores in four European Countries. Journal of Wound Care 4(4):192–195

Olson B 1989 Effects of massage for prevention of pressure ulcers. Decubitus 2(4):32–37

Panel for the Prediction and Prevention of Pressure Ulcers in Adults 1992 Pressure ulcers in adults: prediction and prevention. Clinical practice guideline number 3. AHCPR Publication No. 92–0047. AHCPR, Rockville

Salisbury R E 1985 Transcutaneous PO$_2$ monitoring in bedridden burn patients: a physiological analysis of four methods to prevent pressure sores. In: Lee B Y (ed.) Chronic ulcers of the skin. McGraw-Hill, New York, pp. 189–196

Shea J D 1975 Pressure sores. Classification and management. Clinical Orthopaedics and Related Research 112:89–100

Szor J, Bourguignon C 1997 Description of pain in patients with pressure ulcers (abstract). 29th Annual Wound, Ostomy and Continence Conference.

Touche Ross 1993 The costs of pressure sores. Report to the Department of Health. Touche Ross & Co, London

van der Cammen T J, O'Callaghan U, Whitefield M 1987 Prevention of pressure sores. A comparison of new and old pressure sore treatments. British Journal of Clinical Practice 41:1009–1011

Versluysen M 1986 Pathogenesis of pressure sores in elderly patients with hip fractures. City and Hackney Health Authority, London

Watts S, Clark M 1993 Pressure sore prevention: a review of policy documents. Final report to the Department of Health. University of Surrey, Guildford

Williams S, Jackson B, Watret L, Pell J 1997 Pilot study of case-mix adjusted incidence of pressure sores. Journal of Tissue Viability 7(1):15–17

Xakellis G C, Frantz R A, Lewis A, Harvey P 1998 Cost-effectiveness of an intensive pressure ulcer prevention protocol in long-term care. Advances in Wound Care 11(1):22–29

8 *Nancy A Stotts*

Assessing a patient with a pressure ulcer

INTRODUCTION

Systematic assessment of the patient with a pressure ulcer is pivotal to developing a plan of care. Comprehensive assessment is critical to care since it establishes a baseline for subsequent comparison, permits differential diagnosis, provides the basis for a treatment plan and facilitates timely referral to other health care providers.

This chapter describes a strategy to assess the person with a pressure ulcer. It builds on our understanding of the aetiology of pressure ulcers and models of risk assessment described in Chapters 3 and 6. Several tools that have been used to evaluate ulcers (Pressure Sore Status Tool, the Sessing Scale and the Sussman Scale) are described and their validity and reliability in clinical practice is addressed. The use of history and physical examination for assessment of risk for ulcers and the person with a pressure ulcer is discussed. Staging and detailed assessment of the ulcer itself is described. Criteria are proposed to identify normal healing, impaired healing and infection. The chapter concludes with a discussion of the documentation of findings.

Understanding risk factors is important when assessing the patient with a pressure ulcer as understanding them provides direction for data gathering during the history and physical examination. It is important to keep in mind that patients who have a pressure ulcer need to have risk assessment performed because there is a high probability of ulcer formation at other sites. Little attention has been paid to the assessment and treatment of persons with multiple pressure ulcers; most of the reports on the issue are case studies.

INSTRUMENTS TO ASSESS PRESSURE ULCER STATUS

Various approaches have been used to assess pressure ulcer status and healing, including the Pressure Sore Status Tool (Bates-Jensen et al 1992, Bates-Jensen 1997), the Sessing Scale (Ferrell et al 1995) and the Sussman Tool (Sussman & Swanson 1997). In addition, pressure ulcer condition has been evaluated with staging and by use of the classic history and physical examination.

Pressure Sore Status Tool (PSST)

Bates-Jensen and colleagues (1992) developed the Pressure Sore Status Tool (PSST) as a 13-item paper and pencil tool to record pressure ulcer condition. Items on the PSST are size, depth, edges, undermining, necrotic tissue type, necrotic tissue amount, exudate type, exudate amount, skin colour surrounding the wound, peripheral tissue oedema, induration, granulation, and epithelialization (Fig. 8.1). Items are rated on a Likkert Scale and summed to reach a total score of 13–65. A lower score reflects a better ulcer condition. Content validity was established with a panel of experts and demonstrated a high overall content validity index (0.91). Inter-rater reliability was high between two raters at two times ($r = 0.91$ and 0.92, respectively). Intra-rater reliability for the two raters was high ($r = 0.99$ and 0.96, respectively) (Bates-Jensen et al 1992).

NAME: _____

Complete the rating sheet to assess pressure ulcer status. Evaluate each item by picking the response that best describes the wound and entering the score in the item score column for the appropriate date.

LOCATION: Anatomical site. Circle, indentify right (R) or left (L) and use 'X' to mark site on body diagrams:

_____ Sacrum & coccyx	_____ Lateral ankle
_____ Trochanter	_____ Medial ankle
_____ Ischial tuberosity	_____ Heel _____ Other site

SHAPE: Overall wound pattern; assess by observing perimeter and depth. Circle and *date* appropriate description:

_____ Irregular	_____ Linear or elongated
_____ Round/oval	_____ Bowl/boat
_____ Square/rectangle	_____ Butterfly _____ Other shape

Item	Assessment	Date	Date	Date
		Score	Score	Score
1. Size	1 = Length x width < 4 cm² 2 = Length x width 4–16 cm² 3 = Length x width 16.1–36 cm² 4 = Length x width 36.1–80 cm² 5 = Length x width > 80 cm²			
2. Depth	1 = Nonblanchable erythema on intact skin 2 = Partial-thickness skin loss involving epidermis &/or dermis 3 = Full-thickness skin loss involving damage or necrosis of subcutaneous tissue; may extend down to but not through underlying fascia; &/or mixed partial- & full-thickness &/or tissue layers obscured by granulation tissue 4 = Obscured by necrosis 5 = Full-thickness skin loss with extensive destruction, tissue necrosis, or damage to muscle, bone or supporting structures			
3. Edges	1 = Indistinct, diffuse, none clearly visible 2 = Distinct, outline clearly visible, attached, even with wound base 3 = Well defined, not attached to wound base 4 = Well defined, not attached to base, rolled under, thickened 5 = Well defined, fibrotic, scarred or hyperkeratotic			
4. Undermining	1 = Undermining < 2 cm in any area 2 = Undermining 2–4 cm involving < 50% wound margins 3 = Undermining 2–4 cm involving > 50% wound margins 4 = Undermining > 4 cm in any area 5 = Tunnelling &/or sinus tract formation			
5. Necrotic tissue type	1 = None visible 2 = White/grey nonviable tissue &/or nonadherent yellow slough 3 = Loosely adherent yellow slough 4 = Adherent, soft, black eschar 5 = Firmly adherent, hard, black eschar			
6. Necrotic tissue amount	1 = None visible 2 = < 25% of wound bed covered 3 = 25–50% of wound covered 4 = > 50% and < 75% of wound covered 5 = 75–100% of wound covered			
7. Exudate type	1 = None or bloody 2 = Serosanguineous: thin, watery, pale red/pink 3 = Serous: thin, watery, clear 4 = Purulent: thin or thick, opaque, tan/yellow 5 = Foul purulent: thick, opaque, yellow/green with odour			

Figure 8.1 The Pressure Sore Status Tool.

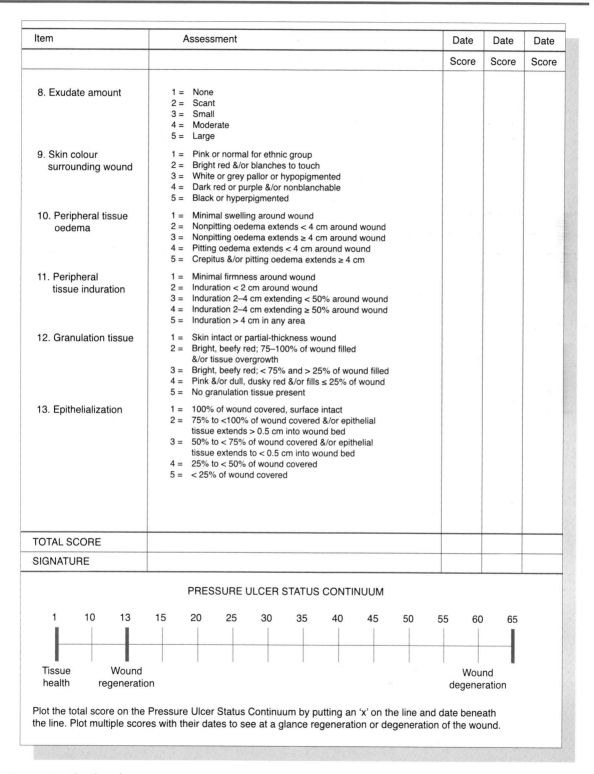

Item	Assessment	Date	Date	Date
		Score	Score	Score
8. Exudate amount	1 = None 2 = Scant 3 = Small 4 = Moderate 5 = Large			
9. Skin colour surrounding wound	1 = Pink or normal for ethnic group 2 = Bright red &/or blanches to touch 3 = White or grey pallor or hypopigmented 4 = Dark red or purple &/or nonblanchable 5 = Black or hyperpigmented			
10. Peripheral tissue oedema	1 = Minimal swelling around wound 2 = Nonpitting oedema extends < 4 cm around wound 3 = Nonpitting oedema extends ≥ 4 cm around wound 4 = Pitting oedema extends < 4 cm around wound 5 = Crepitus &/or pitting oedema extends ≥ 4 cm			
11. Peripheral tissue induration	1 = Minimal firmness around wound 2 = Induration < 2 cm around wound 3 = Induration 2–4 cm extending < 50% around wound 4 = Induration 2–4 cm extending ≥ 50% around wound 5 = Induration > 4 cm in any area			
12. Granulation tissue	1 = Skin intact or partial-thickness wound 2 = Bright, beefy red; 75–100% of wound filled &/or tissue overgrowth 3 = Bright, beefy red; < 75% and > 25% of wound filled 4 = Pink &/or dull, dusky red &/or fills ≤ 25% of wound 5 = No granulation tissue present			
13. Epithelialization	1 = 100% of wound covered, surface intact 2 = 75% to <100% of wound covered &/or epithelial tissue extends > 0.5 cm into wound bed 3 = 50% to < 75% of wound covered &/or epithelial tissue extends to < 0.5 cm into wound bed 4 = 25% to < 50% of wound covered 5 = < 25% of wound covered			
TOTAL SCORE				
SIGNATURE				

PRESSURE ULCER STATUS CONTINUUM

1   10   13   15   20   25   30   35   40   45   50   55   60   65

Tissue health   Wound regeneration   Wound degeneration

Plot the total score on the Pressure Ulcer Status Continuum by putting an 'x' on the line and date beneath the line. Plot multiple scores with their dates to see at a glance regeneration or degeneration of the wound.

Figure 8.1 *Continued*

Subsequent inter-rater reliability established between 15 practitioners who were trained in the use of the scale was 0.78. Reliability between the 15 practitioners and the wound expert was 0.82. Intra-rater reliability was 0.89. Depth on the PSST was compared with what was recorded on the patient's chart (the gold standard for depth) on the same day and the findings yielded a coefficient of 0.91 (Bates-Jensen & McNees 1995).

The PSST has been incorporated into the Wound Intelligence System, a computerized system for wound assessment. Data on over 990 patients produced 7084 wound assessments using the PSST. In this sample, the majority of ulcers were stage II (52.8%) and stage III (34.3%). Some were stage I (4.6%) and stage IV (8.3%) (Bates-Jensen 1997). Preliminary factor analysis showed that the PSST had four factors – size, depth, wound edges and undermining – which accounted for 64% of the variance. The amount of variance accounted for by each of the factors was not reported. The PSST provides a comprehensive assessment. Its limitation is that it is relatively long and therefore is time-consuming to complete. Further exploration of developing these four factors into a simpler model has not been reported.

Sessing Scale

The Sessing Scale was developed as an outcome measure for the evaluation of standardized pressure ulcer care (Fig. 8.2). It was designed to be inexpensive and easy to use to measure the progression of pressure ulcer healing in various settings (Ferrell et al 1995). Six stages are used, ranging from normal skin that is at-risk of ulcer development to the most serious cases. A panel of clinical nurse specialists assessed face validity of the scale and rated the content validity as 100%. Concurrent validity was established by comparing it with the Shea Scale and surface area by planimetry (calculating the surface area by tracing the perimeter of the wound). The Shea Scale was the earliest staging Scale (Shea 1975) and is generally accepted as the standard when instrument validity is tested. Moderately strong relationships have been shown among initial

Stage	Description
0	Normal skin, but at risk
1	Skin completely closed May lack pigmentation or be reddened
2	Wound edges and centre are filled in Surrounding tissues are intact and not reddened
3	Wound bed filling with pink granulating tissue Slough present Free of necrotic tissue Minimum drainage and odour
4	Moderate to minimal granulating tissue Slough and minimal necrotic tissue Moderate drainage and odour
5	Presence of heavy drainage and odour, eschar and slough. Surrounding skin reddened or discoloured
6	Breaks in skin around primary ulcer Purulent drainage, foul odour, necrotic tissue and/or eschar. May have septic symptoms

Figure 8.2 The Sessing Scale.

Sessing stage, initial Shea stage and ulcer diameter ($r = 0.52$, $P < 0.0001$; $r = 0.35$, $P < 0.001$; $r = 0.62$, $P < 0.0001$). When changes in the Shea and the Sessing Scales were correlated, there was a strong relationship between them ($r = 0.90$, $P < 0.0001$). Inter-rater reliability was high ($\kappa = 0.80$) as was test–retest reliability ($\kappa = 0.90$ on two consecutive days). Subsequent testing has not been reported.

Sussman Scale

The Sussman Wound Healing Tool was developed to track the effectiveness of physical therapy wound healing technologies and predict healing. It is a 10-item scale, based on an acute wound healing model (Fig. 8.3). The wound attributes, e.g. necrosis and undermining, are complemented with 11 demographic variables. Each attribute item is rated dichotomously, i.e. present or absent. The instrument has been tested in long-term care by physical therapists

Attribute	Rating
Necrosis	Present or not present
Undermining	Present or not present
Maceration	Present or not present
Erythema	Present or not present
Hemorrhage	Present or not present
Fibroplasia-significant reduction in depth	Present or not present
Appearance of contraction	Present or not present
Sustained contraction	Present or not present
Adherence at wound edge	Present or not present
Epithelialization	Present or not present

Figure 8.3   The Sussman Wound Healing Tool.

and physical therapy assistants. Inter-rater reliability is not reported. Data show that the Sussman Wound Healing Tool has predictive validity for healing for the 21 variables. Further testing for the instrument has been planned (Sussman & Swanson 1997).

STAGING OF PRESSURE ULCERS

Pressure ulcer staging has been used to describe the depth of the ulcer (NPUAP 1989). Initially described by Shea (1975), modification has been proposed by various individuals and groups (Parish et al 1983, IAET 1986, NPUAP 1989). It has been standardized in the United States since the Agency for Health Care Policy and Research (AHCPR) accepted the NPUAP (1989) consensus definition for staging (Box 8.1). Since that time, there has been publication and wide dissemination of the AHCPR Pressure Ulcer Prevention and Treatment Guidelines (AHCPR 1992, 1994). In this model, stage I is characterized by nonblanchable erythema. Stage II demonstrates damage that extends into the dermis. Some authors suggest that stage I and II pressure ulcers are the result of friction and shear – pressure that is exerted parallel to the skin (Maklebust &

BOX 8.1   STAGES OF PRESSURE ULCERS

I   Nonblanchable erythema of intact skin; the heralding lesion of skin ulceration.

II   Partial-thickness skin loss involving epidermis and/or dermis. The ulcer is superficial and presents clinically as an abrasion, blister or shallow crater.

III   Full-thickness skin loss involving damage or necrosis of subcutaneous tissue that may extend down to, but not through, underlying fascia. The ulcer presents clinically as a deep crater with or without undermining of adjacent tissue.

IV   Full-thickness skin loss with extensive destruction, tissue necrosis or damage to muscle, bone or supporting structures. Undermining and sinus tracts may be associated with stage IV pressure ulcers.

Sieggreen 1996). Stage III ulcers extend into the subcutaneous tissue but not through the fascia. Stage IV ulcers are the deepest, involving muscle and bone, tendon or ligament. Vertical pressure is thought to be the primary cause of Stage III and IV ulcers. When tissues are compressed between a bed or chair surface and bony prominences, the greatest pressure is felt in the muscle next to the bone. The pressure causes ischaemia and the muscle becomes necrotic. Because the muscle is deep in the body, beneath the skin and subcutaneous tissue, a stage III or IV ulcer is not visible until the necrosis extends into the skin (Maklebust & Sieggreen 1996).

Originally designed as a measure of depth, staging has inappropriately been adapted as a measure of healing. However, the National Pressure Ulcer Advisory Panel (NPUAP) has recommended that staging not be used to measure healing of pressure ulcers because staging does not accurately describe repair as the ulcers heal (Maklebust 1997). Specifically, ulcers heal by filling in destroyed tissue with scar: lost tissue is not replaced with muscle or subcutaneous tissue.

They recommend that ulcers be staged to describe the degree of injury, but that it should not be used to measure healing. Healing is usually measured using the wound size and characteristics of the wound, for example tissue type.

The NPUAP also recognized that stage I pressure ulcers were somewhat difficult to measure in persons with darkly pigmented skin. As a result, they have proposed a new definition of stage I ulcer as 'nonblanchable erythema of intact skin, the heralding lesion of skin ulceration. In individuals with darker skin, warmth, oedema, induration, or hardness, may also be indicators' (Henderson et al 1997). This definition remains to be tested.

REFERRAL CRITERIA

One important clinical issue is when to refer patients with a pressure ulcer to the advanced practice wound care nurse or for consultation with plastic or general surgery. A general rule is that referral is not needed if the wound is clean and making consistent progress. However, referral is indicated if there is a delay in healing or a sudden negative change.

HISTORY AND PHYSICAL EXAMINATION

The traditional history and physical examination format is appropriate for persons with a pressure ulcer. It provides a comprehensive picture of the person, their overall health and focused information about their pressure ulcer(s). Understanding the patient's health status, concurrent underlying pathology and the factors that contribute to the pressure ulcer allow the health care team to make a differential diagnosis and develop a rational plan of care (Seidel et al 1999).

Initial survey

Generally, the provider begins with an initial survey of the patient and the pressure ulcer. The survey is rapid and is an appraisal of the overall situation. The patient's general condition, overall physical status and responses are judged. The location of the ulcer is noted and, when possible, the general condition of the tissue around and within the ulcer is assessed. In the first minute the provider usually has an initial impression of whether the ulcer is healing or not healing. If the ulcer is covered with necrotic tissue or slough, it cannot be staged. Later, after the initial evaluation is completed, the ulcer is debrided. The wound is then systematically evaluated and documentation is generated about each dimension of the wound. In a situation where debridement cannot be performed, the wound is evaluated and data are recorded with the clearest data available.

History

The history provides 80% of the information about a patient and so is pivotal to accurate diagnosis and subsequent treatment. The nurse obtaining a history must attend to all the usual dimensions, including present illness, past medical history and family history, and then review of systems to stimulate recall of any events that have not previously been reported (Table 8.1).

Several dimensions of the history and physical examination are especially important in patients with wounds because they have been shown to be cofactors in healing. These are nutrition, oxygenation and perfusion and concomitant conditions, including diabetes, immunosuppressive conditions, cardiovascular disease and cancer. In addition, various medications have been implicated in impaired healing, including chemotherapeutic drugs, steroids and anticoagulants. Other routine medications need to be elicited and their contribution to healing appraised, for example anti-hypertensives. The use of over-the-counter drugs should be explored as patients may be taking mega-doses of vitamins or using herbs that may need to be factored into the plan of care.

Previous records should be used to obtain information as is necessary. The social history and living situation provide the information that allows the nurse to tailor the treatment to the situation.

Table 8.1 Comprehensive and specific history for the patient with a pressure ulcer

Pressure ulcer-specific history	Comprehensive history questions
Age	Chief complaint
History of present illness	Present problem/illness
Past medical history: diabetes, coronary artery disease, peripheral vascular disease, hypertension, deep-vein thrombosis, venous insufficiency, history of clots/coagulopathies, smoking history	Past medical history: general health, childhood illness, adult illnesses, immunizations, surgery, functional status, medications/allergies, transfusions, emotional status
Medications/allergies	Family history
Living situation: home care, nursing home, lives alone, family support	Personal and social history: habits, sexual history, home conditions, occupation, environment
Activity: ambulates, moves all extremities, non-mobile, chairbound	Review of systems
Activity of daily living	
Nutritional status	
Hygiene: incontinent, clean/dry skin, bathes daily	
Previous pressure ulcer? If yes, what treatment	

A portion of patients with pressure ulcers have impaired cognitive functioning. At times, these patients are unable to provide accurate information about the present or past history. Available data can be supplemented with information from family.

Examination of the pressure ulcer

A systematic and consistent approach should be used in pressure ulcer evaluation so that each time the provider approaches a patient the same format is used. Such an approach reduces the tendency to omit aspects of the examination. The examination includes measuring the wound size, pressure ulcer tissue and the various properties of partial and full-thickness ulcers as described above (Figs 8.1–8.3, Box 8.1). Finally, the tissue surrounding the ulcer is evaluated.

Size

Size is one of the most important factors to include in ulcer assessment. With pressure ulcers, length, width and depth are measured. Clinically, this can be done with a disposable ruler (Brown-Etris 1995). These parameters are documented in centimetres to the nearest millimetre. One of the issues in measurement of size is which dimension

should be used to measure surface area – head to foot and side to side versus the greatest length and the greatest width that is perpendicular to it. This seemingly minor point is important because wounds do not contract or epithelialize at an equal rate along all edges of the perimeter. The areas that are most superficial and those held most loosely by the underlying tissue move toward the centre of the wound most rapidly. Thus, when measurement is of the longest and widest portion of the wound, the caregiver may not be measuring the same spot consistently. This inconsistency augments the error inherent in the calculation of size based on length × width. Such error may result in an over-optimistic assessment of the wound and delay in the re-evaluation of the treatment plan and implementation of beneficial treatment. To mitigate this problem, the head to foot and perpendicular measurements should be used. Those who believe that the greatest length and the perpendicular width should be used do not feel that the inherent error outweighs the ease of this approach. A consistent approach needs to be used in any facility.

Depth Depth is measured in stage II or greater depth pressure ulcers at the deepest spot, using an applicator. This method is somewhat inconsistent because depth varies and positioning of the patient may determine how the tissues lie and where the deepest point is. This approach is inconsistent but easy to use (Brown-Etris 1995) and probably has enough precision for clinical care.

Measuring surface area and volume There is some controversy about whether surface area (length × width) or wound volume (length × width × depth) provides the best picture of wound status. Volume is argued by some to be a better measure of wound status than surface area because some sores are shaped like a cone, with the top of the cone being the skin surface. When this is the case, the skin has contracted more rapidly than granulation tissue has filled the base. However, in clinical practice, all of these parameters (length, width and depth) are usually measured. Volume is not normally calculated in routine patient care.

The evaluation of area is based on the assumption that the wound is a rectangle (length × width). With volume, the assumption is that the wound is a cube (length × width × depth). In clinical practice, however, the wound edges on the surface are rarely uniformly in a rectangular or square shape, nor is the depth uniform on the base of the pressure ulcer. Consequently, when wound size is estimated with surface area (length × width) or volume (length × width × depth), it is an overestimation of the size.

There are several more accurate approaches to measuring volume, none of which are practical in routine daily care. One approach is to cover the pressure ulcer with a transparent dressing and then fill the cavity with saline. The volume of saline reflects the volume of the wound. This works well with deep wounds. In those that are shallow or traverse a heel or an elbow, this method lacks precision because of the difficulties in estimating the usual contour of the skin over the part.

Dental impression material can also be used to measure volume. It is mixed according to directions, inserted into the wound, allowed to set and then removed. The mould is weighed and its weight transformed into a volume. Alternatively, its volume can be obtained by water displace-

ment. Use of dental impression material to measure volume is good for deep wounds but has the same problems of accuracy that the use of water does in shallow wounds and also those over heels and elbows. In addition, if the weight of the alginate is not determined soon after the mould is created, the accuracy of the volume measurement will depend on how the mould is stored (Stotts et al 1996).

The third approach to measurement of volume is with stereophotogammetry, where a pair of slides is taken simultaneously with two cameras positioned at a fixed distance to form a triangle with the wound. A microcomputer takes the images and calculates wound surface area dimensions, depth and volume (Frantz & Johnson 1992). This is an ideal non-invasive system that is appropriate for research purposes.

Approaches to wound measurement and recording

Kundin Wound Gauge Several other approaches have been used to measure wound size. Kundin has proposed the use of the Kundin Wound Gauge to measure healing. This is a paper ruler that is used to measure width, depth and length. Kundin's approach allows calculation of area and volume. Her formulae are based on the assumption that the wound is an ellipse (Kundin 1985).

Photographs Photographs can also be used to document the presence and gross characteristics of pressure ulcers. When they are taken with a Polaroid camera an immediate image is obtained. Photographs provide a visual reference of the ulcer but may not provide fine detail. They cannot provide information about areas that are undermined. When photographs are taken for research purposes, a 35-mm system is used with a minimum of a 50-mm macro lens. In this case, computerized planimetry may be used to determine surface area (Brown-Etris 1995).

Tracing Tracing of the surface of the sore also may be used (Fig. 8.4). Thomas & Wysocki (1990) compared acetate tracing, photographs and the

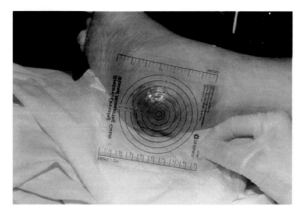

Figure 8.4 The acetate is in place for wound tracing.

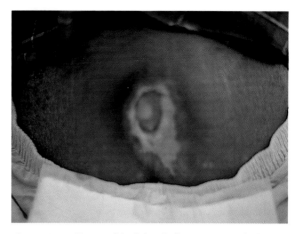

Figure 8.5 Note epithelial tufts between 9 o'clock and 11 o'clock and again at 6 o'clock.

Kundin Wound Gauge to measure venous stasis ulcers (n = 37) and pressure ulcers (n = 36). There was a high correlation between the methods (r = 0.93, P < 0.001); however, they were significantly different. The Kundin Wound Gauge markedly underestimated wound size. The authors recommended the acetate, recognizing that to interpret the data requires measuring of the area with planimetry or scanning into a computer. However, acetate tracing also provides a model of surface area and symmetry that can be compared over time. Digitizing either photographs or acetate tracings has been shown to have very high correlation (r = 0.97) when lower extremity ulcers were evaluated (Brown-Etris et al 1994).

Tissue in the pressure ulcer

Evaluation of the tissue in the pressure ulcer requires appreciation of the types of tissue that are present and the various factors that can affect repair. Accurate evaluation provides the basis for determining therapy and subsequently evaluating whether healing is taking place.

Partial-thickness pressure ulcers

Stage I and II ulcers are partial thickness; they do not extend beyond the epidermis and dermis. In partial-thickness injuries, the majority of healing occurs through regeneration of the epithelium. The new epithelium comes from the skin edges and the skin appendages (glands and hair foll-

icles). The skin edges migrate toward the denuded area and the epithelium moves up the shafts of the glands and hair follicles onto the surface of the tissue (Fig. 8.5). New epithelium in the centre of the wound looks like tufts of cotton candy that are dispersed among denuded areas. The tufts of tissue quickly coalesce because of the wide distribution of glands and hair follicles in the skin. The tissue in partial-thickness injury is moist but not wet. Moisture allows cells to migrate most rapidly and so closure occurs more rapidly than in a dry environment. A dry wound bed results in dehydration of cells and death of tissue.

Full-thickness pressure ulcers

Stage III and IV ulcers are full-thickness injuries, which means that the epidermis and dermis of the skin are denuded. With full-thickness injury, healing occurs through the development of new granulation tissue, epithelialization and contraction. Each process contributes to repair and occurs in a predictable pattern.

Granulation tissue Early after injury, granulation tissue begins to be laid down. New capillaries are formed and collagen is laid down over them. This is visible in the base of the wound as pale tissue and becomes deeper pink and 'beefy' red as the capillary bed builds. The wound usually fills in from the bottom and so depth

107

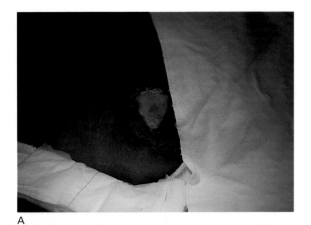

A

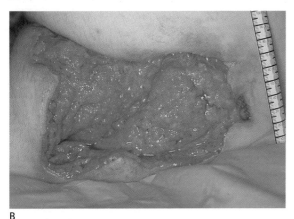

B

Figure 8.6 (A) Good granulation tissue. (B) Poor-quality granulation tissue.

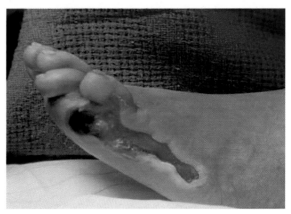

Figure 8.7 Rounded epithelial edge indicates old wound.

decreases first and then wound area decreases. Granulation tissue is characterized by a grainy surface appearance caused by loops of capillaries that are visible on the wound surface (Fig. 8.6).

Epithelialization The epithelial edge surrounds the wound and is the source of epithelial cells to cover the wound (Fig. 8.7). It should be intact and optimally is continuous with the sides and base of the ulcer. When a pressure ulcer has not healed for a period of time, the edge sometimes becomes rolled and, in that case, coverage of the wound is delayed. As the epithelial edge ages, it changes from a pearly pink to pearly as it loses vascularity.

Deep structures Stage IV ulcers extend through the fascia into the muscle and tendons, ligaments and bone may be visible. Normal tendons and ligaments are moist and pearly coloured. Bone is covered with a clear thin membrane called the periosteum. When any of these structures are dehydrated, they cannot be rehydrated and so function is lost. They may be replaced with scar tissue as healing occurs or removed by a health care provider when they become ischaemic and/or infected. When they become infected, these structures are also hard to treat and damage may be irreversible. In either case, it is important to identify the structures present so that critical structures are not inadvertently sacrificed and function lost. Foot ulcers and those of the sacrum are especially challenging.

Tunnelling and undermining Tunnelling and undermining occur in full-thickness pressure ulcers. Tunnelling is an invagination or a blind opening into the tissue. It is caused by the ischaemia that created the ulcer. The tunnel depth is measured as well as the diameter of its opening. The wound is probed for tunnelling. It is important in measuring tunnelling between two areas to use an applicator that is smaller than the tunnel to probe the wound so it does not enlarge the tunnel. All measurements are recorded immediately after they are made to ensure accuracy. In caring for a wound containing tunnelling, it is important to allow the tunnel to close from the most distal portion to the most proximal so that an abscess does not form.

With undermining, the pressure ulcer is larger at the base of the wound than at the skin surface (Fig. 8.8). Undermining is evaluated by inserting a probe or applicator between the skin and the subcutaneous tissue and measuring the farthest point. Undermining will often extend varying distances under the skin and this can be documented using a diagram or by describing the distance as on the face of a clock. Undermined areas are colonized by both Gram-positive and Gram-negative organisms. Anaerobes live especially well in this environment, although Sapico and colleagues (1986) have shown that both aerobic and anaerobic organisms live in undermined areas. When necrotic tissue is present, their numbers are significantly higher. The anaerobes are significantly related to the presence of necrotic tissue in undermined areas and in most cases are associated with foul odour. The odour disappears when the anaerobic bioburden is reduced.

Necrosis and slough Necrotic tissue is dead tissue. It is an integral part of pressure ulcer pathology and so often necrotic tissue is visible in the ulcer (Fig. 8.9). When the necrotic tissue begins to be broken down it turns to slough. Slough is a combination of fibrous tissue and exudate. Slough is the firmer portion and exudate is the liquid/semi-liquid portion that is the byproduct of bacterial metabolic activity. Both the necrotic material and the slough are dead and support infection. Their presence and distribution need to be assessed so that treatment can be instituted. Healing progresses more rapidly when they have been removed from the pressure ulcer.

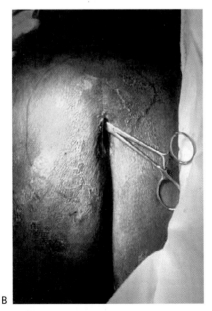

A

B

Figure 8.8 (A) Appearance of sacral ulcer prior to examination. (B) Degree of undermining of a sacral ulcer indicated by the black outline.

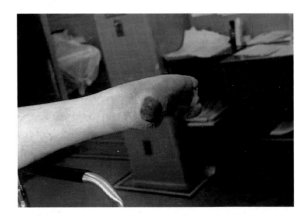

Figure 8.9 Necrotic pressure ulcer.

ASSESSMENT OF THE TISSUE SURROUNDING THE PRESSURE ULCER

The condition of the tissue surrounding the pressure ulcer is assessed. It is compared with that on the opposite side of the body. Observing the condition of the peri-ulcer skin may provide clues as to whether the nursing care provided is sufficient to prevent pressure and subsequent ischaemia. Data may be used to determine the need for pressure-relieving devices and alterations in the turning schedule.

Appreciation of the condition of the peri-ulcer tissue gives the provider a perspective on the extension of the wound. When there is discoloration, open skin or macerated tissue, the provider needs to be alert to the possibility that the wound may extend into the healthy peri-ulcer tissue.

KEY POINTS

♦ The skin is observed for redness and disruption in skin integrity. Skin that is intact and yet friable should be noted. Bruising suggests that there has been bleeding into the tissue and may be due to trauma to the area, with or without alteration in the coagulation cascade

♦ In patients who have had a muscle flap repair, incision lines may be visible. Surgery may have reconfigured the natural contour of the area. Sites of prior skin grafts should also be observed and noted. Healed pressure areas are noted since they are especially vulnerable to reinjury

♦ Concurrent skin disease needs to be differentiated from pressure areas, e.g. psoriasis or pemphigus. Often, more than one skin condition exists in a given patient and the combination of conditions provides a challenge to the patient's provider

♦ The area is palpated for warmth and induration. The presence and degree of oedema is assessed.

EVALUATING HEALING IN PRESSURE ULCERS

The most common way to evaluate healing is monitoring wound size (Brown-Etris 1995). The limitation of this measure of healing is that it is not sensitive to change (Thomas et al 1997). This can be a problem, especially in large wounds where changes may be only a few millimetres per week and, in this case, the question is often whether healing or measurement error has occurred. One of the issues here is whether surface area or volume is most accurate and, for the most part, surface area is seen as an adequate measure of healing. As with all rules, the caveat here is that undermined wounds that have contracted at the wound surface prior to filling with granulation tissue leave a small opening and a track that may require considerable time to heal.

Many clinicians (and researchers) supplement size with other parameters. Clinically often used measured are type of tissue present, the amount of drainage and whether there is undermining or tunneling (Maklebust & Sieggreen 1996, Bale & Jones 1997, Stotts & Cavanaugh 1999).

Several instruments have been proposed to measure healing, including the PSST, Sessing Scale, the Sussman Wound Healing Tool and the Pressure Ulcer Scale for Healing. The PSST (Fig. 8.1) is a well validated measure of healing. The Sessing Scale (Fig. 8.2) and Sussman Wound Healing Tool (Fig. 8.3) have undergone limited testing in the measurement of healing; both show adequate validity. The Pressure Ulcer Scale for Healing is an instrument designed to measure healing in open stage II–IV sores. It has three dimensions: tissue type, exudate quantity and ulcer size (Fig. 8.10). Preliminary testing indicates its validity (Thomas et al 1997).

CHARACTERISTICS OF IMPAIRED HEALING

Impaired healing in pressure ulcers is seen most frequently as slowed or delayed healing. While the timeline for healing is not well established, there is a broad range of 'usual healing' of ulcers, perhaps in part due to the variability in their size.

PATIENT NAME: _____

ID #: _____

ULCER LOCATION: _____

DATE: _____

DIRECTIONS:
Observe and measure the pressure ulcer. Categorize the ulcer with respect to the surface area, exudate and type of wound tissue. Record a sub-score for each of these ulcer characteristics. Add the sub-scores to obtain the total score. A comparison of total scores measured over time provides an indication of the improvement or deterioration in pressure ulcer healing.

	0	1	2	3	4	5
Length x width	0 cm²	< 0.3 cm²	0.3–0.6 cm²	0.7–1.0 cm²	1.1–2.0 cm²	2.1–3.0 cm²
		6	7	8	9	10
		3.1–4.0 cm²	4.1–8.0 cm²	8.1–12.0 cm²	12.1–24.0 cm²	> 24 cm²
Exudate amount	0 None	1 Light	2 Moderate	3 Heavy		
Tissue type	0 Closed	1 Epithelial tissue	2 Granulation tissue	3 Slough	4 Necrotic tissue	

Length x width: Measure the greatest length (head to toe) and the greatest width (side to side) using a centimetre ruler. Multiply these two measurements (length x width) to obtain an estimate of surface area in square centimetres (cm²). **Caveat:** Do not guess! Always use a centimetre ruler and always use the same method each time the ulcer is measured.

Exudate amount: Estimate the amount of exudate (drainage) present after removal of the dressing and before applying any topical agent to the ulcer. Estimate the exudate (drainage) as none, light, moderate or heavy.

Tissue type: This refers to the types of tissue that are present in the wound (ulcer) bed. Score as a '4' if there is any necrotic tissue present. Score as a '3' if there is any amount of slough present and necrotic tissue is absent. Score as a '2' if the wound is clean and contains granulation tissue. A superficial wound that is re-epithelializing is scored as a '1'. When the wound is closed, score as a '0'.

    4 – Necrotic tissue (eschar): Black, brown or tan tissue that adheres firmly to the wound bed or ulcer edges and may be either firmer or softer than the surrounding skin.

    3 – Slough: Yellow or white tissue that adheres to the ulcer bed in strings or thick clumps, or is mucinous.

    2 – Granulation tissue: Pink or beefy red tissue with a shiny, moist, granular appearance.

    1 – Epithelial tissue: For superficial ulcers, new pink or shiny tissue (skin) that grows in from the edges or as islands on the ulcer surface.

    0 – Closed/resurfaced: The wound is completely covered with epithelium (new skin).

Figure 8.10 The Pressure Ulcer Healing Scale.

Table 8.2 Characteristics of impaired healing in partial and full-thickness ulcers	
Partial-thickness ulcers	Full-thickness ulcers
Wound size is increasing	Wound size is increasing
Epithelial tufts are not visible throughout the wound at the site of hair follicles and glands	Epithelial edge is not continuous around the wound and is not moving into the wound bed
Exudate, slough, or eschar is present	Exudate, slough or eschar
Malodorous drainage	The development of a tunnel, undermining or fistula
	Malodorous drainage
	Pain or change in sensation

In partial-thickness ulcers (stage II), lack of granulation tissue in the base, a paucity of epithelial tufts present in the wound bed, or the presence of eschar, exudate, odour or slough characterize impaired healing. In full-thickness sores (stage III or IV), large quantities of exudate, exudate that is extremely thick or thin and exudate that is serosanguineous or coloured yellow or green may alert the practitioner to impairment in healing. Unusual odour and the development of tunnels, undermining or fistulas also characterize impaired healing. Tissue that is covered with eschar or slough or poor-quality granulation tissue is noted. An epithelial edge that is not continuous or does not move into the wound suggests disruption in healing. Pain in the area or a change in sensation, although more subtle than the objective wound signs, may signal impaired healing (Stotts & Cavanaugh 1999) (Table 8.2).

Local infection

Infection is perhaps the most common cause of delayed healing. It is clear that all pressure ulcers are contaminated, i.e., bacteria are present on the surface of the ulcer, and so the risk of infection is ever-present. When those bacteria that are present multiply, colonization is said to be present. Infection occurs when bacteria that are present on the surface and/or colonize the ulcer, actually invade the tissue. Infection is one of the most significant events that delays healing.

When bacteria invade the tissue, a classic inflammatory response is initiated and neutrophils are mobilized. If the body's immune system is not adequate to resist the invasion, the microorganisms multiply in the tissue and eventually infection occurs.

Infection in pressure ulcers is characterized by inflammation, increased amounts of exudate, pain and malodorous discharge. There may be a systemic response that includes fever, increased production of immature white blood cells (a shift to the left) and a positive wound culture. The shift to the left is characterized by an increase in the number of neutrophils (Stotts & Hunt 1997, Robson et al 1999).

The wound may need to be cultured to confirm the clinical diagnosis and to determine the antibiotic that the organism(s) is sensitive to. The three most frequently used approaches to culturing are tissue biopsy, swab and aspiration. Regardless of which of these is selected, the culture needs to be taken from healthy-looking tissue. If exudate or eschar is present, it needs to be removed so that the tissue that appears healthy is visible. The pressure ulcer also needs to be cleansed with a non-antimicrobial solution prior to obtaining the culture. Regardless of the technique used, the specimen should be obtained using sterile technique and transported to the laboratory in a sterile container.

The gold standard for culture is a wound biopsy (Robson et al 1999). With this method, a small piece of tissue is removed from the pressure ulcer and sent to the laboratory under sterile conditions. The limitation of the technique is that tissue is taken from the wound and this may delay healing. It may also be a painful procedure since most authors recommend not using local anaesthetic because this will dilute the organisms in the tissue that is biopsied.

The swab technique involves moving an applicator across a 1 cm² area of the wound surface until the tip of the applicator is moistened with wound fluid. This method is easy to use but is criticized because it overestimates the number of organisms compared with tissue biopsy (Stotts & Hunt 1997).

Aspiration involves inserting a needle attached to a 10 cm^3 syringe into the tissue next to the pressure ulcer. Negative pressure is applied to the plunger and the needle is moved back and forth in several directions to obtain wound fluid in the tissues. Understanding the anatomy of the wound area is important so the inserted needle does not cause structural damage. This method underestimates the number of organisms present compared with tissue biopsy (Stotts & Hunt 1997).

A Gram stain usually is the first culture result reported. It identifies whether infection is present and whether the infection is Gram-positive or Gram-negative. These very early data allow antibiotic treatment to be initiated. At 24 h, a preliminary report is issued that identifies the organisms and at 48 h a final report indicates the organism(s) present and their sensitivity to various antibiotics.

DOCUMENTATION

Every institution should have a policy for documenting assessment of patients, including pressure ulcers. At minimum, documentation should follow the policy.

For pressure ulcers, there should be a risk assessment scale or risk calculator that is used at specified intervals. A history and physical examination are documented that address the overall patient and focus on pressure ulcer-related issues (Table 8.1). Detailed pressure ulcer assessment is important as it provides the basis for determining the effectiveness of the current treatment regimen. The nursing process (assessment, diagnosis, treatment and evaluation) should be inherent in the charting. Outcomes increasingly are emphasized so, if in one's evaluation healing is occurring, it is important to describe the basis of the conclusion. For example, if it is stated that healing is progressing, indicate that this is based on a decrease in ulcer size and development of new granulation tissue. When consistent documentation has been done, it is possible to work with the patient's care team to alter the plan to effect positive and timely outcomes. It will also

protect the nurse from undue liability (Mastering documentation 1999).

A form is often used to enhance consistency. As computerized charting increases, prompting of the nurse to address specific dimensions of the wound may enhance the completeness and accuracy of the data about the pressure ulcer over time.

The case studies illustrate common pressure ulcer presentations and healing trajectories.

CASE STUDY 8.1

Doreen White is a 38-year-old female admitted to the hospital for removal of a brain tumour. The surgery lasted 22 h and after transfer to the intensive care unit (ICU), she became septic, developed adult respiratory distress syndrome, and acute tubular necrosis. On postoperative day 2, a sacral pressure ulcer covered with eschar was discovered. Surgical debridement with anaesthesia cover was carried out at the bedside because the patient was not stable enough to be transferred to the operating room. The decision was made to undertake the debridement because the pressure ulcer was a potential nidus of the sepsis. Debridement revealed a stage IV ulcer that was 4 × 4 cm and 3 cm deep. The cavity was filled with necrotic tissue that was debrided. The surgical debridement was followed by 4 days of enzymatic debridement to ensure that any remaining necrotic material was removed. After 4 days, the base and walls of the ulcer had good granulation tissue present. By postoperative day 7, the patient was extubated, the sepsis and renal failure were resolved, and the patient was transferred to the ward. At that time, the ulcer was 3.8 × 3.5 cm and 2.5 cm deep. The ulcer was packed with loose gauze moistened with normal saline. Two days later, Doreen was discharged home, ambulating, alert and oriented. She was instructed not to sit or lie on the ulcer, except at mealtime when she used a foam cushion on her chair. When the wound became shallow, a hydrocolloid dressing was applied until the ulcer was entirely closed.

1 Why was surgical debridement so appropriate in this case? (See Ch. 11)

2 (a) Note the wound dressing regimens employed over time in relation to the changing local problems at the wound site.

  (b) For each phase of healing recorded here, note the best options available and the advantages and disadvantages of each (See Ch. 10)

3 (a) How would you have involved Doreen White in her care planning? (See Chs 9 and 14)

  (b) What are likely to be the long term-care planning goals?

CASE STUDY 8.2

Jim Davidson is an 80-year-old nursing home resident, with insulin-dependent diabetes mellitus, who was undergoing radiation therapy for cancer of the gastrointestinal tract when a pressure ulcer of the sacrum and both ischia occurred. The patient spends most of his day in the wheelchair and this has an appropriate seat cushion. When in bed he sits upright with his legs crossed. The ischial ulcers were identified on bath day and were stage II, 2 × 3 cm and 0.5 cm deep. These were clean ulcers with granulation tissue in the base and the edges were intact and continuous. Local care for the ulcers focused on maintaining a moist wound bed, and a foam dressing was used for that purpose. The patient was instructed in positioning in bed and was compliant with using a side-lying (< 30 degrees) or prone position while in bed. His time in the wheelchair was limited to 1 h, alternating between being up 1 h and in bed 1 h during the day, except when he went for his radiation therapy. The patient's nutritional status was evaluated. He had gradually lost weight during his radiation therapy, (1.8 kg last month and 1.4 kg in the current month). Blood results showed that his glucose was running in the 350s and all else was normal except his albumin, which was 2.8 g/dl. Insulin and a high-protein diet were initiated in an effort to normalize his glucose and improve his nutritional status. With the change in the regimen, the blood glucose ranged from 140 to 210. Over the month after the ulcers' appearance, Mr Davidson lost 0.9 kg and completed his radiation therapy. The three ulcers gradually decreased in size and were healed at 3 months after their initial appearance.

1 What are the factors that are likely to lead to delayed wound healing for this patient? (See Ch. 9)

2 (a) How would you assess Mr Davidson's nutritional status? (See Ch. 13)

   (b) What role does nutrition play in optimizing wound healing?

3 (a) What factors put Mr Davidson at particular risk of developing pressure sores and how would you assess this risk? (See Ch. 6)

   (b) Review the issues relating to providing Mr Davidson with an appropriate support surface while in bed and in his wheelchair. (See Ch. 7)

   (c) Review the regimens used in this case. What is the rationale behind their choice?

SELF-ASSESSMENT QUESTIONS

1 Identify two assessment parameters that indicate that healing is not progressing normally.

2 If you were going to use the Pressure Sore Status Tool (PSST) to guide your assessment, how could you tell if the wound was not progressing normally?

REFERENCES

Agency for Health Care Policy and Research 1992 Pressure ulcers in adults: prediction and prevention. AHCPR Publication No 92–0047. US Department of Health and Human Services, Rockville, MD

Agency for Health Care Policy and Research 1994 Treatment of pressure ulcers. AHCPR Publication No. 94–0652. US Department of Health and Human Services, Rockville, MD

Bale S, Jones V 1997 Wound care nursing: a patient-centered approach. Baillière Tindall, London

Bates-Jensen B M 1997 The Pressure Sore Status Tool a few thousand assessments later. Advances in Wound Care 10(5):65–73

Bates-Jensen B, McNees P 1995 Toward an intelligent wound assessment system. Ostomy/Wound Management 41(7A):20–28

Bates-Jensen B M, Vredevoe D L, Brecht M L 1992 Validity and reliability of the Pressure Sore Status Tool. Decubitus 5(6):80S–86S

Brown-Etris M 1995 Measuring healing in wounds. Advances in Wound Care 8(4):(Suppl.) 53–8

Brown-Etris M B, Pribble J, LaBrecque J 1994 Evaluation of two wound measurement methods in a multi-center, controlled study. Wounds 6(3):107–111

Ferrell B A, Artinian B M, Sessing D (1995) The Sessing Scale for assessment of pressure ulcer healing. Journal of the American Geriatric Society 43:37–40

Frantz R A, Johnson D A 1992 Stereophotography and computerized image analysis: a three-dimensional method of measuring wound healing. Wounds 4(2):58–62

Henderson C T, Ayello E A, Sussman C, Leiby D M, Bennett M A, Dungog E F, Sprigle S, Woodruff L 1997 Draft definition of stage I pressure ulcers: inclusion of persons with darkly pigmented skin. NPUAP Task Force on Stage I Definition and Darkly Pigmented Skin. Advances in Wound Care 10(5):16–9

International Association for Enterostomal Therapy (IAET) 1986 Standards for pressure ulcer care. IAET, Irvine

Kundin J I 1985 Designing and developing a new measuring instrument. Periop Nurs Q 1:40–45

Maklebust J 1997 Policy implications of using reverse staging to monitor pressure ulcer status. Advances in Wound Care 10(5):32–35

Maklebust J, Sieggreen M 1996 Pressure ulcers: Guidelines for prevention and nursing management, 2nd edn. Springhouse Corporation, Springhouse, PA

Mastering documentation 1999 2nd edn. Springhouse Corporation, Springhouse, PA

National Pressure Ulcer Advisory Panel (NPUAP) 1989 Pressure ulcer incidence, economics, risk assessment. Consensus development conference statement. Decubitus 2(2):24–28

Parish L C, Witkowski J A, Crissey J T 1983 The decubitus ulcer. Masson Pub, New York

Robson M C, Mannari R J, Smith P D, Payne W G 1999 Maintenance of wound bacterial balance. American Journal of Surgery, Nov, 178(5):399–402

Sapico F L, Ginunas V J, Thornhill-Joynes M, Canawatu H N, Capen D A, Klein N E, Khawam S, Montgomerie J Z 1986 Quantitative microbiology of pressure sores in different stages of healing. Diagn Microbiol Infect Dis 5:31–38

Seidel H M, Ball J M, Dains J E, Benedict G W 1999 Mosby's guide to physical examination, 4th edn. Mosby, St Louis

Shea J D 1975 Pressure sores: Classification and management. Clin Orthop 12:89–100

Stotts N A, Cavanaugh C E 1999 Assessing the patient with a wound. Home Healthcare Nurse 17(1):27–36

Stotts N A, Hunt T K 1997 Pressure ulcers. Managing bacterial colonization and infection. Clinics in Geriatric Medicine, 13(3):565–73

Stotts N A, Salazar M J, Wipke-Tevis D, McAdoo E 1996 Accuracy of alginate molds for measuring wound volumes when prepared and stored under varying conditions. Wounds 8(5):158–164

Sussman C, Swanson G 1997 Utility of the Sussman Wound Healing Tool in predicting wound healing outcomes in physical therapy. Advances in Wound Care 10(5):78–81

Thomas A C, Wysocki A B 1990 The healing wound: A comparison of three clinically useful methods of measurement. Decubitus 3(1):18–25

Thomas D, Rodeheaver G T, Bartolucci A A, Frantz R A, Sussman C, Ferrell B A, Cuddigan J, Stotts N A, Maklebust J 1997 Pressure Ulcer Scale for Healing: Derivation and validation of the PUSH Tool. Advances in Wound Care 10(5) 96–101

9 *Moya J Morison, Jane Harris and Jo Corlett*

Planning the care of a patient with a pressure ulcer

INTRODUCTION

Pressure ulcers are commonly encountered in both hospital and community settings and can easily develop into complex lesions of the skin and underlying tissues with inappropriate care. This is, in part, due to the vulnerability of the people who tend to develop pressure ulcers.

Immobility, altered consciousness, greater age and nutritional deficiencies are important risk factors (Ch. 2). The particular vulnerability of those with spinal cord injuries and the elderly admitted with a fractured neck of femur is well known, but there are other high-risk groups such as the previously healthy critically injured survivors of serious trauma (Baldwin & Ziegler 1998), patients undergoing lengthy surgery, such as cardiac surgery (Lewicki et al 1997), the terminally ill (Sopata et al 1997) and children in intensive care (Olding & Patterson 1998). Wound healing in the neonate and in the elderly is qualitatively different from that of the younger adult (Desai 1997a,b), and in all age groups healing is likely to be impaired by concurrent medical conditions such as diabetes mellitus, circulatory and respiratory disorders. It is the variety of factors that can lead to delayed healing that can make planning the care of patients with pressure ulcers so challenging.

As in all aspects of patient care, the findings from an ongoing process of assessment should form the basis for rational decision making (van Rijswijk & Braden, 1999). In the case of wound care, it is all too easy for the assessment process to focus on the wound itself, to the detriment of wider issues. Throughout this book it is suggested that it is essential that the emphasis be shifted from the wound towards the patient with a wound and to acknowledge the environmental and social factors that may influence the healing process. This change in emphasis reflects the trends in nursing, over the last 40 years, towards:

- *a more holistic approach*, which takes cognisance of social, psychological and spiritual aspects of health and well-being, as well as physical factors
- *a more client-centred approach*, which acknowledges the individual's rights to autonomy and self-determination, and moves away from the notion that 'the health care professional knows best' to the notion of client empowerment.

This chapter builds on the knowledge reviewed and summarized in previous chapters, in particular Chapters 3, 7 and 8. Key issues such as the selection of dressings, the use of new technologies (such as laser therapy), surgical interventions, nutritional support and patient education are highlighted here but are explored in more depth in subsequent chapters. The present chapter aims to provide a framework which integrates the theoretical knowledge which has gone before with the practical advice on effective, evidence-based clinical practice that follows.

A MODEL TO FACILITATE CARE PLANNING FOR PATIENTS WITH PRESSURE ULCERS

The basic principles of caring for a patient with a pressure ulcer have been known for several centuries. The surgeon Ambrose Paré lived in France in the sixteenth century and he articulated principles which form the basis of much medical/surgical practice today. He stressed the importance of first removing the cause of the wound. He then advocated a sound nutritional plan, treatment of any underlying disease, local wound debridement, the application of a dressing and psychological support (Levine 1992). These same principles apply today.

A conceptual schema to aid with more detailed care planning is illustrated in Figure 9.1, and was inspired by Braden & Bergstrom's (1987) schema for studying the aetiology of pressures ulcers. At an individual level, pressure ulcers develop as a result of the interaction of a number of factors and care planning involves eliminating or ameliorating their effects, as far as is possible. This model stresses the importance of removing the causes of the wound by relieving pressure and improving tissue tolerance, removing more general causes of delayed healing, optimizing the local wound environment and involving patients and their carers in care planning and implementation.

In the last decade there have been a number of national and international initiatives to establish and disseminate best practice relating to pressure ulcer prevention and treatment in the form of consensus statements, systematic reviews, policy documents and clinical guidelines. Rodeheaver (1995) described the process whereby guidelines were developed in the USA. In the recommendations that follow, particular attention is paid to the outstanding work of the National Pressure Ulcer Advisory Panel (NPUAP 1989) and the Agency for Health Care Policy and Research (AHCPR) Panel for the Prevention and Prediction of Pressure Ulcers in Adults (AHCPR 1992a,b, Bergstrom et al 1994) in the USA, to the European Pressure Ulcer Advisory Panel (EPUAP 1998, 1999) and to the work of the National Health Service (NHS) Centre for Reviews and Dissemination (CRD) at York, in the UK.

The model illustrated in Figure 9.1 provides a framework for the discussion that follows.

Relieving pressure and optimizing tissue tolerance

Maximizing mobility and activity

The diminished ability to change and control body position increases the likelihood that a patient will be exposed to prolonged and intense pressure and will subsequently develop a pressure ulcer (Kosiak 1959) (Chs 2 and 3). For patients with pressure ulcers, improving activity levels, mobility and range of movement is an appropriate goal for most individuals. The beneficial effects of maximizing mobility and activity probably extend beyond the release of pressure from vulnerable areas of the skin and may include improvements in respiratory function, cardiac output and venous return, the maintenance of muscle mass (Braden & Bergstrom 1987) and an enhanced sense of self-efficacy, competence and well-being. As the patient's condition improves, the potential for improving mobility and activity exists and an active rehabilitation programme should be initiated whenever possible. The particular vulnerability of those with spinal injuries is well documented (Chs 2 and 3). Protocols developed in specialist centres address the particular needs of those with marked sensory deficits (Gunnewicht 1996).

Planning for patient positioning, transferring and turning

Whenever possible, it is important to avoid positioning the patient directly on to a pressure ulcer, or directly on to a bony prominence, unless this is contraindicated by other treatment objectives which necessitate that an appropriate pressure-relieving device should be employed (EPUAP 1999). The EPUAP (1998) recommend that correct positioning, or devices such as pillows or foam wedges, should be used to keep bony prominences from direct contact with one another and

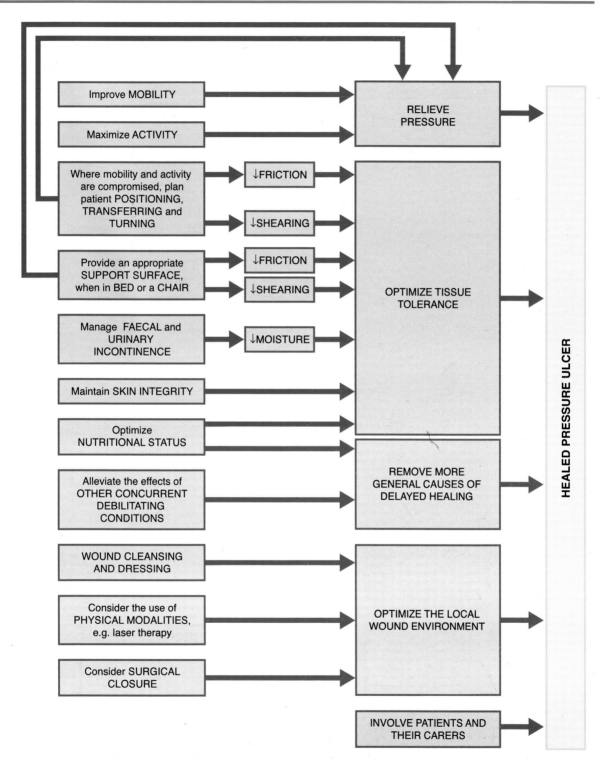

Figure 9.1 A conceptual schema to facilitate care planning for a patient with a pressure ulcer (inspired by Braden & Bergstrom's schema for the study of the aetiology of pressure ulcers, 1987, p. 9).

that care should be taken to ensure that these do not interfere with the action of any other pressure-relieving support surfaces in use.

There is strong evidence to suggest that friction increases the skin's susceptibility to pressure damage, and it is thought that skin damage due to friction and shearing forces can be minimized through correct patient positioning and transferring techniques, using devices to assist manual handling in accordance with EU or US regulations. Postural alignment, distribution of weight, balance, stability and pressure ulcer risk reduction should be considered when positioning patients or selecting equipment (EPUAP 1999). This is especially important when the patient is in a sitting position, whether in bed or a chair.

Any person who is acutely ill and is at risk of developing a further pressure ulcer should avoid uninterrupted periods of sitting out of bed. The EPUAP (1998, 1999) recommend that, in general, this period should not exceed 2 h. Wherever possible, individuals should be encouraged to reposition themselves at frequent intervals to redistribute pressure.

Although many guidelines recommend that any individual in bed who is assessed to be at risk of developing pressure ulcers should be regularly repositioned there remain many unanswered questions relating to the effectiveness of this practice (Cullum et al 1995), the frequency with which repositioning should be undertaken (Knox et al 1994) and the positions in which patients should be placed (Clark 1998) (Ch. 7). Furthermore, local practice is very variable, with regular repositioning by nurses having been supplanted, in many cases, by the use of pressure-redistributing support surfaces.

Providing an appropriate support surface when in bed or a chair

Although a multitude of pressure-reducing products are on the market, and a number of decision-making guides have been published (Dealey 1995, Stewart 1997), few well-designed studies support the claims of manufacturers (Maklebust 1999). Benefits can be derived from the use of a variety of pressure ulcer prevention devices but information on patient outcomes and the cost effectiveness of most devices is scarce (Hitch 1995, EPUAP 1999).

Clark & Cullum (1992) conducted a series of pressure ulcer prevalence surveys within one health district over a 4-year period. The prevalence of pressure ulcers increased from 6.8% (1986) to 14.2% (1989) while the available stocks of pressure-relieving mattresses increased from 69 (1987) to 186 (1989). These results appear to cast doubt on the common assumption that successful pressure ulcer prevention can be achieved through expanding the stocks of pressure-relieving mattresses and beds.

Price et al (1999) have challenged the assumption that low-unit-cost support systems are ineffective for very high-risk patients, and health economists and others are encouraging managers to be more sophisticated in their decision making when purchasing equipment, by including considerations of efficiency, reliability, depreciation and operating costs (Conine & Hershler 1991, Price 1999).

Following a systematic review of the literature, Cullum et al (1995) concluded that:

- the standard hospital mattress is less effective at preventing pressure ulcers than some low-pressure foam mattresses
- most of the equipment available for the prevention and treatment of pressures ulcers has not been reliably evaluated, and no 'best buy' can be recommended
- patients at risk of developing a pressure ulcer should be provided either with an evaluated low-pressure foam mattress or, if at higher risk, with a large-celled alternating-pressure mattress or a proven low-air-loss or air-fluidized bed; however, there is insufficient research evidence on clinical or cost effectiveness to guide equipment choice.
- randomized controlled trials accompanied by economic analysis could provide decision makers with reliable evidence on the relative cost effectiveness of different intervention strategies within a relatively short time.

The lack of reliable equipment data was restated by Cullum et al (1999a,b) following a further review of the evidence.

Managing faecal and urinary incontinence

The presence of excessive moisture has been linked to pressure ulcer aetiology in a number of classic epidemiological studies (Norton et al 1962, Barbenel et al 1977) but there is now a debate about the role of incontinence in pressure ulcer development and whether it is a primary causative factor, a symptom of ill health or acts by enhancing local friction and shear forces (Bliss 1993) (Ch. 3). Whatever the mechanism by which urinary and faecal incontinence may exert their effects, it is important that the underlying cause of the incontinence is sought, and whenever possible corrected. Referral to a clinical nurse specialist in incontinence may be indicated in intractable cases.

Maintenance of skin integrity

Every effort should be made to optimize the condition of the patient's skin (EPUAP 1998). Skin condition should be inspected and documented daily and any changes should be recorded as soon as they are observed. It is important to avoid excessive rubbing over bony prominences as this does not prevent pressure damage and may cause additional damage.

Skin irritants such as starch, soap and detergent residues, which may be present in sheets, are implicated in pressure ulcer development but have been little researched (Alberman 1992, Bridel, 1993) (Ch. 2).

Optimizing nutritional status

A person's nutritional status has frequently been implicated as a risk factor in pressure ulcer development (Ch. 2) and it has long been recognized that malnutrition is often second only to a failure to alleviate the effects of pressure in leading to delayed wound healing (Agarwal et al. 1985); yet nutritional assessment and nutritional support are often overlooked. While thought of as primarily a problem for hospitalized patients, poor nutritional intake has also been identified among patients in the community (Green et al 1999). Following assessment, which may need to involve the dietician, a plan

of appropriate nutritional support should be developed for nutritionally compromised individuals, as described in Chapter 13.

Removing more general causes of delayed wound healing

A large number of intrinsic patient factors found to be associated with pressure ulcer development exert their influence through affecting tissue perfusion. These factors are thought to include smoking, vascular disease and altered body temperature (Bergstrom & Braden 1992). However, the situation is not clear cut and the interplay of a number of factors may be important (Ch. 3).

Many factors can adversely affect wound healing, as illustrated in Figure 9.2, and those factors amenable to correction need to be addressed as part of a comprehensive care plan. Some issues relating to providing the optimum local environment for healing, which overcome any adverse local conditions, are described below.

Optimizing the local wound environment

Wound cleansing and dressings

Over the last 20 years, there has been a proliferation of new wound dressing products (Ch. 10), many with similar physical and therapeutic properties. Ovington (1999) has carried out an extensive review of dressings and adjunctive therapies, in order to update the recommendations in the 1994 AHCPR guidelines (Bergstrom et al 1994). General principles for dressing selection are summarized in Box 9.1, based on the EPUAP recommendations.

Where the wound contains devitalized tissue, debridement is usually indicated in order to remove a medium for infection, to facilitate uncomplicated healing and to enable the extent of tissue damage to be assessed. Methods of wound debridement are discussed in detail in Chapter 10, but some important principles are summarized in Box 9.2.

Wounds should be cleansed, as necessary, with tap water or with water that is suitable for drinking or with saline, using minimal mechanical force

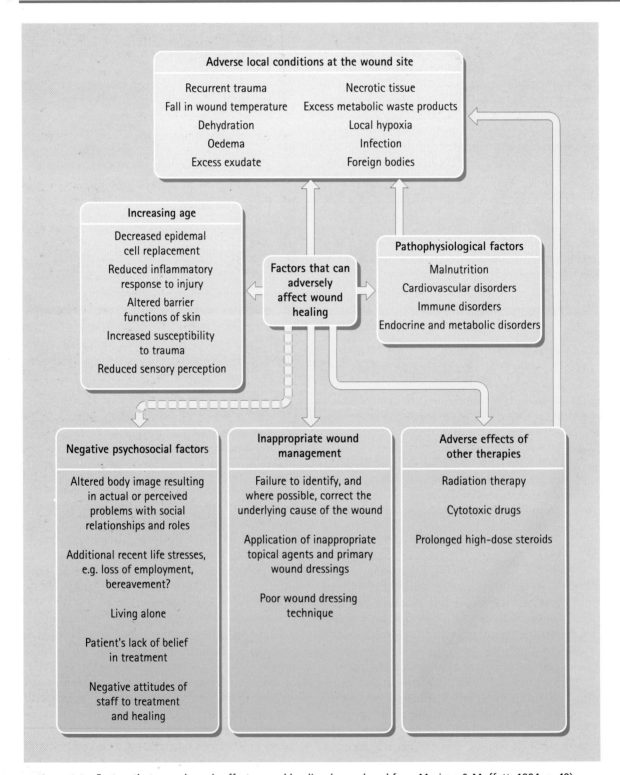

Figure 9.2 Factors that can adversely affect wound healing (reproduced from Morison & Moffatt, 1994, p. 49).

BOX 9.1 EUROPEAN PRESSURE ULCER ADVISORY PANEL GUIDELINES ON THE USE OF WOUND DRESSINGS (EPUAP 1999)

- Use a dressing which maintains a moist environment at the wound/dressing interface

- Determine the condition of the wound and establish treatment objectives before selecting a dressing (see Chs 8 and 10)

- Maintain dressings *in situ* for as long as is clinically appropriate and in line with manufacturers' recommendations. Frequent dressing removal can damage the wound bed

- If there is leakage or 'strike through' of exudate the dressing should be changed, as this causes a break in the barrier that the dressing provides to external contamination. If strike through occurs frequently it may be appropriate to reconsider the choice of dressing

- The use of wound protocols, based on sound evidence, can help to avoid unnecessary changes of dressing

- Regular observation of the wound enables progress with healing to be monitored, and can alert the clinician to the need to change treatment objectives.

BOX 9.2 EUROPEAN PRESSURE ULCER ADVISORY PANEL GUIDELINES ON WOUND DEBRIDEMENT (EPUAP 1999)

Debridement is defined as the removal of devitalized tissue from a wound

- remove devitalized tissue in pressure ulcers when appropriate for the patient's condition and consistent with the patient's goals

- methods of debridement include surgical, enzymatic, autolytic, larvae (myasis) or a combination

- surgical methods range from scissors and scalpel used at the bedside by a competent nurse to surgical debridement performed by a surgeon in the operating theatre

- pain associated with surgical debridement should be prevented or managed

- surgical, enzymatic and/or autolytic debridement techniques may be used when there is no urgent clinical need for drainage or removal of devitalized tissue

- if there is urgent need for debridement, as with advancing cellulites or sepsis, surgical debridement should be used and must be performed by a competent person

- with terminally ill patients, overall quality of life should be taken into account when deciding whether to debride the wound and the manner in which it should be accomplished

- dry eschar need not be debrided if oedema, erythema or drainage are not present

- dry eschar may be removed with dressings (such as hydrocolloids and hydrogels) which provide a moist environment to encourage autolysis

- assess these wounds daily to monitor for complications.

(EPUAP 1999). Irrigation can be useful for cleaning a cavity ulcer. Allowing the patient to take a shower is often appropriate, and can be therapeutic in a broader sense by enabling the person to be and feel socially and hygienically clean.

The place of antiseptics in wound management has been the subject of intense debate, while certain historical approaches, such as the use of larval therapy and honey, are experiencing a resurgence of interest and are being re-evaluated for both efficacy and clinical effectiveness (Thomas et al 1998, Cooper & Molan 1999, Naylor 1999). The EPUAP (1999) recommend that antiseptics should not be routinely used to clean wounds but may be considered when clinical assessment suggests that bacterial loads need to be controlled. Ideally, antiseptics should only be used for a limited time, until the wound is clean and surrounding inflammation is reduced.

New challenges are being presented by the epidemic methicillin-resistant *Staphylococcus aureus* (EMRSA) in hospital settings (Perry 1996) and there is almost certainly the potential for further restricting the use of topical antibiotics in chronic wounds (Tammelin et al 1998), which led to the rapid emergence of MRSA in the 1980s.

Of the new generation of products, growth factors are currently stimulating intense interest, because of their potential to actively stimulate wound healing by modulating endogenous repair processes (Graham 1998a,b). Until the processes involved in normal and abnormal wound healing are more fully understood their use can, however, be somewhat haphazard.

Local wound management products are an adjunct to rather than a replacement for therapeutic regimens aimed at tackling the underlying causes of the wound and the threats to the tissue's tolerance of pressure.

The use of physical modalities

Other therapies that are proving of value today include hyperbaric oxygen therapy (Donlin & Bryson 1995), pulsed electromagnetic energy (PEME) therapy (Buswell 1992), vacuum-assisted wound closure (Deva et al 1997, Kalailieff 1998, Banwell, 1999) and ultrasound. The merits, indications and contraindications for these therapies are discussed in Chapter 12. While many of the published studies involve only a limited number of cases, and the European Pressure Ulcer Advisory Panel (EPUAP 1999) caution that, at present, insufficient research has been completed to recommend their general use, these physical modalities provide exciting possibilities for the future and deserve closer attention and evaluation now, especially for intractable wounds.

Surgical options for wound closure

The ultimate goal in the treatment of pressure ulcers is to obtain a closed, healed wound that resists recurrence (LaRossa & Bucky 1997). Surgical reconstruction may be the treatment of choice for some patients (Khanna et al 1994, Akguner et al 1998). The indications for surgery

and the challenges of postoperative care are described in Chapter 11. An example of a pathway-based care protocol is given by Brown & Smith (1999).

Involving patients and their carers

The value of theories and models to facilitate a holistic approach to care planning

There has been a proliferation of nursing theories since the 1950s driven, in part, by a need to understand what makes nursing unique as a professional enterprise. One of the aims of theories is to aid decision making in practical situations; however, when different theories appear to be pointing in different directions they can, at first, make the situation seem more complex rather than more straightforward. The application of theories in nursing is still in its infancy (Hunink 1995, Fitzpatrick & Whall 1996).

Many theories implicitly or explicitly make use of 'the nursing process', which involves four steps: patient assessment, care planning, implementation and the evaluation of the consequences of the care given. However, many nurses argue that such an approach contradicts the concepts of shared responsibility, mutuality and client autonomy that characterize a client-centred approach (Lindsey & Hartrick 1996). In this chapter, a middle way is adopted which pragmatically acknowledges the value of a systematic approach to patient assessment, care planning and implementation (Christensen & Kenney 1990) and yet seeks to move beyond this model by viewing clients as their own experts, rather than as passive recipients of advice and care.

The patient's central role

Many patients with chronic non-healing wounds such as pressure ulcers can appear to be apathetic and may seem to health care professionals to have little motivation to help themselves. Pressure ulcers often develop at a time when the patient is least able to help themselves because of illness or disability, and when a chronic wound is slow to heal, patients can come to believe that they are helpless to influence the situation in a positive way. However, when a client-centred approach is adopted, the individual's rights to autonomy and self-determination are fully acknowledged, the nurse and the client share responsibility for care planning and the focus shifts from the individual's deficits to facilitating the client's potential for self-help. The principles of patient education, methods of creating a therapeutic environment for learning, and maximizing the patient's commitment and involvement in care are discussed in detail in Chapter 14. The application of Orem's (1991) self-care deficit theory to the care of a patient with a pressure ulcer is illustrated here, with the help of a case study (Case study 9.1, Table 9.1).

Involving the patient's lay carers

A task that is often neglected is the education and support of lay carers. For every person aged 65 years and older admitted to some form of institutionalized care there are twice as many people of equal disability living at home, whose carers are intimately involved in every aspect of care giving, often with little or no professional support (Baharestani 1994).

Educational programmes relating to the prevention and management of pressure ulcers should be structured, organized and comprehensive, and made available at all levels of health care providers, patients and family or caregivers (AHCPR 1992a,b, EPUAP 1998). The categories of information which should be considered for inclusion are summarized in Box 9.3. Clearly, the content, level and methods of presenting the programme should be modified to suit the audience (Beitz 1998). There is a growing literature targeted specifically at lay carers, as exemplified by the AHCPR patients' guide to pressure ulcer prevention published in 1992 (AHCPR 1992b). An increasing number of carers now have easy access to information written especially for them via the Internet. This source of information is, however, inaccessible to many of the poorest members of our society, to the 'IT illiterate' and to those who are socially excluded. Direct contact with a health care professional from an outreach service can provide invaluable help to people in such vulnerable groups.

CASE STUDY 9.1

Orem's self-care deficit theory applied to a patient with a pressure ulcer

Mrs Betty Andrews is a 78-year-old widow who has been admitted to hospital from a nursing home in the community with a stage IV sacral pressure ulcer. She has lived in a nursing home for several years since experiencing a left-sided cerebrovascular accident which left her with a right-sided weakness. She is able to engage in some self-care activities, but her mobility is very restricted. She spends long periods of time lying in bed, or sitting in her chair. She is occasionally urine incontinent.

Orem's concept of nursing is clearly applicable to a patient with a pressure ulcer. The patient has been unable to prevent the pressure ulcer from developing, and she has been unable to meet the universal self-care requisite of preventing a hazard to human life, functioning and well being. Mrs Andrews now has a health deviation requisite in that a pressure ulcer exists which needs to be treated and she is unlikely to be able to meet this demand. The pressure ulcer also makes it more difficult for Mrs Andrews to achieve other self-care demands, such as engaging in social activities (inability to balance solitude and social interaction).

Orem's model directs the nurse towards assessing the patient in three of the major areas associated with pressure ulcer development: prolonged pressure on tissues as a result of immobility (inability to balance activity and rest), poor nutrition and hydration (maintaining food and water intake) and incontinence (maintaining appropriate elimination processes). Mrs Andrews has lost both her partner and her home, which may well be contributing to her lack of motivation to maintain self-care activities. The self-care deficits which have resulted in a demand for help with self-care are likely to be long-term problems and the nurse needs to identify an appropriate system of nursing and methods of helping the patient to overcome them, if the existing pressure ulcer is to heal and further tissue breakdown is to be prevented. The nurse would need to function within the partially compensatory system, described by Orem, acting for the patient in performing local wound care, ensuring that any incontinent episodes are dealt with promptly to prevent further deterioration of the skin, and providing appropriate pressure-relieving devices and nursing interventions aimed at regular relief of pressure from compromised tissues. The nurse should attempt to teach the patient and significant others about the importance of a nutritious diet and maintaining adequate fluid intake and will also have to support Mrs Andrews in re-establishing her motivation for self-care.

An outline care plan inspired by Orem's model is given in Table 9.1.

Table 9.1 Care plan for Betty Andrews based on Orem's (1991) self-care deficit theory of nursing

Universal self-care requisites	Self-care ability	Self-care deficit (actual)	Self-care deficit (potential)	Nursing actions
Maintain sufficient intake of air	Normally able to maintain an adequate intake of air	None at present	An inability to maintain adequate air intake could result in insufficient perfusion of tissues with oxygen	Monitor respiratory patterns for indication of insufficient air intake (**acting for**)
Maintain sufficient intake of water	Can hold a cup with assistance and swallow fluids without difficulty	Unable to obtain fluids independently Unwilling to drink due to fear of incontinence	Potential risk of dehydration of integumentary tissues increases risk of skin breakdown	Educate patient of the need to drink fluids (**teaching**) Provide fluids and offer assistance with these on a regular basis (**acting for**) Monitor fluid intake (**acting for**) Provide toileting facilities promptly (**developmental**)
Maintain sufficient intake of food	Can feed herself independently and is able to chew and swallow food	Unable to obtain or prepare food for herself Unable to cut food into manageable mouthfuls Uninterested in eating and has a poor dietary intake	Poor nutritional status increases risk of skin breakdown and delays healing of existing wounds	Educate patient of the need to maintain adequate nutritional input (**teaching**) Provide appetising food which has a high nutrition content (**acting for**) Provide assistance with eating Monitor food intake (**acting for**) Provide dietary supplements if necessary (**acting for**)
Elimination processes	Continent of faeces	Occasionally incontinent of urine Unable to use toilet facilities independently	Urine traps moisture next to the skin and causes irritation, increasing the risk of skin breakdown	Offer toileting facilities on a regular basis (**developmental**) Provide prompt assistance with toileting (**acting for**) Cleanse and dry the skin promptly if incontinence occurs (**acting for**)
Balance between activity and rest	Sits for long periods in a chair, or lies in bed	Physical activity and mobility is very restricted	Prolonged pressure on tissues, prevents adequate perfusion, increasing risk of pressure ulcer development and further deterioration of existing wounds	Provide pressure-relieving devices (**acting for**) Encourage movement and mobility to relieve pressure (**supporting**) Monitor condition of skin regularly (**acting for**)

Table 9.1 *Continued*

Universal self-care requisites	Self-care ability	Self-care deficit (actual)	Self-care deficit (potential)	Nursing actions
Maintain balance between solitude and social interaction	Enjoys socializing with other inmates of nursing home		Loss of usual social contacts and feelings of isolation may result in loss of motivation to engage in self-care activity	Encourage interaction with other patients (**supporting**) Encourage visits by family and friends (**supporting**)
Prevention of hazards to life, functioning and well-being	Has the ability to understand how pressure ulcers develop and how to prevent them	Lacks ability to take preventative actions independently Lacks ability to care for existing pressure ulcer	Further deterioration of existing pressure ulcer and development of new ones	Provide preventative actions and encourage self-care with these where possible (**supporting/acting for**) Provide appropriate wound care of existing pressure ulcer (**acting for**)
Normalcy		Restricted physical activity results in a limited living environment	Loss of motivation to engage in self-care activity	Encourage physical activity where possible and contact with others to maximize living environment (**supporting**)
Developmental self-care requisites	Elderly lady with no close family, but one niece who visits occasionally	Elderly lady unable to meet universal self-care requisites and engage in self-care activities	Loss of motivation to engage in self-care activity	Encourage self-care and independence where possible (**supporting**) Encourage visits by family and friends (**supporting**)
Health deviation self-care requisites	Is aware of the need to seek help in dealing with pressure ulcer and willing to comply with nursing interventions	Unable to perform wound care independently		Provide wound care as appropriate (**acting for**)

Seeing the patient in a wider social context

Although the focus of this chapter is predominantly on the individual, there are many hints in the literature to suggest that society's view of health and health care, and the attitudes of family members, friends and health care professionals in the local community have an impact on the nature of the individual's experience of a wound. As illustrated in Figure 9.3, individuals are members of families, who are in turn embedded within a local community, set in a wider society. The term 'system' describes 'an integrated whole' in which the parts are interconnected in a complex web of relationships (Fig. 9.3). Systems theory is reflected in a number of models of nursing such as Neuman's systems model, where the client is seen as a unique individual, decision making is shared

BOX 9.3   EUROPEAN PRESSURE ULCER ADVISORY PANEL GUIDELINES ON INFORMATION TO INCLUDE IN EDUCATIONAL PROGRAMMES FOR HEALTH CARE PROVIDERS, PATIENTS AND FAMILY/CAREGIVERS (EPUAP 1998)

◆ pathophysiology and risk factors for pressure damage

◆ risk assessment tools and their application

◆ skin assessment

◆ selection and instruction in the use of pressure-redistributing and other devices

◆ development and implementation of individualized programmes of care

◆ principles of positioning to decrease risk of pressure damage

◆ documentation of processes and patient outcome data

◆ clarification of responsibilities for all concerned

◆ health promotion

◆ development and implementation of guidelines

The educational programme should be updated on a regular basis, based on the best available evidence. The content of programmes should be modified according to the audience.

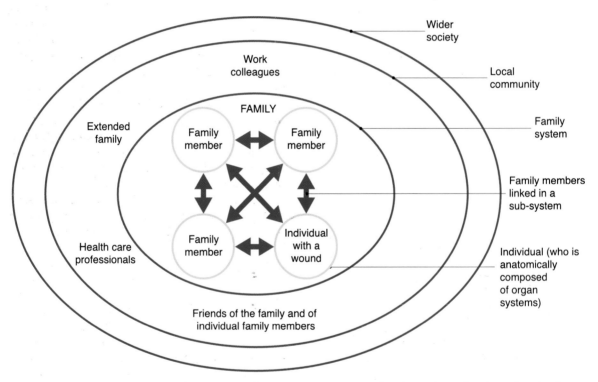

Figure 9.3   The conceptualization of the individual with a pressure ulcer, embedded within a family, set in a local community, and encompassed by a wider society (based on Morison, 1995, p. 98)

and diversity is valued and respected (Neuman 1995), and in the models of King (1981) and Roy & Andrews (1991). Family systems theory under-pins the present move towards the practice of family nursing (Wright & Leahey 1994, Robinson & Wright 1995, Whyte 1997).

The aim of care planning should be to take a holistic approach to understanding the unique context within which each individual's wound is to be managed, and to understanding the interaction of a multiplicity of variables on many system levels.

THE CONTEXT OF CARE

The context of care comprises an intricate blend of components which are unique to each individual and have a profound effect on their care experience and quality of life. Government policy, demography and the structure of care provision systems are as relevant to the care context as patient health beliefs and family systems.

Central to the context is the care setting. This may range from the more structured and predictable environment of the hospital, to the broad diversity of settings in the community, including residential or nursing homes and the person's own home. In the UK, health care reform since the early 1990s (Department of Health 1990) has shifted the emphasis away from hospital care to care in the community for certain client groups. Consequently, community-based care is provided for many people who are elderly or disabled, often with chronic health problems, and those who are acutely ill. The fact that these patients are at greatest risk of pressure ulcer development poses a number of challenges to professional and lay carers, particularly when the patient is cared for at home.

Home care can provide the ideal setting for individualized and holistic care. Burnard (1998) identified the value of interpersonal one-to-one care which community nurses can provide. However, two vital components of care in the community setting must be emphasized. First, although nursing may take the lead, the care and support of vulnerable patients relies upon a network of services from the statutory, voluntary and private sectors. Multidisciplinary collaboration and teamwork are central to the coordination of services to provide the quality and continuity of care required by the dependent patient at home. Secondly, the concept of family

nursing, discussed by Wright & Leahey (1987, 1994) acknowledges roles and relationships within families and their response, both positive and negative, to changes in life events such as illness and ageing. The detrimental effects of caregiving on the physical and psychological health of the family carer are well documented (Nolan et al 1990, Baharestani, 1994). Clearly, individualized care therefore relates to meeting the needs of the whole family and not just the needs of the patient.

Nursing care for patients with wounds requires a different approach at home from the more carefully controlled residential or hospital environment. For example, role definition has a different orientation, with the need for professional carers to accept the family as partners and key members of the caring team rather than assistants to the professional care givers. A number of practical issues must also be considered. For example, the intermittent nature of home visits means that continuous care and monitoring of the patients condition is not possible. Care is oriented towards patient independence and participation and support for family carers. It includes strategies such as structured care planning, teaching and education for the patient and carers and mechanisms to enhance continuity of care, such as accurate and comprehensive documentation.

Resources such as support surfaces for beds and chairs may be difficult to obtain or adapt for home use. Lifting and repositioning of patients at home may be difficult for lone carers, either lay or professional, and the installation and use of lifting devices may be problematic. Young (1992) cites acceptability to the patient and carer as an important consideration when selecting equipment; most families do not wish their home to look like a hospital ward. Acknowledgment of the limitations which may accompany home care enables the nurse to work closely with the patient, family and other agencies and plan care accordingly.

Until recently, in the UK, a limited selection of wound care products was available to nurses working in the community. However, additions to the drug tariff, which lists all items prescribable by general practitioners, as outlined by Morgan (1999), now offer community nurses a wider range of options. Flexibility and responsiveness to the needs of patients in the community have been further enhanced by legislation allowing initial prescribing of a wide range of wound care items by district nurses (Department of Health 1992).

However, as Franks & Moffatt (1999) have shown, patients with pressure ulcers treated in the community experience a number of problems, including social isolation and poor mobility, which compromise their quality of life. The provision of truly holistic care for the patient with a pressure ulcer and their family is dependent on an understanding of the multidimensional nature of the context of care and recognition of the significance of its elements for each patient. The development of organizations such as the AHCPR and EPUAP, which aim to improve prevention and management of pressure ulcers through a comprehensive and multifactorial approach, reflect the complexity and importance of meeting patient's needs.

THE IMPLEMENTATION OF EVIDENCE-BASED PRACTICE AND MULTIDISCIPLINARY CARE PLANNING

There are many published examples of the implementation of evidence-based practice guidelines within organizations (Hopkins et al 1998, Shipperley 1998), and the implementation process is reviewed in Chapter 15. Impressive reductions in the occurrence of pressure ulcers have been reported in the USA following implementation of the AHCPR guidelines (Regan et al 1995, Xakellis et al 1998), although it must be said that there were concurrent organizational changes in the units studied, which may have influenced the results. Whether the implementation of guidelines leads to cost savings is even less clear cut, as discussed in Chapter 5.

Tremendous benefits can accrue when health care professionals collaborate to develop interdisciplinary patient care plans. Dzwierzynski et al (1998) found that the implementation of a pathway for surgical reconstruction of pressure ulcers decreased the length of hospital stay, and the use of medication, laboratory tests and radiology services, saving almost $11 000 per patient.

Clinical nurse specialists in tissue viability clearly have an important role to play as advanced practitioners, researchers and educators (Hutton 1997). One of their roles is effectively to liaise with other professionals such as physiotherapists (McCulloch 1998), dieticians (Liebmann 1998) and occupational therapists (Aldersea 1997).

CONCLUSION

Many of the practices undertaken to prevent and treat pressure ulcers are contentious, based on estimates and guesses rather than evidence (Clark 1999). This chapter has highlighted important gaps in our knowledge, which require further research, and some paradoxes brought to light through research, especially in relation to patient support systems.

More reliable economic data are also required. West & Priestly (1994) suggest that an ideal economic assessment of pressure ulcers would include the cost of prevention for different patient groups, the rate of conversion of different risk groups into actual pressure ulcers and the relative cost effectiveness of different methods of treatment.

While there have been many important technical advances in local wound management over the last 20 years there are still a number of unanswered questions, especially in relation to the use of growth factors and adjunctive physical therapies such as vacuum-assisted closure.

It is important not to lose sight of the prime focus of our care and concern, and that is the patient. For many, pressure ulcers are associated with pain and discomfort, lowered self-esteem and altered body image (Rintala 1995) (Ch. 4) and for some complications such as sepsis and osteomyelitis can be life-threatening. Baharestani (1994) found that the consequences for carers included increased fatigue, limited socialization and often financial hardship. The social support required by elderly patients and their carers living in the community has been greatly underestimated (Keeling et al 1997) and should be seriously considered when planning care. In conclusion, in relation to establishing evidence-based practice and clinical effectiveness in the treatment of pressure ulcers we clearly still have a long way to go.

CASE STUDY 9.3

Select a patient with a pressure ulcer who has multiple and complex needs and who is currently in your care.

1 Review your care plan for this patient with reference to the conceptual schemas illustrated in Figures 9.1 and 9.2.
   a. How comprehensive is your care plan?
   b. Does it fully address your patient's needs?

2 On reflection, do you perceive a need to change any aspects of your current care planning system? If not, what are the particular strengths of your approach to care planning?

CASE STUDY 9.2

Return to the Case Study 9.1 (on p. 125)

1 Draw up a care plan for this patient, using a model of your choice.

2 Compare your plan with the plan given in Table 9.1
   (a) What are the similarities?
   (b) In what ways does your plan differ?
   (c) Evaluate the strengths and limitations of Orem's model, in this context, compared with the model that you have used.
   (d) What are the strengths and limitations of applying a 'generic' model, such as Orem's model, to a particular clinical context?
   (e) Do you think that the application of a nursing model is compatible with multidisciplinary care planning?

SELF-ASSESSMENT QUESTIONS

1 In what ways do you currently involve patients and their lay carers in care planning? Are there any ways in which they could become more involved?

2 What are the advantages of multi-disciplinary care planning? Are there any practical problems associated with this approach, and if so how could they be overcome?

FURTHER READING

Bergstrom N, Bennett M A, Carlson C E et al 1994 Pressure ulcer treatment. Clinical practice guideline No. 15, AHCPR Publ. No. 95–0653. US Department of Health and Human Services/Public Health Service, Rockville

Cullum N, Deeks J, Sheldon T A, Song F, Fletcher A W 1999 Beds, mattresses and cushions for pressure sore prevention and treatment. Updated software, issue 3 edn. The Cochrane Library, Oxford

European Pressure Ulcer Advisory Panel (EPUAP) 1999 Guidelines on treatment of pressure ulcers. European Pressure Ulcer Advisory Panel Review 1(2):1–6

Maklebust J 1999 An update on horizontal patient support

surfaces. Ostomy/Wound Management 45(Suppl 1A):70S–77S

Ovington L G 1999 Dressings and adjunctive therapies: AHCPR guidelines revisited. Ostomy/Wound Management 45(Suppl 1A):94S–106S

Price P 1999 The challenge of outcome measures in chronic wounds: a review of measures of efficacy, efficiency and effectiveness. Journal of Wound Care 8(6):306–308

Van Rijswijk L, Braden B J 1999 Pressure ulcer patient and wound assessment: an AHCPR clinical practice guideline update. Ostomy/Wound Management 45 (Suppl 1A): 56S–67S

REFERENCES

Agarwal N, Del Guercio L R M, Lee B Y 1985 The role of nutrition in the management of pressure sores. In: Lee B K (ed.) Chronic ulcers of the skin. McGraw-Hill, New York, pp. 133–145

Agency for Health Care Policy and Research (AHCPR) 1992a Pressure ulcers in adults: prediction and prevention: clinical practice guideline number 3, AHCPR No. 92-0047. US Department of Health and Human Services, Rockville

Agency for Health Care Policy and Research (AHCPR) 1992b Preventing pressure ulcers: a patient's guide. US Department of Health and Human Services, Rockville

Akguner M, Karaca C, Atabey A, Menderes A, Top H 1998 Surgical treatment for ischial pressure sores with gracilis myocutaneous flap. Journal of Wound Care 7(6): 276–278

Alberman K 1992 Is there any connection between laundering and the development of pressure sores? Journal of Tissue Viability 2(2):55–56

Aldersea P 1997 Sore points. Nursing Times 93(40):63–66

Baharestani M M 1994 The lived experience of wives caring for their frail home-bound elderly husbands with pressure ulcers. Advances in Wound Care; 7(3):40–52.

Baldwin K M, Ziegler S M 1998 Pressure ulcer risk following critical traumatic injury. Advances in Wound Care 11(4):168–173.

Banwell P E 1999 Topical negative pressure therapy in wound care. Journal of Wound Care 8(2):79–84.

Barbenel J C, Jordan M M, Nicol S M 1977 Incidence of pressure-sores in the Greater Glasgow Health Board Area. Lancet ii:548–550

Beitz J M 1998 Education for health promotion and disease prevention: convince them, don't confuse them. Ostomy/Wound Management; 44(3A Suppl):71S–77S

Bergstrom N, Braden B 1992 A prospective study of pressure sore risk among institutionalized elderly. Journal of the American Geriatrics Society 40:747–758

Bergstrom N, Bennett M A, Carlson C E 1994 Pressure ulcer treatment (Clinical Practice Guideline 15), AHCPR No. 95–0653. US Department of Health and Human Services/Public Health Service, Rockville

Bliss M R 1993 Aetiology of pressure sores. Reviews in Clinical Gerontology 3:379–397

Braden B J, Bergstrom N 1987 A conceptual schema for the study of the etiology of pressure sores. Rehabilitation Nursing 12(1):8–12

Bridel J 1993 The aetiology of pressure sores. Journal of Wound Care 2(4):230–238

Brown D L, Smith D J 1999 Bacterial colonization/infection and the surgical management of pressure ulcers. Ostomy/Wound Management 45(1A Suppl):109S–120S

Burnard P 1998 Listening is a personal quality. Journal of Community Nursing 12(2):36–38

Buswell W 1992 Treating a pressure sore with PEME. Journal of Wound Care; 1(2):14–18

Christensen P J, Kenney J W 1990 The nursing process: application of conceptual models, 3rd edn. Mosby, Toronto

Clark M 1998 Repositioning to prevent pressure sores – what is the evidence? Nursing Standard 13(3):58–64

Clark M 1999 Beds and mattresses. Journal of Wound Care 8(7):323

Clark M, Cullum N 1992 Matching patient need for pressure sore prevention with the supply of pressure-redistributing mattresses. Journal of Advanced Nursing 17:310–316

Conine T A, Hershler C 1991 Effectiveness: a neglected dimension in the assessment of rehabilitation devices and equipment. International Journal of Rehabilitation Research 14: 117–122

Cooper R, Molan P 1999 The use of honey as an antiseptic in managing *Pseudomonas* infection. Journal of Wound Care 8(4):161–164

Cullum N, Deeks J, Fletcher A, Long A, Mouneimne H, Sheldon T 1995 The prevention and treatment of pressure sores: how effective are pressure-relieving interventions and risk assessment? Effective Health Care Bulletin 2(1):1–16

Cullum N, Deeks J, Sheldon T A, Song F, Fletcher A W 1999a Beds, mattresses and cushions for pressure sore prevention and treatment. Updated software, issue 3 edn. The Cochrane Library, Oxford

Cullum N, Deeks J, Sheldon T A, Song F, Fletcher A W 1999b Beds, mattresses and cushions for pressure sore prevention and treatment. Journal of Tissue Viability 9(4):138

Dealey C 1995 Mattresses and beds: a guide to systems available for relieving and reducing pressure. Journal of Wound Care 4(9):409–412

Department of Health 1990 The NHS and Community Care Act. HMSO, London

Department of Health 1992 Medicinal Products Prescription by Nurses etc. Act. HMSO, London

Desai H 1997a Ageing and wounds, part 1: foetal and postnatal healing. Journal of Wound Care 6(4):192–196

Desai H 1997b Ageing and wounds, part 2: healing in old age. Journal of Wound Care 6(5):237–239

Deva A K, Siu C, Nettle W J S 1997 Vacuum-assisted closure of a sacral pressure sore. Journal of Wound Care 6(7):311–312

Donlin N J, Bryson P J 1995 Hyperbaric oxygen therapy. Journal of Wound Care 4(4):175–178

Dzwierzynski W W, Spitz K, Hartz A, Guse C, Larson D L 1998 Improvement in resource utilization after development of a clinical pathway for patients with pressure ulcers. Plastic and Reconstructive Surgery 102(6):2006–2011

European Pressure Ulcer Advisory Panel (EPUAP) 1998 A policy statement on the prevention of pressure ulcers from the European Pressure Ulcer Advisory Panel. British Journal of Nursing 7(15):888–890

European Pressure Ulcer Advisory Panel (EPUAP) 1999 Guidelines on treatment of pressure ulcers. European Pressure Ulcer Advisory Panel Review 1(2):1–6

Fitzpatrick J, Whall A L 1996 Conceptual models of nursing: analysis and application, 3rd edn. Appleton & Lange, Stamford

Franks P J, Moffatt C J 1999 Quality of life issues in chronic wound management. British Journal of Community Nursing 4(6):283–289

Graham A 1998a The use of growth factors in clinical practice (Part 1). Journal of Wound Care 7(9): 464–466

Graham A 1998b The use of growth factors in clinical practice (Part 2). Journal of Wound Care 7(10): 536–540

Green S M, Winterberg H, Franks P J, Moffatt C J, Eberhardie C, McLaren S 1999 Nutritional intake in community patients with pressure ulcers. Journal of Wound Care 8(7):325–330

Gunnewicht B R 1996 Management of pressure sores in a spinal injuries unit. Journal of Wound Care 5(1): 36–39

Hitch S 1995 NHS Executive Nursing Directorate – strategy for major clinical guidelines: prevention and management of pressure sores, a literature review. Journal of Tissue Viability 5(1): 3–24

Hopkins A, Gooch S, Danks F 1998 A programme for pressure sore prevention and management. Journal of Wound Care 7(1):37–40

Hunink G 1995 A study guide to nursing theories. Campion Press, Edinburgh

Hutton D J 1997 The clinical nurse specialist in tissue viability services. Journal of Wound Care 6(2): 88–90

Kalailieff D 1998 Vacuum-assisted closure: wound care technology for the new millennium. Perspectives 22(3):28–29

Keeling D, Price P, Jones E, Harding K G 1997 Social support for elderly patients with chronic wounds. Journal of Wound Care 6(8):389–391

Khanna A, Henderson H P, Beg M S A 1994 Closure of an ischial pressure sore with a sartorius musculocutaneous flap. Journal of Wound Care 3(2):76–78

King I M 1981 A theory of nursing: systems, concepts, process. John Wiley, New York

Knox D M, Anderson T M, Anderson P S 1994 Effects of different turn intervals on skin of healthy older adults. Advances in Wound Care 7(1): 48–52

Kosiak M 1959 Etiology and pathology of ischaemic ulcers. Arch Phys Med Rehabil 40: 62–68

LaRossa D, Bucky L P 1997 Surgical management. In: Parish L C, Witkowski J A, Crissey T (eds) The decubitus ulcer in clinical practice. Springer Verlag, Berlin, pp. 84–113

Levine J M 1992 Historical notes on pressure ulcers: the cure of Ambrose Paré. Decubitus 5(2): 23–27

Lewicki L J, Mion L, Splane K G, Samstag D, Secic M 1997; Patient risk factors for pressure ulcers during cardiac surgery. AORN Journal 65(5):933–942

Liebmann L J 1998 Patterns of nursing home referrals to consultant dieticians. Geriatric Nursing 19(5):284–285

Lindsey E, Hartrick G 1996 Health-promoting nursing practice: the demise of the nursing process? Journal of Advanced Nursing 23:106–112

Maklebust J 1999 An update on horizontal patient support surfaces. Ostomy/Wound Management 45 (1A Suppl): 70S–77S

McCulloch J M 1998 The role of physiotherapy in managing patients with wounds. Journal of Wound Care 7(5):241–244

Morgan, D A 1999 Wound management products in the Drug Tariff. Pharm J 263 (7072), 820–825

Morison M J 1995 Family perspectives on bed wetting in young people. PhD thesis, Queen Margaret College, Edinburgh

Morison M J, Moffatt C 1994 A colour guide to the assessment and management of leg ulcers, 2nd edn. Mosby, London

National Pressure Ulcer Advisory Panel (NPUAP) 1989 Pressure ulcers prevalence, cost and risk assessment: consensus, development, statement. Decubitus 2(2):24–28

Naylor I L 1999 Ulcer care in the Middle Ages. Journal of Wound Care 8(4):208–212

Neuman B 1995 The Neuman systems model, 3rd edn. Appleton a& Lange, Norwalk

Nolan M, Grant G, Ellis N 1990 Stress is in the eye of the beholder: reconceptualising the measurement of carer burden. Journal of Advanced Nursing 15:544–555

Norton D, McLaren R, Exton-Smith A N 1962 An investigation of geriatric nursing problems in hospital. Churchill Livingstone, Edinburgh

Olding L, Patterson J 1998 Growing concern. Nursing Times 94(38):74–79

Orem D E 1991 Nursing: concepts of practice. Mosby, St Louis

Ovington L G 1999 Dressings and adjunctive therapies: AHCPR guidelines revisited. Ostomy/Wound Management 45(1A Suppl):94S–106S

Perry C 1996 Methicillin-resistant Staphylococcus aureus. Journal of Wound Care 5(1):31–34

Price P 1999 The challenge of outcome measures in chronic wounds: a review of measures of efficacy, efficiency and effectiveness. Journal of Wound Care 8(6):306–308

Price P, Bale S, Newcombe R, Harding K 1999 Challenging the pressure sore paradigm. Journal of Wound Care 8(4):187–190

Regan M B, Byers P H, Mayrovitz H N 1995 Efficacy of a comprehensive pressure ulcer prevention program in an extended care faciity. Advances in Wound Care 8(3):51–55

Rintala D H 1995 Quality of life considerations. Advances in Wound Care 8(4):28.71–28.83

Robinson C A, Wright L M 1995 Family nursing interventions: what families say makes a difference. Journal of Family Nursing 1(3):327–345

Rodeheaver G T 1995 The US model for national standards of care: a description of how guidelines for the management and prevention of pressures sores were established. Journal of Wound Care 4(5):238–240

Roy C, Andrews H 1991 The Roy adaptation model. Appleton & Lange, Norwalk

Shipperley T 1998 Guidelines for pressure sore prevention and management. Journal of Wound Care 7(6): 309–311

Sopata M, Luczak J, Glocwacka A 1997 Managing pressure sores in palliative care. Journal of Wound Care 6(1):10–11

Stewart T P 1997 Support systems. In: Parish L C, Witkowski J A, Crissey J T (eds) The decubitus ulcer in clinical practice. Springer Verlag, Berlin; pp. 145–168

Tammelin A, Lindholm C, Hambraeus A 1998 Chronic ulcers and antibiotic treatment. Journal of Wound Care 7(9):435–437

Thomas S, Andrews A, Jones M 1998 The use of larval therapy in wound management. Journal of Wound Care 7(10):521–524

van Rijswijk L, Braden B J 1999 Pressure ulcer patient and wound assessment: an AHCPR clinical practice guideline update. Ostomy/Wound Management 45 (1A Suppl): 56S–67S

West P, Priestly J 1994 Money under the mattress. Health Service Journal 104(5398): 20–22.

Whyte D A 1997 Explorations in family nursing. Routledge, London

Wright L M, Leahey L M 1987 Families and life-threatening illness. Springhouse, Springfield

Wright L M, Leahey M 1994 Nurses and families: a guide to family assessment and intervention, 2nd edn. Davis, Philadelphia

Xakellis G C, Frantz R A, Lewis A, Harvey P 1998 Cost-effectiveness of an intensive pressure ulcer prevention protocol in long-term care. Advances in Wound Care 11(1): 22–29.

Young J 1992 The use of specialised beds and mattresses. Journal of Tissue Viability 2(3): 79–81

10 *Liza Ovington*

Wound management: cleansing agents and dressings

INTRODUCTION

Wound healing is a complex and highly ordered series of biochemical processes that is the culmination of the actions of different types of cell in response to different cellular environments involving oxygen, temperature, pH, growth factors, enzymes, etc. (Kindlen & Morison 1997). When the various cells are healthy and efficient and their environments are within normal homeostatic parameters, the healing process proceeds predictably and without incident. When those cells and their environments are compromised by alterations in local or systemic conditions, the healing process is impaired and the wound does not close in an orderly or timely fashion.

Management of the non-healing wound requires co-ordinated action at many levels (Fig. 10.1). The environments that impact on wound management include the sociopolitical environment of the patient's home, the care setting and the health care system, the systemic environment of the body and the local environment of the wound. The health care system in general, as well as the specific setting in which care is rendered, may affect what treatments and therapies are available for use by the medical community (Heenan 1999). The availability or absence of support in the home from a spouse or family member can influence certain product selections or regimens for elderly or debilitated patients. Systemic conditions include nutritional status, blood glucose levels and immune function. A variety of disease processes and oral medications may also have a significant impact on

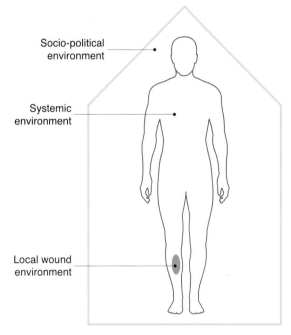

Figure 10.1 Environments affecting wound management.

wound healing and must be considered in the overall plan for management (Ch. 9). Finally, the local environment of the wound itself plays a critical role in determining certain aspects of wound management. The status of the exposed tissues and structures, condition of the surrounding skin, level and nature of exudate and microbial status influence decisions related to topical management. There is a dynamic interplay at many system levels – the cellular, organ, systemic, individual, social, organizational and political –

which can present health care professionals with enormous technical and personal challenges.

LOCAL WOUND MANAGEMENT

This chapter focuses on local wound management, specifically the use and selection of cleansing agents and dressings. However, it is important to remember that local management is a necessary but not in itself sufficient part of caring for a patient with a non-healing wound (Fig. 10.2). Non-healing wounds are usually the visible manifestation of one or multiple underlying pathologies. It is exceedingly rare that local management alone will effect a transformation from non-healing to healing. Medical and/or surgical management of these underlying pathologies and management or minimization of complicating factors are the most critical aspects of care and these issues are addressed in Chapters 7, 9, 11 and 13. Education of the patient and family regarding both the care and the cause of the wound is vital not only for optimal healing but also for health maintenance and prevention of wound recurrence (this is addressed in Ch. 14).

REMOVAL OF IMPEDIMENTS TO HEALING

The majority of activities involved in topical wound management, using wound cleansing and dressings, focus on removing impediments or barriers to the healing process rather than actively

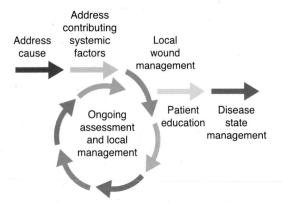

Figure 10.2 The wound management cycle.

accelerating it beyond its normal, optimal biochemical pace, with the possible exception of exogenous growth factors. Optimization of the local wound environment is the goal, and reports of 'accelerated' healing due to a topical agent or dressing are most often relative to a non-optimal environment. Parameters for local optimization by topical agents and dressings include bacterial burden, presence of necrotic tissue and physiological levels of moisture, pH and temperature.

Products and processes for wound cleansing, which aim to optimize the local environment in terms of levels of bacteria and necrotic tissue are addressed first. It is inherently logical to begin local wound management with attention to these two parameters of the local wound environment because they are indisputable impediments to healing and can culminate in infection. Without preliminary attention to these parameters, attempts to optimize others are likely to have little effect.

MICROBIAL STATUS OF TISSUE

Before discussing cleansing products, it is of value first to examine the target to be cleansed – the wound. There are three microbiological states that are possible in a wound: contamination, colonization and infection (Gilchrist 1997) (Fig. 10.3). Contamination is characterized as the simple presence of microorganisms in the wound but without proliferation. It is generally accepted that all wounds, regardless of aetiology, are contaminated. Humans have at least 10^{14} microorganisms living in or on our bodies (Williams & Leaper 1998), making a sterile wound impossible.

Colonization is characterized as the presence and proliferation of microorganisms in the wound but without a host reaction. Colonization is a common condition in chronic wounds such as venous ulcers and pressure ulcers and does not necessarily delay the healing process. In fact, there are data to suggest that colonization by certain bacteria actually encourages the healing process (Levenson 1983, Laato et al 1988, Kilcullen et al 1998). Controlled experiments in a rat incisional wound model using subcutaneously implanted sponges inoculated with solutions containing live

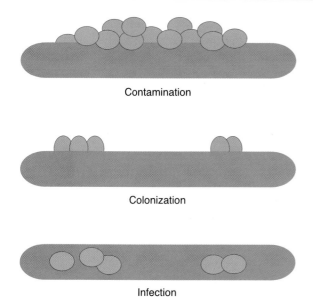

Contamination

Colonization

Infection

Figure 10.3 Microbial states of wounds.

Staphylococcus aureus (1×10^2 organisms/ml) accelerated wound healing, as measured by increases in granulation tissue components (Laato et al 1985, 1988). The proposed mechanisms of the positive effects of low-level bacterial colonization include increased local blood flow and enhanced recruitment of macrophages and fibroblasts, leading to increased angiogenesis and granulation. A component in the cell wall of bacteria (peptidoglycan) has been shown to be chemotactic for macrophages and neutrophils and is also thought to be chemotactic for fibroblasts (Kilcullen et al 1998).

When bacteria invade healthy tissues and continue to proliferate to the extent that their presence and by-products elicit or overwhelm the host immune response, this microbial state is known as infection. The classic signs and symptoms of infection include local redness, pain and swelling, fever and changes in the amount and character of wound exudate.

WOUND CLEANSING AND DEBRIDEMENT

In presenting a broad summary of wound cleansing and debridement it is appropriate to begin with a historical quotation: 'The germ is nothing; it is the terrain in which it grows that is everything' (Pasteur 1880). Pasteur's caveat about 'terrain' is important to a discussion of bacterial levels and wound infection. The wound terrain comprises the environmental conditions that will enable or discourage the 'germ' or microorganism that is inevitably present in the wound to successfully colonize the wound surface and perhaps to eventually invade viable tissue. Acute and chronic wounds offer distinctly different environments for colonization. Chronic wounds are often characterized by an impaired vascular supply and varying amounts of devitalized tissue that offers a nutritional supply to microorganisms, as well as a varied topography of cracks, crevices, undermining and tunnels that can represent a 'safe harbour' for proliferation. Surgically made acute wounds, by comparison, are in general relatively free of debris and are well vascularized but acute traumatic wounds can, in some cases, be heavily contaminated. For these reasons, wound cleansing and debridement are important processes related to preventing infection in chronic wound management. Cleansing is the first line of defence in removal of microorganisms and foreign materials and certain types and amounts of devitalized tissue from the wound. Debridement can be considered 'a special type of cleansing' that is called for when devitalized tissue of a specific nature is present in larger amounts.

A discussion of wound cleansing agents should begin with an accurate definition of the process. Cleansing, or cleaning in general, is a process of physically removing dirt or other foreign materials such as particulates or microorganisms from a site, be it a wound or an inanimate work surface. Cleaning one's laundry consists of agitating the clothes in aqueous solution to loosen dirt and remove it by draining and rinsing the solution. The addition of soaps or detergents to the wash simply helps with the loosening process. Cleansing a wound similarly encompasses loosening and rinsing away dirt and foreign materials or microorganisms. Cleansing does not require the 'killing' of anything. Once the action of killing is introduced or desired, then the process is not merely cleansing but disinfection or antisepsis. Disinfection is defined as killing of microorganisms on inanimate surfaces such as floors or surgical instruments, while antisepsis is defined as killing of micro-organisms on a living surface such as the skin or a wound.

CLEANSING MATERIALS AND METHODS

These semantics are important because the three processes or concepts have been confusingly inter-mingled in terms of products used and developed for wound cleansing. The primary objective of cleansing a wound is to remove foreign materials and reduce the bioburden. Topical products commonly used in the name of wound cleansing include antiseptics, antibiotics, detergents, surfac-tants, saline and water.

Intact skin is a formidable barrier to micro-organisms and chemicals due primarily to the tough, keratinized (and non-living) stratum corneum layer and secretions from sebaceous and sweat glands. When this barrier is breached, viable tissues are exposed and are vulnerable to both desiccation and infection. The use on an open wound of many solutions considered safe on intact skin may be damaging. While cleansing has been defined as a physical process of removal, many clinicians feel the need to use an antiseptic solution as a cleansing agent in an effort to kill potential pathogens in the wound and thereby stave off infection. Interestingly, it has been shown that even the surface of intact skin cannot be ren-dered bacteria-free by any antiseptic. Bacteria exist deep in adnexal structures and are brought to the skin surface by secretions of sweat and sebum. Even if one's hands are scrubbed with 70% ethanol to achieve a 99.7% reduction of surface bacteria, subsequent immediate washing with soap and water results in a significant increase in surface bacteria (Laufman 1989). It is thought that the friction induces shedding of epithelial squames that harbour viable bacteria.

TISSUE TOXICITY ISSUES

Another historical quotation is pertinent when considering the use of antiseptics as wound cleansing products: 'It is necessary in the estima-tion of the value of an antiseptic to study its effect on the tissues more than its effect on the bacteria' Fleming (1919).

Most antiseptics work by destruction of bacte-rial cell walls; however, this mechanism does not spare non-bacterial cells such as wound fibro-blasts and macrophages (Hellewell et al 1997). The heterogeneous environment of a wound is also challenging for antiseptic efficacy. For example, alcohols are in general excellent broad-spectrum antimicrobial agents, especially on inanimate surfaces where they outperform most other antiseptics. However, their effectiveness in a wound environment is compromised by the presence of organic materials such as blood, mucus and connective tissue proteins (Mertz & Ovington 1993). Alcohols also evaporate rapidly and are drying to the tissues.

Sodium hypochlorite solutions are excellent surface disinfectants and debriding agents but are toxic to cultured fibroblasts, white blood cells and endothelial cells and have been shown to impair and halt blood flow of the microcirculation in animal models. They are chemically unstable solutions and are inactivated by contact with organic materials such as those found in the envi-ronment of an open wound. Hydrogen peroxide is also frequently used for wound cleansing. It has no measurable antimicrobial effect but it has been shown to be toxic to fibroblasts in culture. Hydrogen peroxide releases oxygen bubbles on contact with tissues, where it is broken down by the catalase enzyme. These bubbles provide a physical agitation of the wound surface that may loosen debris or microorganisms; however, they have also been shown to cause air-filled bullae and to disturb new epithelium when hydrogen peroxide is used to treat split-thickness skin graft donor sites (Gruber et al 1975).

Iodine is another popular and effective broad-spectrum antiseptic used in wound cleansing. An informative review of the discovery, uses and evolution of iodine and its compounds as anti-septics and the development of povidone iodine is provided by Lawrence (1998). The key issues are discussed here.

Pure iodine is caustic and almost insoluble in water (0.355 g/L). It must be chemically complexed with an iodophor (usually a polymer or protein) that renders it soluble in an aqueous solution where it then slowly releases free iodine as the active antiseptic agent. Povidone iodine is an iodophor that uses a polyvinylpyrrolidone polymer to complex iodine and it is available in several formulations, including an aqueous solution, an ointment, a cream and a surgical scrub (which includes a detergent). In-vivo and in-vitro studies of povidone iodine solution and scrub have demonstrated toxicity to cells such as fibroblasts, red blood cells and neutrophils as well as detrimental effects on wound breaking strength. The toxicity of the scrub has been attributed primarily to the detergent ingredient. Clinical data suggest that iodine may at best be ineffective in an open wound and at worst might actually impair the endogenous phagocytic response to infecting microorganisms. In a study performed in head and neck surgical wounds, investigators found that 28% of wounds irrigated with povidone iodine postoperatively became infected compared with zero control wounds irrigated with saline (Becker 1986). Another study examined the bioburden via quantitative tissue biopsy in pressure ulcers treated with silver sulphadiazine (SSD), saline gauze or povidone iodine (Kucan et al 1981). The investigators found that SSD was 100% effective in keeping the tissue bioburden below 10^5, saline gauze was 79% effective and povidone iodine was only 64% effective.

However, it appears that the formulation of the iodophor is a vital aspect of utilizing iodine safely as a wound-cleansing agent. Povidone iodine cream has been shown to reduce bacterial counts and enhance healing in inoculated blister wounds in humans (Stahl-Bayliss et al 1990). The enhancement of healing is likely to be due to the occlusive nature of the cream vehicle. A particular formulation of iodine in a hydrophilic starch powder has been studied in eight randomized controlled clinical studies in venous, diabetic and decubitus ulcers (Moberg et al 1983) where it exhibited not only antimicrobial and debriding effects but also enhanced healing when compared with controls.

The use of topical antibiotics to reduce bacterial numbers in the wound bed is also controversial. One reason is that the widespread and indiscriminate use of antibiotics in general has contributed to the evolution of resistant bacterial species. The randomized controlled study mentioned previously (Kucan et al 1981) did document a beneficial effect of SSD cream in the reduction of levels of bacteria in pressure ulcers. However, there is a general paucity of trial data to confirm the effectiveness of topical antibiotic use in chronic wounds as opposed to acute wounds. Generally positive results have been reported for topical antibiotic use in acute wounds, although sensitization to certain products has been reported. Notwithstanding this, a recent randomized controlled trial comparing the postoperative topical use of bacitracin and white petrolatum in 884 patients undergoing minor ambulatory surgical procedures revealed no differences in either development of infection or in healing (Smack et al 1996).

Detergents or surfactants are chemicals that assist in cleansing by reducing surface tension between particulates and a surface. They may possess either a positive (cationic) or negative (anionic) chemical charge, both a positive and a negative charge (amphoteric), or no charge at all. This last type is known as non-ionic. Non-ionic surfactants or detergents have proven to be the only variety that is not harmful to the cells involved in the wound healing process. Non-ionic surfactants are often added to commercial aqueous-based cleansing solutions to potentiate their physical cleansing effects.

It has become a general consensus among many wound care practitioners that normal saline represents the safest and most physiological cleansing agent for chronic wounds that do not have significant amounts of devitalized tissue or signs of clinical infection. There have even been arguments for the use of regular tap water as a safe cleansing solution (Riyat & Quinton 1997, Moscati et al 1998). In one randomized controlled study of 705 consecutive emergency room patients, the infection rate in wounds irrigated with sterile saline was 10.3% compared with 5.4% in wounds irrigated with tap water (Angeras et al 1992). An update on irrigating fluids and their effects on wounds is given by Lawrence (1997).

TISSUE DELIVERY ISSUES

As important as the choice of cleansing solution, is the temperature of the solution and the method of delivery of the solution to the wound surface. Cleansing solutions that are refrigerated or even at room temperature can reduce the surface temperature of the wound, resulting in local hypothermia. It is known from the surgical experience that tissue hypothermia can result in decreased mitogenesis and decreased phagocyte activity. It can take as long as 40 min for a wound to regain its original temperature after cleansing and several hours for cellular activities to normalize (Flannagan 1997).

Cleansing solutions must also be delivered to the wound surface with sufficient volume and force to loosen and wash away microorganisms and debris. However, excessive force may drive the loosened material into viable tissue rather than out of it (Rodeheaver et al 1975). A safe range of effective irrigation pressures has been established as 27.6–103.5 kPa (4–15 psi). A 35-ml syringe fitted with a 19-gauge angiocatheter tip delivers a stream of liquid at a pressure of 55.2 kPa (8 psi). Increasing the bore of the angiocatheter or decreasing the size of the syringe results in higher pressure streams, whereas decreasing the bore or increasing the size of the syringe results in lower pressures.

A wound is not a static entity or an inanimate surface, but a complex, fragile and dynamic milieu of viable endogenous cells and structures, exogenous microorganisms, labile chemicals and chemical reactions, devitalized cells and microorganisms, and potential foreign particulate matter from the external environment. The differential impact of cleansing solutions and methods on all of these components of the wound must be weighed in terms of overall benefit to the healing process.

DEBRIDEMENT VERSUS CLEANSING

If a significant amount of devitalized tissue is present in the wound bed, it will not only physically delay healing, it will predispose the wound to colonization and subsequent infection by providing a site of attachment and source of nutrients for bacteria. Therefore, the expedient removal of devitalized tissue or debridement is advisable for optimal healing. Devitalized or necrotic tissue may have a variety of appearances, from loosely adherent yellow slough to tightly adherent, leathery black eschar. Removal or debridement can be achieved by various methods depending on the amount and nature of the necrotic tissue and the patient's overall status. Surgical debridement is the most expedient method but requires special expertise (Vowden & Vowden 1999a); some patients may not be candidates for surgical debridement. Sharp debridement using a scalpel or scissors may be performed in an out-patient setting, but also requires training. Mechanical debridement through the use of wet-to-dry dressings, whirlpool, high-pressure irrigation, or scrubbing with gauze or sponge is easier to perform but is less selective and may damage viable tissue. Enzymatic treatment is more selective and requires more time but may be facilitated by the use of moisture-retentive dressings. However, the efficacy of enzymatic agents is considered questionable by some. A small randomized controlled trial comparing the efficacy of an enzymatic debriding agent with that of an amorphous hydrogel in removing eschar from full-thickness pressure ulcers found no significant differences in performance (Martin et al 1996). Finally, autolytic debridement through the use of moisture-retentive dressings to retain endogenous enzymes at the wound surface to digest devitalized tissues is the most selective, least invasive, albeit slowest method. Non-sharp techniques for wound debridement are reviewed by Vowden & Vowden (1999b).

PROMOTION OF TISSUE VIABILITY AND PROLIFERATION

Once the wound environment has been optimized in terms of removing impediments to healing by cleansing and/or debridement, attention should be turned towards maintaining the viability of the healthy tissue and establishing conditions that facilitate the proliferation of new tissues to close the wound. Important systemic factors that promote healing include adequate blood supply and nutrition; however, the focus in this chapter is on local factors – specifically those that are impacted by wound dressing materials.

TISSUE HYDRATION EFFECTS

Perhaps the single most pertinent parameter of the local wound environment relative to tissue viability and proliferation is that of tissue hydration. Cells and tissues are viable only within a narrow range of hydration. One of the critical functions of intact skin is therefore to maintain functional hydration levels of the underlying tissues by acting as a barrier to moisture loss to the atmosphere. When skin is intact, the stratum corneum is the seat of this barrier function. Moisture loss from intact skin (i.e. through the stratum corneum) can be measured as the moisture vapour transmission rate (MVTR) and varies slightly with anatomical location or thickness. An averaged value for the MVTR of intact skin is around 200 g of moisture vapour/m^2/day (Lamke et al 1977). The MVTR of skin that is devoid of stratum corneum or of a superficial wound is almost 40 times as high, at 7874 g/m^2/day (Rovee et al 1972).

The impact that wound dressing materials could have on replacing this moisture barrier function of the stratum corneum was not fully recognized and introduced to practice until the latter half of the twentieth century. In the early 1960s, studies in both animal and human models documented increasing healing rates for wounds maintained in a physiologically moist local environment relative to wounds exposed to air and allowed to desiccate (Winter 1962, Hinnman & Maibach 1963). Since that time, research data have suggested that a physiologically moist local wound environment also contributes to diminution of pain and enhancement of cosmesis relative to a dry desiccated wound environment (Nemeth et al 1991; Hedman 1988).

Multiple mechanisms have been suggested for the effects of a moist local environment on healing. Histological studies of wounds healing in a moist environment versus wounds healing in a dry environment have revealed that the dry environment results in further tissue death beyond the original cause of the wound. This is sometimes referred to as dehydration necrosis (Rovee et al 1972, Winter 1962). It has also been shown that resurfacing epithelial cells move farther and faster in a moist environment, whereas a dry environment can effectively retard their progress (Winter 1962). Further studies of wounds healing in a moist environment have shown that the fluid that is retained at the wound surface by a semi-occlusive dressing contains proteolytic enzymes and functional growth factors (polypeptides that promote cellular movement or proliferation) that enhance the healing process (Chen et al 1992). In dry wounds, these enzymes and proteins may be present, only deeper in the tissue and in lower concentrations. Another proposed mechanism for the reduced healing times associated with moist wound healing involves the 'current of injury' or a naturally occurring electrical potential that exists between the layers of the skin after an injury. This current flows in a moist wound but is 'turned off' when the wound is allowed to dry out (Jaffe & Vanable 1984). This endogenous electrical current may play a role in the enhancing of healing by promoting cell migration and also by causing cells to express more receptors for growth factors (Falanga et al 1987). Finally, maintenance of stable wound temperature may be a further benefit of semi-occlusive dressings. When moisture vapour is allowed to escape freely from a wound, the evaporative process results in a local cooling of the tissues, with the previously discussed effects on cellular mitosis and phagocyte efficiency. A dressing that slows the evaporative process may therefore reduce temperature loss from the tissues. Certain dressings such as foams and hydrocolloids have been demonstrated to have an insulating effect on wound tissues relative to air exposure or gauze (Thomas 1990).

The basic concept of maintaining or establishing a physiologically moist local wound environment is inherently logical. Cells and tissues subsist and function in a moist milieu beneath the intact stratum corneum of unwounded skin.

Yet in the case of a wound, the conventional wisdom of both the lay person and the surgeon is to allow or even encourage the exposed tissues to desiccate. The underlying motive that drives this response is perhaps the fear of infection. Indeed, when Winter's early studies were presented in a medical forum, the first questions in an ensuing discussion were related to a fear of infection. There was concern that the moist environment (or materials that created it) that apparently enhanced the healing rate might also enhance the infection rate by encouraging the survival and growth of undesirable microorganisms in the wound. A number of retrospective and prospective studies of wounds managed topically by materials that sustain a moist environment and by conventional materials (gauze and saline) have documented that this fear is unwarranted. Observed rates of infection have actually been lower for wounds dressed with semi-occlusive dressings than with gauze.

The development of materials that sustain a moist wound environment for optimal healing has become a thriving industry. Such materials are largely synthetic polymers that are fashioned into fibres, mats, wafers, or membranes that are semipermeable to gases such as oxygen and carbon dioxide and moisture, yet often impermeable to liquids. This characteristic earns them the general term 'semi-occlusive'. The term semi-occlusive is often used interchangeably with the term occlusive, which implies a total lack of permeability to either liquids or gases. Few of the newer synthetic dressings are truly occlusive and semi-occlusive is the more appropriate term used to denote dressings that promote moist healing. These different types of semi-occlusive dressings create or maintain a moist local environment by capturing transpired water vapour or liquid drainage from the wound and holding it at the surface. The most frequently used alternative to these dressings is that ubiquitous natural fibre dressing cotton gauze. It is possible to use gauze and saline to establish and maintain a continuously moist wound environment; however, gauze has been shown to require substantially more dressing changes, labour and overall cost than the polymeric, semi-occlusive materials.

THE ROLES OF DRESSINGS: FORM VERSUS FUNCTION

Semi-occlusive wound dressings are commonly categorized, discussed and reviewed from the standpoint of their composition. Describing what a wound dressing consists of from a materials point of view is informative and it has been done well and in great detail by many authors (Turner 1989, Thomas 1990, Ovington 1998). However, such discussions are not always instructive in terms of selecting a wound dressing for clinical use. What the product is made of or what it contains is only part of the selection criteria. While this information is still useful in some early navigation through the myriad of dressings currently available (Fig. 10.4, Table 10.1), equally vital information needed is that of the function or performance of the dressing, regardless of its composition. Rather than presenting a description of physical form and characteristics of generic dressing categories such as transparent films, foams, alginate fibres, hydrocolloid wafers, amorphous hydrogels, collagen sheets and newer speciality materials, this section will attempt to weave this information into the broader context of dressing functions and performance parameters.

A performance-based approach to dressing use

Performance is the way in which something functions, or the action for which a thing is espe-

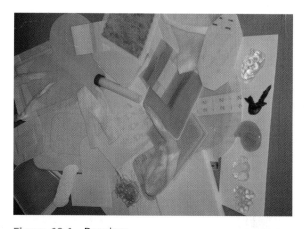

Figure 10.4 Dressings.

Table 10.1 Currently available dressing products in the USA. Data from Ostomy Wound Management 1998 Buyer's Guide, July 1998, 44(7):109–145

Wound dressings (material categories)	Number of types marketed
Alginates	26
Biosynthetics	9
Collagen	9
Composites	20
Contact layers	7
Foams	26
Gauzes (woven and nonwoven)	33
Gauzes (impregnated)	25
Gauzes (nonadherent)	13
Gauzes (packing/debriding)	17
Gauzes (roll/wrapping)	18
Elastic support bandages	17
Hydrocolloids	41
Hydrofibres	2
Hydrogels (amorphous)	30
Hydrogels (wafers)	19
Hydrogels (impregnated gauze)	14
Compression bandages and systems	24
Specialty absorptives	17
Transparent films	21
Wound fillers	10
Wound cleansers	28

cially *suitable* or employed. Most licensed dressing products are suited to wound healing in terms of their safety. However, some products are more suitable than others for a specific phase of wound healing or for specific wound conditions (Fig. 10.5). Despite this, many dressings are often promoted as being the only product required for varying types of wounds of differing conditions and causes. Dressings often have marketing claims or indications for certain wound aetiologies, such as pressure ulcers, diabetic ulcers or donor sites. However, a pressure ulcer could be clean, shallow and granulating with minimal drainage, or deep and undermined with heavy drainage and large areas of necrosis. These two different pressure ulcer scenarios have clearly different management needs and the optimal dressings for each are unlikely to be the same (Fig 10.5). Since a dressing almost never addresses or corrects the underlying pathology of a wound, it should not be selected on the basis of wound aetiology but on local wound needs determined by a thorough assessment of the wound

and periwound skin. The wound needs are criteria for dressing function or performance, which then becomes the basis of product selection.

This type of performance-based approach to product selection is already a familiar concept in prescribing drugs. First the desired performance is identified, then the specific types of available products with that function are examined. For example, if a patient is clinically depressed, the clinician determines that an antidepressant is needed. From that point the decision is between specific drug categories, including tricyclics, monoamineoxidase inhibitors or serotonin reuptake inhibitors. Drugs can be classified based on their structures but clinical selection of a particular drug usually begins with its classification by function. With respect to wound dressings, the focus has been more on their categories rather than their functions. Recent discussions have surfaced in the literature that take note of this situation. Krasner (1997) calls for a paradigm shift in decision making about dressings. The shift is described as the interactive and active utilization of dressing materials in the same way as drugs; with specific actions, interactions, contraindications, indications and side effects. Other characteristics of dressings to consider include the frequency of dressing changes, the unit cost of the dressing and the cost of its application in terms of nursing time, ease of application and removal and effects on the quality of life for the patient, including pain relief. van Rijswijk & Beitz (1998) present arguments for classification of dressings based on clinically valid functions as opposed to categorization based on product components in order to increase clinical utility.

Some dressing manufacturers have realized that their products would be better utilized if they were viewed in terms of their functions and have attempted to convey functions of their products in their advertising. One range of products began using red, yellow and black dots on their product packaging in an attempt to correlate the use of the product to the status of the tissues in the wound bed. The red dot indicated clean, granulating wounds, yellow indicated wounds with necrotic slough and black indicated dry, eschar-covered wounds. Other

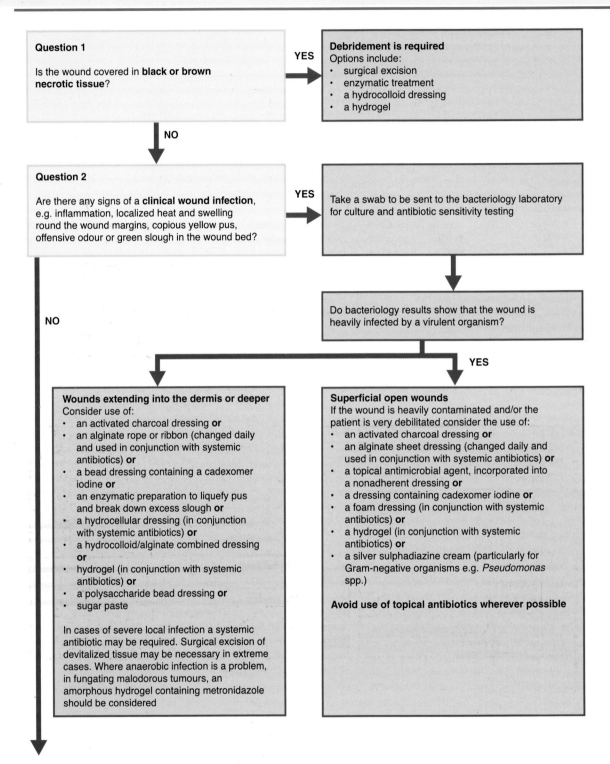

Question 1

Is the wound covered in **black or brown necrotic tissue**?

YES →

Debridement is required
Options include:
- surgical excision
- enzymatic treatment
- a hydrocolloid dressing
- a hydrogel

NO ↓

Question 2

Are there any signs of a **clinical wound infection**, e.g. inflammation, localized heat and swelling round the wound margins, copious yellow pus, offensive odour or green slough in the wound bed?

YES →

Take a swab to be sent to the bacteriology laboratory for culture and antibiotic sensitivity testing

NO ↓

Do bacteriology results show that the wound is heavily infected by a virulent organism?

YES →

Wounds extending into the dermis or deeper
Consider use of:
- an activated charcoal dressing **or**
- an alginate rope or ribbon (changed daily and used in conjunction with systemic antibiotics) **or**
- a bead dressing containing a cadexomer iodine **or**
- an enzymatic preparation to liquefy pus and break down excess slough **or**
- a hydrocellular dressing (in conjunction with systemic antibiotics) **or**
- a hydrocolloid/alginate combined dressing **or**
- hydrogel (in conjunction with systemic antibiotics) **or**
- a polysaccharide bead dressing **or**
- sugar paste

In cases of severe local infection a systemic antibiotic may be required. Surgical excision of devitalized tissue may be necessary in extreme cases. Where anaerobic infection is a problem, in fungating malodorous tumours, an amorphous hydrogel containing metronidazole should be considered

Superficial open wounds
If the wound is heavily contaminated and/or the patient is very debilitated consider the use of:
- an activated charcoal dressing **or**
- an alginate sheet dressing (changed daily and used in conjunction with systemic antibiotics) **or**
- a topical antimicrobial agent, incorporated into a nonadherent dressing **or**
- a dressing containing cadexomer iodine **or**
- a foam dressing (in conjunction with systemic antibiotics) **or**
- a hydrogel (in conjunction with systemic antibiotics) **or**
- a silver sulphadiazine cream (particularly for Gram-negative organisms e.g. *Pseudomonas* spp.)

Avoid use of topical antibiotics wherever possible

Figure 10.5   Which wound care product? Deciding priorities in the local management of open wounds (based on Morison & Moffatt, 1994, pp. 77–81). Note that this algorithm is intended only as a guide; it is not fully comprehensive or exclusive.

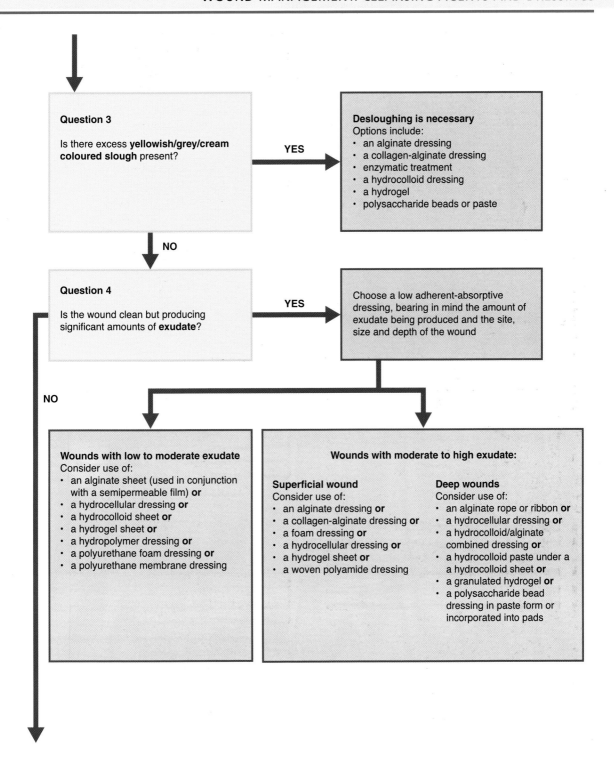

Question 3

Is there excess **yellowish/grey/cream coloured slough** present?

YES →

Desloughing is necessary
Options include:
- an alginate dressing
- a collagen-alginate dressing
- enzymatic treatment
- a hydrocolloid dressing
- a hydrogel
- polysaccharide beads or paste

NO ↓

Question 4

Is the wound clean but producing significant amounts of **exudate**?

YES →

Choose a low adherent-absorptive dressing, bearing in mind the amount of exudate being produced and the site, size and depth of the wound

NO

Wounds with low to moderate exudate
Consider use of:
- an alginate sheet (used in conjunction with a semipermeable film) **or**
- a hydrocellular dressing **or**
- a hydrocolloid sheet **or**
- a hydrogel sheet **or**
- a hydropolymer dressing **or**
- a polyurethane foam dressing **or**
- a polyurethane membrane dressing

Wounds with moderate to high exudate:

Superficial wound
Consider use of:
- an alginate dressing **or**
- a collagen-alginate dressing **or**
- a foam dressing **or**
- a hydrocellular dressing **or**
- a hydrogel sheet **or**
- a woven polyamide dressing

Deep wounds
Consider use of:
- an alginate rope or ribbon **or**
- a hydrocellular dressing **or**
- a hydrocolloid/alginate combined dressing **or**
- a hydrocolloid paste under a a hydrocolloid sheet **or**
- a granulated hydrogel **or**
- a polysaccharide bead dressing in paste form or incorporated into pads

Figure 10.5 *Continued*

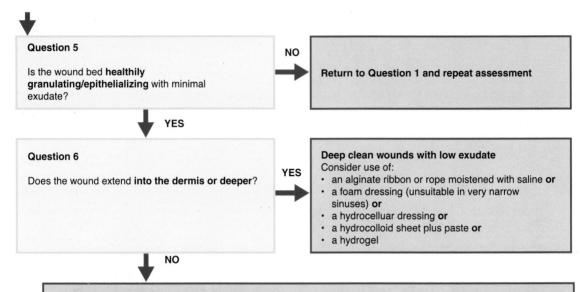

Question 5

Is the wound bed **healthily granulating/epithelializing** with minimal exudate?

NO → Return to Question 1 and repeat assessment

YES ↓

Question 6

Does the wound extend **into the dermis or deeper**?

YES → **Deep clean wounds with low exudate**
Consider use of:
- an alginate ribbon or rope moistened with saline **or**
- a foam dressing (unsuitable in very narrow sinuses) **or**
- a hydrocelluar dressing **or**
- a hydrocolloid sheet plus paste **or**
- a hydrogel

NO ↓

Superficial clean wounds with low exudate
There is a wide range of dressings available for the treatment of healthy superficial, granulating/epithelializing wounds, including:
- an alginate island dressing **or**
- a semipermeable film dressing **or**
- a foam dressing **or**
- a hydrocellular dressing **or**
- a hydrocolloid sheet dressing **or**
- a hydrogel **or**
- a hydropolymer dressing **or**
- an absorbent low-adherent dressing **or**
- a woven polyamide dressing **or**
- a polyurethane membrane dressing **or**
- a silicone dressing **or**
- a knitted viscose dressing

In addition to the nature of the wound bed, many other factors should be considered before a dressing is selected, including:
- the site of the wound and ease or otherwise of applying the dressing
- the size of the wound
- the frequency of dressing changes required
- comfort and cosmetic considerations
- where and by whom the dressing will be changed
- the availability of the dressing, in the size required – not all dressings are available to patients whose wounds are being managed in the community, and where the dressing is available on the community Drug Tariff it may not be available in all sizes.

Where all other considerations are equal, choose the cheapest dressing.

Before using any wound care product for the first time **ALWAYS** consult the manufacturer's recommendations, contraindications, precautions and warnings. This information can change, so it is worth re-reading the manufacturer's instructions at frequent intervals. For 'prescription only' wound care products the relevant product data sheets **MUST** first be consulted prior to use.

If there is still any doubt about the suitability of any dressing the patient's doctor should be consulted and further advice obtained from the local pharmacist.

Figure 10.5 *Continued*

companies have devised charts that categorize products in their range based on the absorbent capacity of each. Graphic icons indicating a product's functional category as skin care, exudate absorption, hydration, cleansing or compression have also been used. However, there is a need to go beyond these single-company approaches: what is needed is more than a guide to a particular range of products, such as an approach to thinking differently about all available dressing products.

A more general performance-based approach to using wound dressings might be guided by six basic questions (Table 10.2):

- What does the wound need?
- What does the product do?
- How well does the product perform?
- What does the patient need?
- What is available in this setting?
- What is practical?

Answers to what the wound needs are found by thorough local assessment of the wound in terms of its three dimensions, the type or types of tissue present in the wound bed (granulation, epithelial, slough, eschar), quality and quantity of drainage, condition of the periwound skin and microbial status. This assessment must not only be performed initially but also at each dressing change. Wounds are not static entities; their needs change as they progress, or as they deteriorate. A dressing that was appropriate in the early, exudative inflammatory phase of wound healing becomes inappropriate for optimal healing during the later, less exudative phase of re-epithelialization. As the wound evolves in either direction, dressing choices must similarly evolve to meet local needs. Ongoing assessment of the wound is critical for successful management (see Ch. 8).

Answers to what the product does should be sought from many sources, including marketing materials, data from controlled clinical trials and objective data from in-vitro evaluations. Other important sources of information are the product package insert and labelling, since a product may not perform as expected if not used as directed. Product material safety data sheets (MSDSs) are available upon request from manufacturers and contain detailed information on composition and handling. If there are concerns about components of a dressing related to allergic reactions, this is a valuable document to have on file.

Answers to how well a product performs in relation to others in the same material category or of similar function ideally are found in randomized controlled clinical trials that examine head-to-head comparisons. Unfortunately such trials are relatively few in number and it would be almost impossible from a logistical and cost standpoint to compare all products of a category or function to all others through a randomized trial. There may be a trial comparing Dressing A with Dressing B, and a second trial comparing Dressing B with Dressing C, but because clinical trials of wound healing involve so many variables, and because there is no consensus on which healing end points are valid and how to measure them, it is rarely possible to then link

Table 10.2 Performance-based approach to using wound dressings	
Questions	Answer source
What does the wound need?	Thorough assessment of the wound and periwound skin
What does the product do?	Product literature; clinical, in-vivo or in-vitro data
How well does the product perform?	Comparative clinical studies (randomized controlled trials) Objective laboratory comparisons
What does the patient need?	Comprehensive medical and psychosocial assessment of patient
What is available in this setting?	Health plan coverage, facility formulary, reimbursement
What is practical?	Case management, goals of treatment (combined with all of the preceding answers)

the two trials and get a comparison of Dressing A with Dressing C. In the absence of controlled clinical data, comparative laboratory data may be of some value in gauging relative product performance. Such laboratory studies of different commercial brands of transparent films, hydrocolloids and hydrogels have suggested that there is indeed variable performance between different brands of a particular category of dressing (Thomas & Loveless 1988, 1997, Sprung et al 1998).

A few important caveats concerning laboratory testing of dressing products are worth mentioning. The testing conditions should model as closely as possible clinically relevant parameters. For example, one particular in-vitro study examined the absorptive capacity of 23 different amorphous hydrogels and used three different test fluids (water, normal saline and wound fluid). A wide variation in absorptive capacity was observed for many products depending on what test fluid was used. In general, it was found that a dressing's water absorption was significantly higher than (and not predictive of) its ability to absorb wound fluid. Normal saline absorption, however, correlated quite well with wound fluid absorption. This difference is likely to be due to the fact that both saline and wound fluid are ionic solutions whereas water is not. The same study examined the effects of fluid temperature on absorption by 17 different hydrocolloid wafers. Saline or water at room temperature and at body temperature was differentially absorbed by all products tested. Some products absorbed more when the test fluid was at room temperature and others absorbed more when the test fluid was at body temperature. This type of data should cause one to stop and think when well-meaning company representatives perform demonstrations of dressing absorption at trade shows and conferences using drinking water at room temperature or even from a chilled container.

Returning to the six questions that may guide performance-based dressing selection, the question of what the patient needs is answered by comprehensive medical and psychosocial evaluation. As mentioned earlier, a dressing cannot address underlying causes or systemic factors that contribute to impaired healing. The question

of what is available pertains to the patient's health care plan and/or the broader health care environment in terms of availability of specific products, payment for products and services, and the cost effectiveness of the product. Finally, the question of what is practical relates to the overall care plan and what the goals of wound treatment are, as well as how complicated the product is to use and whether it will be applied and removed by a health care professional, a family member or the patients themselves.

Dressing performance parameters

Wound needs constitute performance parameters or functions for dressings and the concepts are almost interchangeable. Performance parameters or functions may be either general or wound specific and not every dressing can be expected to do everything well or even at all. The needs for variable performance based on the needs of different wounds or even the same wound throughout its healing course have played a part in the current proliferation of wound dressing products. By adopting a performance-based approach, the clinician attempts to match available dressings and their functions to the needs of a wound. The general areas of dressing function and the categories of dressing materials that meet them will now be reviewed (Table 10.3).

Important functional areas for wound dressings include:

- general optimization of the local wound environment
- the ability to be either adherent or nonadherent to periwound skin
- the ability to conform to either wound depth or challenging anatomical topography
- the ability to absorb wound exudate, or alternatively to promote tissue hydration
- the ability to promote autolytic debridement
- the ability to promote the healing process or to recruit or activate critical cells involved in the healing process
- the ability to influence infection control or odour control
- relative ease of use and range of use.

Table 10.3 Performance parameters of dressings and categories that meet them

Dressing performance parameters	Appropriate dressing material categories
Optimize local environment	Any material if used appropriately
Adherent to skin	Many dressings with adhesive borders or surface coatings
Nonadherent	Tubular products Contact layers
Conformable to topography	Extra-thin versions of hydrocolloids Extra-thin versions of foams Transparent films
Conformable to depth	Amorphous gels Rope versions of alginates Pastes, powders
Absorb excess exudate	Foams Alginates Superabsorbents Textile fibres
Promote tissue hydration	Films Hydrocolloids
Promote autolytic debridement	Gel wafers Amorphous gels
Promote phases/attract cells of the healing process	Collagen Acemannan β-Glucan Certain emulsions
Assist in bacterial control	Materials that provide an impermeable mechanical barrier Silver-containing products Iodine-containing products
Assist in odour control	Absorptive products in general Products containing activated charcoal
Ease of use	Products used in appropriate situations and according to instructions
Range of use	Varies by situation and product

The last area depends primarily on the care setting and the end-user. Each of these functional areas will now be briefly discussed with respect to currently available generic classes of wound dressings.

Optimizing the local wound environment

Optimization of the local wound environment is the most nebulous of the functional areas and the least discriminating – any dressing can accomplish this if used appropriately. The 'if' in this statement is a large one. It has already been stated that even gauze can optimize the local wound environment if care is taken to keep it continually moist. However, this rarely happens (except during clinical trials when saline and gauze is used as a control dressing and everyone involved is paying close attention!). It is also true that any dressing can be used inappropriately. An alginate dressing used on a wound with minimal exudate will not optimize the local wound environment. Rather, it is likely to dry out the wound bed and stick to the surface. A hydrocolloid dressing or other dressing that is adherent to periwound skin and is changed too frequently may strip the periwound skin. An adhesive dressing applied to a newly epithelializing wound may adhere to and destroy the fragile epithelium upon removal. An amorphous hydrogel dressing used on a draining wound may severely macerate the periwound skin.

Adherence

The need for a dressing to remain in place is obvious. The selection of a dressing that is adhesive or nonadhesive may depend in part on the condition of the patient's skin and the frequency of dressing changes. Many dressings have adhesive borders or adhesive coatings, whereas some have no adhesive. Certain dressings are characterized by the tenacity of their adhesive, such as the hydrocolloids, while others are characterized by the gentleness of their adhesive. Certain extra-thin foam products have adhesive applied to their wound-facing surface in a pattern that leaves open areas of no adhesive and tend to be gentler to the skin upon removal. If a dressing has no adhesive system and the patient cannot tolerate adhesives, a range of nonadhesive dressing retention products is available. Such products include tubular nettings and gauzes (in diameters to accommodate, e.g., a finger, a limb, a torso, a head) and self-adherent wraps. Polymeric, perforated wound contact layers are available that are placed in the wound bed to allow passage of wound drainage but prevent adhesion of a secondary dressing placed on top of the wound.

Conformability

The conformability of a dressing plays a role in its ability to remain in place over a bony prominence such as the ankle or elbow or on a challenging site such as the ear or finger. Extra-thin products in general are more conformable than their thicker counterparts. Foams and hydrocolloids are available in extra-thin versions. Transparent films are inherently thin and conformable but may be difficult to handle. A different aspect of conformability is that of three-dimensional shape or wound depth, tunnelling or undermining. It is a general principle that wound dressings should gently fill all spaces in the wound or eliminate dead space. Products such as amorphous hydrogels, hydrocolloid pastes and powders readily take on the shape of whatever they are placed into or on, but in general should be used to line rather than fill up a wound cavity. Rope versions of alginates are also readily conformable to cavities and undermining.

Absorbency

Absorption is the parameter that has driven a huge amount of differentiation in wound dressing products, including foams, alginates, hydrofibres, superabsorbents, gels that absorb and textile-based fibres. Increased absorbency theoretically increases wear time and thereby decreases dressing changes and disturbances to the wound bed. These effects could result in an overall decreased cost of care. Some absorptive materials wick drainage from the wound surface laterally and may contribute to periwound maceration, whereas other materials are characterized by their lack of lateral wicking.

Hydration

Maintenance of hydration levels of healthy granulation tissue or rehydration of desiccated tissues to facilitate debridement can be achieved by using transparent films, hydrocolloids, sheet hydrogels or amorphous gels. If facilitation of autolytic debridement is the objective, amorphous hydrogels that donate moisture to the tissues are the best choice. If there are significant amounts of necrotic tissues, autolytic debridement may not be appropriate and sharp debridement or surgical debridement is more expedient. Aggressive sharp debridement has even been suggested to facilitate healing of diabetic foot ulcers by resetting the balance between excessive levels of wound proteases and their endogenous inhibitors (Steed et al 1996).

Promoting natural healing processes

Certain materials have been shown to recruit and/or activate cells such as macrophages and fibroblasts. Since these cells play instrumental roles in the healing process it is believed that more of them or their increased functioning may enhance the healing process. For example, macrophages can perform debridement activities in the wound bed as well as secrete multiple growth factors that facilitate angiogenesis and recruit fibroblasts. Fibroblasts synthesize components of granulation tissue, including collagen, elastin and glycosaminoglycans. Macrophages are stimulated by complex carbohydrates, such as β-glucan (Wolk & Danon 1985), and by a constituent of aloe, acemannan (Zhang & Tizard 1996). Both of these ingredients can be found in commercially available wound dressings (acemannan hydrogel, β-glucan-coated contact layer). Theoretically, using materials that activate or recruit wound cells as wound dressings or components of wound dressings could increase the formation of granulation tissue, new blood vessels or facilitate wound debridement. However, once an active ingredient is incorporated into a dressing, it must be available from the dressing to the wound tissues in an amount sufficient to elicit the biological effect observed in studies of the free ingredient. No studies are available on the release of the aforementioned ingredients from the dressings and there are no comparisons of the wound healing effects of the dressings with and without the ingredient.

Macrophages in a human wound model have also been shown to be activated by a particular wound dressing emulsion (Coulomb et al 1997). Collagen has been shown to recruit macrophages and fibroblasts, and is available in sheet, powder and gel forms for use as a wound dressing. Collagen may also act as 'scaffolding' to guide the in-growth of new connective tissue and blood vessels (Mian et al 1992).

Infection and odour control

Semi-occlusive dressings may play a role in infection control by means of their physical barrier properties and creation of a moist wound environment, which optimizes endogenous phagocytic activity. Some semi-occlusive dressings contain active antibacterial ingredients such as iodophors and silver ions. By controlling bacterial levels, such dressings may also facilitate odour control. There are several types of wound dressings (foams, alginate, contact layer) that contain activated charcoal in their composition to absorb odour.

KEY POINTS

♦ Cleansing is a physical process of dislodging and removing foreign materials and microorganisms from the wound bed. Wound cleansing is commonly accomplished through fluid irrigation. Effective cleansing requires appropriate selection of irrigation solution and an appropriate method of delivery to the tissues. Clinicians should be mindful of the effects of both the solution and the delivery method on the delicate tissues of the wound

♦ Wound cleansing should be accomplished using non-cytotoxic solutions and irrigation pressures below 103.5 kPa (15 psi). If there are extensive amounts of necrotic tissue in the wound, simple cleansing may not be adequate and a form of debridement may be indicated

♦ Wound dressings can play a vital role in the overall management of pressure ulcers if used appropriately. Dressing selection should be based on a thorough assessment of the wound. The choice of wound dressing should not be static but should evolve as the wound heals

♦ Dressing selection will vary with the characteristics of the wound. At a minimum, the variables of size, depth, location on the body, viability of the wound tissues, amount of exudate and condition of the periwound skin should play a role in selection. The functions and performance of the dressing selected should mirror the needs of the wound.

PRODUCT PRICE VERSUS TREATMENT COSTS

As a final caveat almost all types of semi-occlusive dressings that create or maintain a physiologically moist wound environment will have a unit price higher than that of gauze and clinicians or facilities often make the mistake of believing that they cannot afford to use the higher-priced dressing. It is vital to differentiate between the price of the dressing and the cost of care. Price refers to the money expended to acquire the product by the unit, the box or the case. Cost, on the other hand, refers to the money spent and includes both the price of the product and the price of the various resources consumed in using it. Examples of such resources include but are not limited to ancillary supplies (cleansers, tapes, gloves, pain-controlling medications, etc.), labour costs associated with caregiver time expenditure (windshield time, dressing change time, etc.), and costs associated with length of stay in the health care setting, and even the cost to the patient in terms of lost work days. It is possible for a product to be inexpensive to acquire but expensive to use because it results in delayed wound healing (relative to another treatment) or increased complications. Conversely, a product that is more expensive to acquire may actually be less expensive to use because it achieves more rapid healing with fewer complications. For a detailed discussion of health economics issues see Chapter 5.

CASE STUDY 10.1

A 72-year-old female is admitted to hospital from a nursing home with a full-thickness pressure ulcer over her right trochanter. The wound is packed with gauze that is fully saturated with serosanguineous exudate. Upon removal of the gauze dressing and assessment, the wound measurements are found to be 8 cm long, 5 cm wide and 3 cm deep. Only granulation tissue is noted in the wound bed. Periwound tissues are intact. The patient is placed on a pressure-relieving surface and evaluated for nutritional status.

1 What method of wound cleansing would be appropriate for this wound?
   (a) Hydrogen peroxide rinse
   (b) Normal saline delivered by gravity from a bottle
   (c) Sodium hypochlorite solution delivered by 35-ml syringe fitted with 19 G catheter tip
   (d) Normal saline delivered by 35-ml syringe fitted with 19 G catheter tip

2 Following irrigation of the wound, how should it be dressed?
   (a) Firmly packed with povidone iodine soaked gauze
   (b) Filled with amorphous hydrogel and covered with adhesive film
   (c) Filled with alginate rope and covered with adhesive film
   (d) Covered with an adhesive foam dressing

SELF-ASSESSMENT QUESTIONS

1 Devise a policy for wound cleansing procedures based on the condition of the wound bed (e.g. normal saline irrigation with appropriate pressure for granulating wounds or wounds with little necrosis, debridement methods for wounds with different types or higher levels of necrosis).

2 Select four types of dressings that you would need at a minimum to manage the majority of pressure sores in your care setting, keeping in mind dressing function and wound needs.

REFERENCES

Angeras M H, Brandberg A, Falk A, Seeman T 1992 Comparison between sterile saline and tap water for the cleaning of acute traumatic soft tissue wounds. European Journal of Surgery 158(6–7):347–350

Becker G D 1986 Identification and management of the patient at high risk for wound infection. Head and Neck Surgery Jan/Feb: 205–220

Chen W Y, Rogers A A, Lydon M J 1992 Characterization of biologic properties of wound fluid collected during the early stages of wound healing. Journal of Investigative Dermatology 99(5):559–564

Coulomb B, Friteau, L, Dubertret L 1997 Biafine applied on human epidermal wounds is chemotactic for macrophages and increases the IL-1/IL-6 ratio. Skin Pharmacology 10(5):281–287

Falanga V, Bourguignon G J, Bourguignon L Y 1987 Electrical stimulation increases the expression of fibroblast receptors for transforming growth factor beta. Journal of Investigative Dermatology 88:488

Flannagan M 1997 Wound cleansing. In: Morison M, Moffatt C, Bridel-Nixon J, Bale S (eds), Nursing management of chronic wounds. Mosby, London, pp. 87–101

Fleming A 1919 The action of chemical and physiological antiseptics in a septic wound. British Journal of Surgery 7:99–129

Gilchrist B 1997 Infection and culturing. In; Krasner D, Kane D (eds) Chronic wound care, 2nd edn. Health Management Publ Inc., Wayne, pp. 109–114

Gruber R P, Vistnes L, Pardoe R 1975 The effect of commonly used antiseptics in wound healing. Plastic and Reconstructive Surg 55(4):472–476

Hedman L A 1988 Effect of a hydrocolloid dressing on the pain level from abrasions on the feet during intensive marching. Military Medicine, 153:188–190

Heenan A 1999 Wound dressing and the Drug Tariff. Journal of Wound Care 8(2):69–72

Hellewell T B, Major D A, Foresman P A, Rodeheaver G T 1997 A cytotoxicity evaluation of antimicrobial and non-antimicrobial wound cleansers. Wounds 9(1):15–20

Hinnman C D, Maibach H I 1963 Effect of air exposure and occlusion on experimental human skin wounds. Nature 200:377–378

Jaffe L F, Vanable J W 1984 Electrical fields and wound healing. Clinics in Dermatology 2(3):34–44

Kilcullen J K, Ly Q P, Chang T H, et al 1998 Nonviable Staphylococcus aureus and its peptidoglycan can stimulate macrophage recruitment, angiogenesis, fibroplasis and collagen accumulation in wounded rats. Wound Repair and Regeneration 6(2):149–156

Kindlen S, Morison M 1997 Physiology of wound healing. In: Morison M, Moffatt C, Bridel-Nixon J, Bale S (eds) A colour guide to nursing management of chronic wounds, 2nd edn. Mosby, London, pp. 1–26

Krasner D 1997 Dressing decisions for the twenty-first century: on the cusp of a paradigm shift. In: Krasner D, Kane D (eds) Chronic wound care, 2nd edn. Health Management Publications, Inc., Wayne, pp. 139–151

Kucan J O, Robson M C, Heggers J P, Ko F 1981 Comparisons of silver sulfadiazine, povidone iodine and physiologic saline in the treatment of chronic pressure ulcers. Journal of the American Geriatrics Society 29(5):232–235

Laato M, Niinikoski J, Lundberg C, Gerdin B 1988 Inflammatory reaction and blood flow in experimental wounds inoculated with Staphylococcus aureus. Eur Surg Res 20(1):33–38

Laato M, Lehtonen O P, Niinikoski J 1985 Granulation tissue formation in experimental wounds inoculated with Staphylococcus aureus. Acta Chir Scand 151(4):313–318

Lamke L O et al 1977 The evaporative water loss from burns and water vapor permeability of grafts and artificial membranes used in the treatment of burns. Burns 3:159–165

Laufman H 1989 Current use of skin and wound cleanser and antiseptics. Am J Surg 157:359–365

Lawrence J C 1997 Wound irrigation. Journal of Wound Care 6(1):23–26

Lawrence J C 1998 The use of iodine as an antiseptic agent. Journal of Wound Care 7(8):421–425

Levenson S M, Kan-Gurber D, Gruber C, et al 1983 Wound healing accelerated by Staphylococcus aureus. Archives of Surgery Mar;118(3):310–320

Martin S J, Corrado O J, Kay E A 1996 Enzymatic debridement for necrotic wounds. Journal of Wound Care Jul;5(7):310–311

Mertz P, Ovington L 1993 Wound healing microbiology. Dermatologic Clinics 11(4):739–748

Mian M, Beghe F, Mian E 1992 Collagen as a pharmacological approach in wound healing. International Journal of Tissue Reaction 14(Suppl):1–9

Moberg S, Hoffman L, Grennert M L, Holst A 1983 A randomized trial of cadexomer iodine in decubitus ulcers. Journal of the American Geriatrics Society 31(8):462–465

Morison M, Moffatt C 1994 A colour guide to the assessment and management of leg ulcers. Mosby, London, pp. 77–81

Moscati R M, Reardon R F, Lerner E B, Mayrose J 1998 Wound irrigation with tap water. Acad Emerg Med Nov;5(11):1076–1080

Nemeth A J, Eaglstein W H, Taylor J R, et al 1991 Faster healing and less pain in skin biopsy sites treated with an occlusive dressing. Archives of Dermatology 127:1679–1683

Ovington L G 1998 The well-dressed wound: an overview of dressing types. Wounds Jan/Feb 10 Supplement A:1A–11A

Riyat M S, Quinton D N 1997 Tap water as a wound cleansing agent in accident and emergency. J Accident and Emergency Medicine 14(3):165–166

Rodeheaver G T, Pettry D, Thacker JG, Edgerton MT 1975 Edlich wound cleansing by high pressure irrigation. Surg Gynecol Obstet Sep;141(3):357–362

Rovee D T, Kurowsky C A, Labun J, Downes A M 1972 Effect of local wound environment. In: Rovee D T, Maibach H (eds) Epidermal wound healing. Year Book Medical Publ, Chicago, pp. 159–181

Smack D, Harrington A, Dunn C, Howard R et al 1996 Infection and allergy incidence in ambulatory surgery patients using white petrolatum versus bactracin ointment. JAMA 276:972–977

Sprung P, Hou Z, Ladin D A 1998 Hydrogels and hydrocolloids: an objective product comparison. Ostomy/Wound Management 44(1):36–53

Stahl-Bayliss C M, Grandy R P, Fitzmartin R D, Chelle C, Oshlack B, Goldenheim P D 1990 The comparative efficacy and safety of 5% povidone-iodine cream for topical antisepsis. Ostomy/Wound Management Nov-Dec;31:40–49

Steed D, Donohoe D, Webster M W, Lindsley L 1996 Effect of extensive debridement and treatment on the healing of diabetic foot ulcers. J Am Coll Surg Jul;183(1):61–64

Thomas S 1990 Functions of a wound dressing. In: Thomas S (ed) Wound management and dressings. Pharmaceutical Press, London, pp. 9–19

Thomas S, Loveless P 1988 Comparative review of the properties of six semipermeable film dressings. The Pharmaceutical Journal June:785–788

Thomas S, Loveless P 1997 A comparative study of the properties of twelve hydrocolloid dressings. World Wide Wounds http://www.smtl.co.uk/world-wide-wounds

Turner T D 1989 The development of wound management products. Wounds 1(3):155–171

van Rijswijk L, Beitz J 1998 The traditions and terminology of wound dressings: food for thought. Journal of Wound, Ostomy and Continence Nursing 25:116–122

Vowden K R, Vowden P 1999a Wound debridement Part 2: Sharp technique. Journal of Wound Care 8(6):291–294

Vowden K R, Vowden P 1999b Wound debridement Part 1: Non-sharp technique. Journal of Wound Care 8(5):237–240

Williams N A, Leaper D J 1998 Infection. In: Leaper D J, Harding K G (eds) Wounds: biology and management. Oxford Medical Publications, Oxford, pp 71–87

Winter G D 1962 Formation of scab and the rate of epithelialization of superficial wounds in the skin of the young domestic pig. Nature 193:293–294

Winter G D 1972 Epidermal regeneration studied in the domestic pig. In Rovee D T, Maibach H (eds) Epidermal wound healing. Year Book Medical Publ, Chicago, pp. 71–112

Wolk M, Danon D 1985 Promotion of wound healing by yeast glucan evaluated on single animals. Medical Biology 63(2):73–80

Zhang L, Tizard I R 1996 Activation of a mouse macrophage cell line by acemannan: the major carbohydrate fraction from *Aloe vera* gel. Immunopharmacology 35(2):119–128

11 *Jens Lykke Sørensen, Bo Jørgensen and Finn Gottrup*

Wound management: surgical intervention

INTRODUCTION

A pressure ulcer is a serious or potentially serious condition that always calls for active treatment. The proportion of pressure ulcers suitable for operation is dependent on the patient population, but normally only a few per cent are candidates for surgery. However, among selected groups of patients, such as spinal cord injured with deep grade III or IV pressure ulcers (Bergstrom et al 1994) surgery may be indicated for the majority.

Pressure ulcers are expensive to treat. Costs are estimated to be £1000–20 000 per year per pressure ulcer (NPUAP 1989, Kuhn & Coulter 1992, Frantz et al 1995). Prevention is found to be cheaper than cure (Regan et al 1995) and surgical treatment can be more expensive than conservative treatment (Siegler & Lavaizzo-Mourey 1991).

The crucial questions are who would benefit from surgical intervention, and how should the pressure ulcers be treated? Surgery should improve the patient's situation as a whole, and it is not always the most obvious surgical method that is the best choice for the individual patient. If the resources, including a committed and well-educated staff on all levels, are not present then surgery is likely to fail since insufficient care and postoperative support make recurrence almost inevitable.

SELECTION OF PATIENTS FOR PRESSURE ULCER SURGERY

No unambiguous criteria for selecting pressure ulcer patients for surgery exist, but decision guidelines, etc., have been developed (Linder & Morris 1990, Siegler & Lavaizzo-Mourey 1991, Bergstrom et al 1994, Pressure Ulcer Guideline Panel 1995, Foster et al 1997). Pressure ulcer surgery is for select groups of patients and indications should be strict, treatment protocols clear, treatment goals realistic and there should be improvement in the patient's quality of life.

Identification of pressure ulcers for surgery

Superficial grade I and II pressure ulcers (Bergstrom et al 1994) should be treated conservatively using optimal ulcer treatment (Ch. 10) and by elimination of local and general conditions interfering with healing (Chs 8 and 9). Clean pressure ulcers which can heal by conservative means require no surgical treatment; however, there are exceptions (see section on Surgical repair).

Deep pressure ulcers are usually candidates for surgery. Deep pressure ulcers lack large amounts of soft tissue and if conservative healing succeeds, the resulting area will consist of stiff and scanty scar tissue. If the patient requires a tissue with high mechanical performance, conservative healed tissue is often of an insufficient quality, and there will be no reason to await healing.

The time factor can also be an indication for surgery. Large wounds often take many months to heal by conservative means: healing is much quicker after surgery.

Long-standing pressure ulcers (years) can result in the development of amyloidosis or malignant degeneration of the pressure ulcer into a Marjolin ulcer, a planocellular carcinoma. These factors should also be considered in the indications for surgery.

Underlying infected bone is also an indication for surgery. Osteomyelitis in pressure ulcers is eliminated by surgery (Deloach et al 1992). Debrided osteomyelitic bone must be covered with soft tissue with a good blood supply to ensure healing (Bergstrom et al 1994).

Identification of patients for surgery

All patients with a grade III or IV pressure ulcer should be evaluated for surgical treatment. However, pressure ulcer patients always have other diseases, making access to the whole patient (and not only the pressure ulcer) extremely important. The patient's ability to tolerate an operation and participate in postoperative rehabilitation must be evaluated. Concurrent diseases must be corrected preoperatively (see section on Preoperative preparation). The risk of anaesthesia and surgery must be weighed against the benefit of elimination of the pressure ulcer. It is possible that some patients may be drug addicts or have daily habits or social circumstances that should be changed before surgery can be recommended. A non-cooperative patient is at overwhelming risk of recurrence and if the rehabilitative outcome cannot be anticipated, surgery should be postponed until the circumstances are under control. Setting the indication for surgery should always be a careful and individually based estimation (Box 11.1). In pressure ulcer patients fit for surgery the absence of appropriate care and pressure relief can eliminate the indication for surgery. The indication for surgery can be more or less absolute, as in sepsis emanating from a decubital focus.

Terminal patients with pressure ulcers are never candidates for surgery. Treatment should be limited to symptomatic bedside treatment to reduce odour and other discomfort. In debilitated patients, debridement without subsequent reconstruction may be the optimal treatment. Patients prone to general recovery can also benefit from an isolated debridement, since a clean cavity can heal after the patient is mobilized and the region relieved of pressure. As mentioned, an operation can shorten the course of healing significantly, bringing about earlier rehabilitation of the patient.

Spinal cord injured patients cannot be expected to regain sensibility. They cannot detect pain caused by pressure and ischaemia, and cannot relieve pressure because of paralysis. These patients need tissue of a sufficient magnitude and quality to withstand unphysiological pressure. Reconstruction of deep pressure ulcers with myocutaneous flaps will usually be indicated for these patients. In other groups, such as patients with sclerosis disseminata in advanced stages, the intellect and frame of mind of the patients must be assessed in order to evaluate the future compliance.

Multitrauma patients easily develop pressure ulcers. They often will recover and the pressure ulcers will heal when the risk factors are eliminated. If nothing is lost by awaiting spontaneous healing and no deeper structures are affected, major surgery is not indicated.

Informed consent of the patient is an obvious prerequisite and is of the utmost importance because of the high rates of complications and recurrences associated with surgery (Garg et al 1992, Bergstrom et al 1994, Evans et al 1994, Foster et al 1997, Niazi & Salzberg 1997).

BOX 11.1 IDENTIFICATION OF PATIENTS FOR SURGERY

1 Identify pressure ulcer patient.

2 Evaluation of pressure ulcer: conservative treatment? Surgery?

3 Evaluation of patient's physical state: concurrent medical diseases? Medical treatment? Fit for anaesthesia and operation?

4 Evaluation of patient's mental state: cooperative? Informed? Motivated? Realistic? Patient's wishes?

5 Evaluation of future: outcome? Rehabilitative possibilities? Social network? Control?

KEY POINTS

◆ Carefully select patients for surgery. Surgery should only be offered to patients who can cooperate and who would benefit from operation

◆ All pressure ulcers must be vigorously treated

◆ Only deep, grossly necrotic or infected pressure ulcers are candidates for surgery

◆ Use the simplest, most effective and least traumatic surgical method

◆ Assessment, prevention, education and control are indispensable parts of surgical pressure ulcer treatment.

SURGERY

The surgical treatment of pressure ulcers consists of debridement and usually some kind of reconstruction with soft tissue padding into the defect. A variety of methods are available (see Surgical repair later in this section).

If patients are subjected to major debridement or reconstructive procedures, they should be transferred to a department for plastic and reconstructive surgery. Minor surgical intervention does not entail transfer.

Preoperative preparation

When seen for the first time the pressure ulcer patient often is not ready for surgery. Conditions impairing healing should be controlled preoperatively.

A pressure ulcer develops when the patient has not had sufficient relief from pressure. Obviously, the surgical treatment of a pressure ulcer is useless if problems of pressure, shear, friction and skin care are not solved first (Ch. 7). Pressure ulcer preventive measures (pressure relief, etc.) should be undertaken throughout the course of treatment, including during surgery when pressure sores can also develop.

Most pressure ulcer patients are undernourished (Ch. 13). If the patient is able to receive nutrition orally, infusion of protein is not indicated; however, protein infusion might be indicated for other reasons such as treatment of severe oedema. Obese patients should not be put on a diet before healing of the pressure ulcers is completed.

Depletion of minerals and vitamins occurs slowly (months), but must still be corrected. Supplying additional minerals to pressure ulcer patients has not proven beneficial unless a deficit pre-exists.

Anaemia is closely related to pressure ulcers (Ch. 6). This anaemia is chronic and iron supplements are indicated only in iron deficit. In severe anaemia, blood transfusion is indicated. Blood volume and erythrocyte concentration should be at least close to normal before anaesthesia, surgery and blood loss.

Dehydration and hypovolaemia must be corrected immediately, in all patients. Dehydration seriously interferes with the peripheral circulation and insufficient circulation aggravates pressure ulcer development and hampers healing. Depending on the patient's condition, rehydration can be performed orally or parenterally. Cardiac decompensation and other factors influencing circulation should also be optimized preoperatively (Ch. 6).

Smoking has a negative influence on healing (Jørgensen et al 1998), and is found to be correlated (although not unequivocally) to the development of pressure ulcers (Bergstrom et al 1994, Rodriques & Garber 1994).

Spasticity and contractures in spinal cord injured patients can have a devastating effect on flap reconstruction and sometimes a negative effect on the development and healing of pressure ulcers (Bergstrom et al 1994, Rodriques & Garber 1994). Medical treatment of spasms or elimination of factors provoking spasms (such as avoiding forceful wound cleansing) can often control spasms. Percutaneous nerve block may be indicated. Surgery on peripheral nerves and on the central nervous system have been used to counter persistent spasms. Neurosurgical intervention on the central nervous system is destructive and should be avoided.

Preoperative treatment with muscle-releasing casts or intraoperative tenotomy can be used to release muscle spasms (Rubayi et al 1990).

If surgery is planned where there is a risk of postoperative contamination with urine or faeces, an indwelling urine catheter and lower bowel emptying is indicated (Niazi & Salzberg 1997).

Pressure ulcers are always colonized by bacteria. This is not necessarily a sign of infection (Sapico et al 1986, Rudensky et al 1992, Bergstrom et al 1994), but the rate of failure to heal and levels of bacterial counts have been found to be directly correlated (Sapico et al 1986, Bergstrom et al 1994). However, Sapico et al (1986) found that the healing of myocutaneous flaps was not influenced by preoperative bacterial counts, although the patient sample was small. Osteomyelitis has also been found not to have a negative influence on the rate of postoperative complications (Thornhill-Joynes et al 1986). Pressure ulcer colonization can be managed by wound cleaning and debridement without the support of antibiotics (Rudensky et al 1992, Bergstrom et al 1994). Sepsis from a pressure ulcer focus is especially dangerous and has a high mortality rate (Bergstrom et al 1994).

Bone underlying deep pressure ulcers should always be investigated preoperatively with conventional X-ray for osteomyelitis, although the images are seldom diagnostic. The clinical appearance, laboratory tests and bone cultures usually secure diagnosis. Scanning and scintigraphic investigations are only used in selected cases (Lewis et al 1988).

In the preparatory phase, the nurse is a key figure. The nurse has the most intense and frequent contact with the patient and is responsible for coordination and execution of treatment in concert with the surgeon. The specialist nurse should be engaged in the care and treatment of the patient as soon as possible. The introduction of tissue viability nurses in the UK has reduced the incidence rate of pressure ulcers and improved their treatment through standardization (Bergstrom et al 1994). The teaching programme is introduced to the patient preoper-

atively and physical training is commenced if the patient is capable.

It is stated that most pressure ulcers can be prevented, and the development of pressure ulcers is evidence of insufficient nursing. This is not true. Even the most enthusiastic pressure ulcer prevention by the most diligent nurse can fail because the innumerable pressure ulcer developing factors cannot all be controlled at all times.

Debridement

The first step in pressure ulcer surgery is sufficient debridement. If correct wound cleansing cannot eliminate purulent secretion or odour, or if necrosis is present, debridement is indicated.

If reconstruction of a pressure ulcer is indicated, debridement should be by a one-step procedure prior to the reconstruction. If the patient is not ready for surgery, a stepwise bedside debridement can be performed if necrotic or infected tissue is present. Acute revision is indicated only in progressing cellulitis or sepsis developing from a pressure ulcer (Bergstrom et al 1994). At the bedside, clean instruments are sufficient for changing dressings and wound cleansing, but for debridement, sterile instruments should be used both at the bedside and in the operating theatre (Bergstrom et al 1994).

Enzymatic debridement and mechanical abrasion is less effective and more expensive than surgical debridement. In the presence of masses of devitalized tissue only surgical debridement is effective (Ch. 10).

When debridement is complete, only healthy and well-perfused tissue must be left. All necrotic, scarified or infected tissue, including bone, heterotopic calcifications and old granulation tissue, should be removed. A safe way to make sure that all of the ulcer cavity wall is removed is to dye the cavity (e.g. with methylene blue) and then remove all coloured tissue. Necrotic tissue is harmful and should, as a rule, be removed since it promotes bacterial growth and hampers healing (Sapico et al 1986, Bergstrom et al 1994). However two exceptions exist:

1 In certain uninfected cases an eschar can be left as a biological dressing as an alternative to debridement, which leaves a defect oozing plasma and housing microorganisms.
2 With an eschar on a heel the soft tissue is scarce and rather immobile, and almost inevitably the pressure lesion is extended to the bone. To protect the calcaneum against desiccation by denudation, an eschar can be left.

In diabetic ulcers the borders should be incised to reveal or prevent retention and infection. Since devitalized tissue is without perfusion, systemic antibiotics are ineffective in eliminating microorganisms in necrotic tissue.

After debridement, bone should be left with a smooth non-prominent surface to reduce local pressure on the reconstructed area (Linder & Morris 1990). In osteomyelitis in the ischial tuberosities only the affected part should be debrided. Prophylactic total ischiectomy is never indicated because urethral fistulas and perineal ulcerations can develop (Linder & Morris 1990, Bergstrom et al 1994).

During debridement, specimens for diagnosis of bacterial growth should be obtained. A tissue biopsy is preferable to a swab culture (Sapico et al 1986, Deloach et al 1992, Bergstrom et al 1994). If the pressure ulcer extends to the bone, a biopsy of the bone involved should be obtained (Lewis et al 1988, Bergstrom et al 1994). Many experts prefer non-invasive diagnosis of osteomyelitis if operative debridement is not planned. However, non-invasive methods, such as aspiration of fluid from the ulcer, are considered less satisfactory (Lewis et al 1988, Bergstrom et al 1994). If clinical osteomyelitis is present, the authors' preference is bone biopsy. Osteomyelitis can be expected in the majority of deep pressure ulcers (Deloach et al 1992). By increasing the number of bone biopsies the probability of obtaining a correct microbiological diagnosis is increased.

Debridement reduces the bacterial counts in an ulcer. Treatment with antibiotics is indicated only if infection is present, or if sepsis is a risk after debridement. If reconstruction is performed immediately after the debridement, antibiotics are compulsory. In cases with active osteomyelitis or sepsis, antibiotics are initiated preoperatively (Bergstrom et al 1994).

Haemostasis must be obtained carefully after debridement. Because of the hyperaemia in the sound tissue surrounding an ulcer, pressure ulcer patients have a significant risk of developing haematomas postoperatively. After debridement, the bleeding from minor vessels should be controlled with a dry gauze dressing loosely applied in the cavity until the next change of dressing after 8–24 h. If later reconstruction is planned, the cavity can be loosely packed with a disinfecting bandage, which can be left untouched until reconstruction. Wingate et al (1992) suggested prophylactic desmopressin to reduce perioperative bleeding.

Debridement and wound cleansing of a pressure ulcer should not be painful to the patient. Anaesthesia or sufficient analgesics can solve problems with pain but can also create new problems. If patients are anaesthetized often, or are constantly loaded with major analgesics, their ability to be mobilized or nourish sufficiently will be affected. The source of pain should be eliminated, e.g. by gentle technique, sharp instruments and selection of proper bandages. Anaesthesia is not necessary at every debridement and should be reserved for thorough debridement at infection or for reconstructive procedures. Analgesics should, if needed, be administered at sufficient strength and dose prior to debridement or a change of bandage.

A particular problem is debridement in spinal cord injured patients with spinal lesions above the fifth thoracic segment. In these patients, debridement or other manipulation of the pressure ulcer can provoke autonomic hyperreflexia. This is a potentially dangerous condition with critical elevation of blood pressure as the most important symptom. If autonomic hyperreflexia occurs, manipulation of the patient has to be stopped immediately and the blood pressure decreased by acute reduction of vascular tone. Spinal cord injured patients with complete lesion above the pressure ulcer can usually be operated on without anaesthesia. However, the patient must be prepared for immediate anaesthesia and be carefully observed during the surgical procedure.

In cases where immediate reconstruction is not an option, and where rapid growth of fresh granulation tissue is advantageous, vacuum assisted closure (VAC) is an option (Banwell 1999). Granulation tissue for split-thickness skin grafting is obtained quickly, while secondary healing of pressure ulcers by VAC treatment takes several weeks. The resulting shrinkage of the cavity using VAC is of no advantage if reconstruction is planned. The cavity formed is smaller, but the surrounding tissue is less compliant than untreated debrided tissue.

When reconstruction is considered, it must be decided whether debridement and reconstruction can be performed in one or two sessions. If treatment is split into two separate operations, time will be available to achieve a microbiological diagnosis. Sealing the pressure ulcer defect with a flap can conceal the development of haematoma or infection beneath the reconstructed tissue. This risk may be reduced as these complications will develop before the reconstruction is accomplished. The great advantage of a single-session procedure is the reduction of time and resources. The current trend seems to favour a single-session procedure (Anthony et al 1992, Foster et al 1997). The authors prefer a two-session procedure in pressure ulcers where bone is affected or there is a major bacterial presence.

Surgical repair

Always choose the least demanding procedure available for the goals decided upon for the individual patient (Box 11.2).

Direct closure

Direct closure is a very simple method. Nevertheless it is rarely indicated in pressure ulcer surgery (Bergstrom et al 1994): where a pressure ulcer has developed, the tissue has vanished. Often, the edges of the pressure ulcer surface can be forced together, but this will lead to increased tension in the superficial tissue and a

KEY POINTS

♦ Surgical treatment of pressure ulcers must always be individualized

♦ Direct suture is seldom advisable. It is only to be used where there is an abundance of loose tissue

♦ Split-thickness skin grafting is indicated in granulating superficial pressure ulcers where there is no need to withstand significant pressure or friction

♦ Cutaneous flaps are indicated when no deeper structures are affected and no greater mechanical stresses are expected on the area

♦ Myocutaneous flaps are the treatment of choice for deep pressure ulcers when deep structures are affected, bulk in the cavity is needed or greater mechanical load is expected in the region.

deep cavity – factors participating in the development of pressure ulcers (Chs 3 and 6) – and dehiscence (Anthony et al 1992, Bergstrom et al 1994). In some cases where the lack of tissue is not too great, direct suture might occasionally be possible and advisable. In the authors' experience very few pressure ulcers are suitable for direct closure.

Split-thickness skin grafting

Split-thickness skin grafting is another simple method, but patients must be carefully selected.

About 10–15% of our patients are treated by split-thickness skin grafting. Often, these patients have several or recurrent pressure ulcers.

A skin graft will only take if it is transplanted to a clean well-vascularized bed and immobilized during healing. The skin graft will heal in about 10 days, but it should not be subjected to involuntary mechanical loading for about 3 weeks. Moderate pressure does not hamper healing of a skin graft. If the pressure helps to immobilize the transplant, as with tie-over dressings, it might be desirable. Even a well-healed split-thickness skin graft will never be as good as the original soft tissue cover. The graft consists of epidermis and a part of the dermis without the usual skin adnexas. This makes the transplant thinner and less pliable. Furthermore no extra tissue will be added over time, e.g. subcutaneous tissue will not grow beneath the graft, which makes it unsuitable for covering defects without soft tissue padding underlying the granulation tissue. Skin grafts easily erode if they are subjected to maceration or friction (Smith & Aston 1991).

Split-thickness skin grafting is indicated for large, shallow and well-granulating pressure ulcers, and when the pressure ulcer area can be expected to be protected from non-physiological high-pressure loading in the future. Large surfaces can often be eliminated by split-thickness skin grafting, avoiding oozing of protein and liquid. A split-thickness skin graft has better surface quality than the epithelial cover obtained by conservative healing of a large area.

Cultivated skin products have been developed, but no expertise in the use of these in pressure ulcer surgery currently exists.

Full-thickness skin grafting

Full-thickness skin grafts consist of all the dermal and epidermal elements. This makes the graft thicker and more resistant to loading. However, this thicker graft has higher demands on the recipient bed and, for practical reasons (the donor site cannot heal spontaneously without scarification and must be sutured or covered with a split skin graft), is of limited size. The authors have only infrequently used a full-thickness skin graft in pressure ulcer surgery. The indication is usually a well-granulating superficial pressure ulcer on a surface likely to be subjected to future pressure or friction, such as the heel or other part of the foot. When full-thickness skin grafts are indicated, a flap would often be an equally good alternative.

Local flaps

Flaps can be categorized according to the type of vascular supply or the types of tissue in the flaps (i.e. skin, fascia and muscle). Random flaps have no specific blood supply. Because of lack of well-defined vessels supplying blood throughout the flaps they are of limited dimensions and consist of one or a few tissue layers (skin, subcutis, fascia). Flaps carrying well-defined vessels (axial flaps) have a much wider range of reconstructive abilities regarding size, versatility and tissue constituents (Strauch et al 1990, Smith & Aston 1991).

Skin flaps were used as the standard surgical treatment of pressure ulcers a few decades ago. They are now usually only used as alternatives when better options are unavailable. Skin flaps can literally be raised anywhere on the body, but if the surroundings of the pressure ulcer are not loose and sound, the flap will not solve the problem of insufficient soft tissue; it will only redistribute the inadequacy. In sacral pressure ulcers of limited size with no bone involvement a local skin flap is often the first choice (Linder & Morris 1990, Strauch et al 1990).

Fasciocutaneous flaps have a better blood supply than most random cutaneous flaps. The extra padding supplied by the fascia is of limited significance from the view of pressure distribution. The subcutaneous tissue between the skin and fascia will all be integrated in the fasciocutaneous flaps, but subcutaneous tissue is of limited value in pressure ulcer treatment because of its low resistance to pressure and tear and modest blood supply (Ch. 3). Fasciocutaneous flaps are suitable for the reconstruction of selected grade III or IV pressure ulcers without underlying osteomyelitis and without non-physiological loading. Scrotal flaps have been used to cover perineal pressure sores; it should be advantageous that the skin can slide on a multitude of fascias, but we have not found this type of flap satisfactory.

Myocutaneous flaps are the treatment of choice in reconstructive procedures for deep pressure ulcers (Rubayi et al 1990, Anthony et al 1992, Bergstrom et al 1994, Foster et al 1997, Niazi & Salzberg 1997). The myocutaneous flap offers the best opportunity for supplying the pressure ulcer cavity with sufficient bulk containing both excellent blood supply (muscle) and normal integumental cover (full-thickness skin). Yet, it must be noted that muscle has a low tolerance for ischaemic injury. From an anatomical point of view there is no reason for transposition of muscle into a pressure ulcer cavity, since these pressure point areas do not, under normal circumstances, contain muscle. Experiments indicate that muscle beneath pressure-loaded skin is an advantage (Naito & Ogata 1994). The flap should be designed large enough for reuse in case of recurrence. The donor site can usually be closed directly, which is preferable to skin transplantation or secondary flaps.

The flaps are usually elevated (i.e. freed from their surroundings) until they are attached only by their vascular pedicles, making the flap very pliable. Raising a myocutaneous flap affects or eliminates the function of the muscle, providing a balance between optimal coverage and normal muscular function. Some muscles, such as the tensor fascia latae muscle, are expendable in all patients. Others, such as the gluteus maximus muscle, are essential and should not be used in patients expected to be ambulatory postoperatively. In some instances, e.g. the gluteus maximus muscle and the quadriceps (Strauch et al 1990, Smith & Aston 1991, Hagerty & Gould 1995), the muscle can be split in order to both preserve function and obliterate a pressure ulcer cavity.

Reconstruction with myocutaneous flaps is major surgery, and selection of suitable patients is important to avoid causing harm. Spinal cord injured patients can usually be offered reconstruction with otherwise inexpendable muscles because of the lack of voluntary function of the muscle in question (Kroll & Hamilton 1989, Strauch et al 1990, Smith & Aston 1991, Bergstrom et al 1994). In other situations, the importance of eliminating a pressure ulcer cavity will have a higher priority than the muscle function: osteomyelitis will be most effectively treated by using highly vascularized muscle tissue.

About 80% of our pressure ulcer patients receiving reconstructive procedures are treated with myocutaneous flaps.

BOX 11.2 CHOOSING THE LEAST DEMANDING PROCEDURE

1 Identify pressure ulcers

2 Evaluate each pressure ulcer: location? Grade? Size? Tissue viability? Infection?

3 Treatment options for each pressure ulcer: pressure relief? Wound cleansing? Debridement? Reconstruction?
  — Pressure relief: mobilize patient? Support surface?
  — Wound cleansing: dressing? Technique? Debridement? Antibiotics?
  — Debridement: at bedside? In the theatre? One or more sessions?
  — Reconstruction: direct suture? Skin grafting? Cutaneous flap? Myocutaneous flap? Unconventional procedures? Alternatives?

Advanced and unconventional procedures

Sensate flaps (i.e. flaps containing intact sensory nerves) have been used in spinal cord injured patients to provide skin cover with sensation (Kuhn & Coulter 1992, Niazi & Salzberg 1997) to otherwise anaesthetized skin. Recurrence rates might be reduced with the use of sensate flaps (Kuhn & Coulter 1992, Bergstrom et al 1994), but new sensation can have the form of unpleasant dysaesthesiae. This makes the patients move any loading to just outside the sensate part of the flap, to an insensitive area, and a new pressure ulcer can develop (Kuhn & Coulter 1992). An accessible flap can be raised from areas with intact sensation, such as the tensor fascia latae flap to the pelvic region (Kuhn & Coulter 1992).

Free flaps are muscle or myocutaneous flaps totally freed from the donor side and connected to vessels at the recipient site by microsurgical techniques. Free flaps in pressure ulcer surgery are only rarely described in the literature (Park & Koa 1998). Free flap procedures are time-consuming and resource demanding and probably should be limited to a last recourse.

Tissue expansion has been introduced in the treatment of pressure ulcers as skin expansion (Espositio et al 1991) or expansion of several tissue layers (Gray et al 1990, Bergstrom et al 1994). By expanding the tissue surrounding a pressure ulcer by gradually inflating expanders beneath the tissue in question more local tissue will be available. However, experience in this field is limited.

Reinforcing the tissue covering former or threatening pressure ulcer areas has been attempted using carbon fibre pads. Minns & Sutton (1991) found the method encouraging, with a success rate of 68%.

Flap selection

The anatomical site of the pressure ulcer naturally has a pronounced influence on the selection of flaps. A certain consensus exists about the selection of flaps for the different pressure ulcer locations (Linder & Morris 1990).

Sacral pressure ulcers neighbouring the edges of the gluteus maximus muscles make the gluteus maximus myocutaneous flap the first choice (Fig. 11.1). The muscles, although inexpendable for normal gait can be used in spinal cord injured patients or others without ambulatory function, but should at least be partly preserved in walking patients (Fig. 11.2). Muscle and myocutaneous flaps consisting of only half the muscle can be created (Strauch et al 1990) (Fig. 11.2). A distally based flap is also a possibility. This type of flap has the advantage of being free of suture lines in the area used for sitting (Strauch et al 1990) (Fig. 11.1). A large number of flaps based on the gluteus maximus have been developed (Rubayi

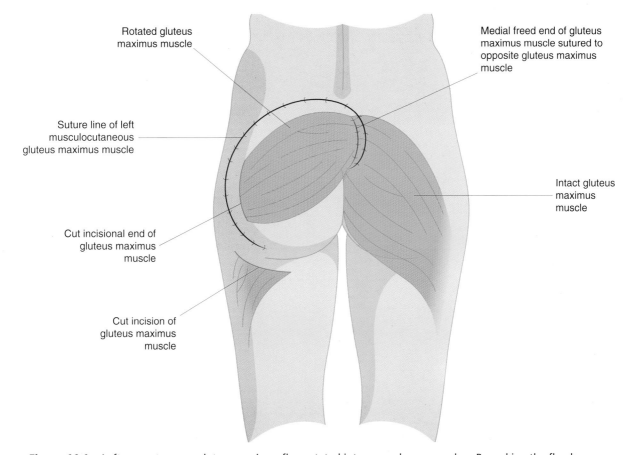

Rotated gluteus maximus muscle

Medial freed end of gluteus maximus muscle sutured to opposite gluteus maximus muscle

Suture line of left musculocutaneous gluteus maximus muscle

Intact gluteus maximus muscle

Cut incisional end of gluteus maximus muscle

Cut incision of gluteus maximus muscle

Figure 11.1 Left myocutaneous gluteus maximus flap rotated into a sacral pressure ulcer. By making the flap large, no split-thickness skin graft was necessary to cover the donor site.

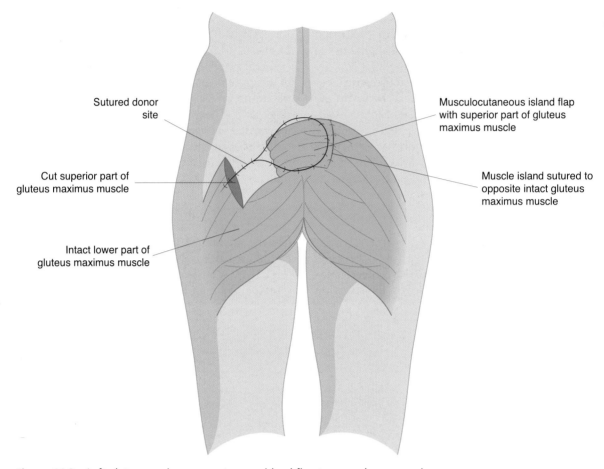

Sutured donor site

Musculocutaneous island flap with superior part of gluteus maximus muscle

Cut superior part of gluteus maximus muscle

Muscle island sutured to opposite intact gluteus maximus muscle

Intact lower part of gluteus maximus muscle

Figure 11.2 Left gluteus maximus myocutaneous island flap to a sacral pressure ulcer.

et al 1990, Strauch et al 1990, Aggrawal et al 1996) (Figs 11.1–11.4). Flaps based on gluteus maximus are safe, but the dissection is often bloody. In patients with old spinal cord injury the atrophy of the muscle may be pronounced, making identification difficult (Bergstrom et al 1994). If the flap is planned correctly, the donor site often can be closed directly. The potential size of the gluteus maximus flap and the symmetrical location usually also makes these flaps usable as a secondary option. Alternatives such as a thoracolumber flap or more distant flaps are available (Strauch et al 1990).

Ischial pressure ulcers are one of the most frequent types of pressure ulcer on the pelvis. Several suitable flaps are available (Kroll & Hamilton 1989, Linder & Morris 1990, Strauch et al 1990, Angrigiani et al 1995, Foster et al 1997). The primary choice for the authors is a flap based on the hamstrings. This is a versatile and safe flap, which can be readvanced a few times (Kroll & Hamilton 1989), which is why it should always be raised primarily in its full length. The proximal part of the flap can be de-epithelialized and swept around the ischial tuberosity as extra padding. By modifying the muscle content, the flap can be used in spinal cord injured patients, who use muscle spasms to ease movement, and in ambulant patients. Our second choice (but for several authors the primary choice) for isolated ischial pressure ulcers is a myocutaneous gluteus maximus flap (Linder & Morris 1990). The tensor fascia latae flap can easily cover an ischial ulcer, and in patients with sensory loss below third

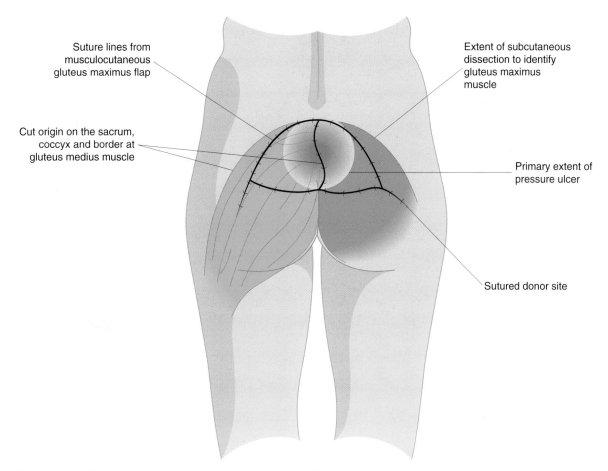

Suture lines from musculocutaneous gluteus maximus flap

Cut origin on the sacrum, coccyx and border at gluteus medius muscle

Extent of subcutaneous dissection to identify gluteus maximus muscle

Primary extent of pressure ulcer

Sutured donor site

Figure 11.3 Bilateral gluteus maximus myocutaneous V–Y flaps to a sacral pressure ulcer. Note the Z-form suture line between the flaps: the upper and lower corners of the flaps neighbouring the pressure ulcer have been used instead of resection of the corners and a straight suture line.

lumbar level this flap can bring sensibility to the ischial area (see Advanced and unconventional procedures earlier in this section; Linder & Morris 1990). We usually only use this flap for closure of an ischial pressure ulcer if it is concomitant with a trochanteric ulcer, and both can be closed with the same flap. This method has the disadvantage that much of the flap closure is in the area used in sitting and the donor site often needs a split-thickness skin graft for closure. A gracilis myocutaneous flap is also accessible, but only for small or moderate-sized ischial defects. Some authors (Foster et al 1997) have found a significantly greater rate of success with the inferior gluteus maximus island flap and the inferior

gluteal thigh flap compared with the hamstring flap and the tensor fascia latae flap.

Trochanteric pressure ulcers can primarily be closed with a tensor fascia latae flap (Siddique et al 1993, Bergstrom et al. 1994, Ercöcen et al 1998). The flap is safe with a good blood supply, the muscle is expendable and, used for the present purpose, the donor defect can normally be closed directly (Fig. 11.5); otherwise the donor site is closed with a split-thickness skin graft. The second choice is the vastus lateralis, the rectus femoris flap or the inferior-based gluteus maximus flap (Linder & Morris 1990, Strauch et al 1990).

Pressure ulcers on the heel are common, but should usually be treated conservatively. When

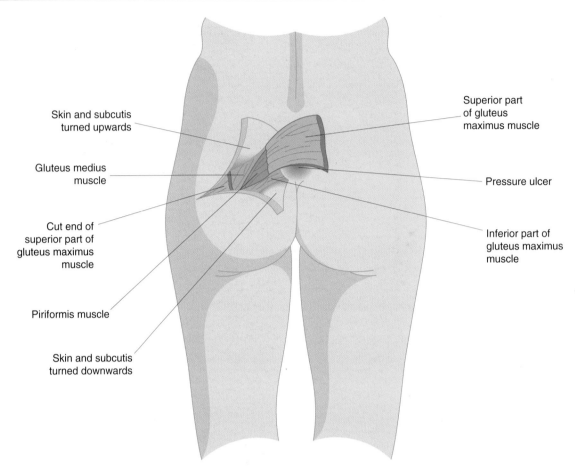

Skin and subcutis
turned upwards

Gluteus medius
muscle

Cut end of
superior part of
gluteus maximus
muscle

Piriformis muscle

Skin and subcutis
turned downwards

Superior part
of gluteus
maximus muscle

Pressure ulcer

Inferior part of
gluteus maximus
muscle

Figure 11.4   Left gluteus maximus muscle flap to a sacral pressure ulcer. The upper part of the muscle is released laterally and turned, much as a page in a book, into the pressure ulcer. The donor site is sutured and the muscle is covered with a split-thickness skin graft.

necessary, heel ulcers can be covered with a suralis fasciocutaneous flap or local muscle flaps (Strauch et al 1990).

Deep pressure ulcers on toes with osteomyelitis are usually best treated with amputation of the toe. The healing potential must be assessed before surgery is commenced.

In addition to the locations already mentioned, less commonly pressure ulcers can develop over any bony prominence on the extremities. The malleoli, the knee, and the elbow are most often affected. Depending on the involvement of bone, local cutaneous, myocutaneous, or possibly pure muscle flaps are available (Strauch et al 1990, Smith & Aston 1991).

In the head, an abundance of flaps are available, but pressure ulcers in this location are not frequent and usually have a short history with intact deep structures. The rich blood supply in the region almost abolishes the need for flap reconstruction.

Several locations on the upper trunk are prone to develop pressure ulcers in at-risk patients (Ch. 3). Local cutaneous or fasciocutaneous flaps are usually sufficient treatment but, when needed, myocutaneous flaps are also available (Strauch et al 1990, Smith & Aston 1991).

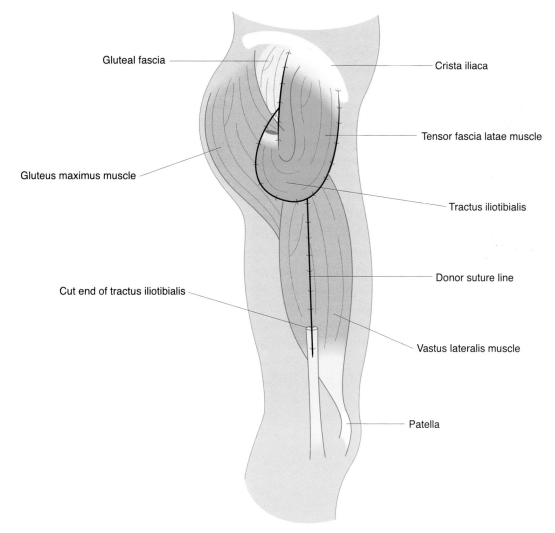

Gluteal fascia

Crista iliaca

Tensor fascia latae muscle

Gluteus maximus muscle

Tractus iliotibialis

Donor suture line

Cut end of tractus iliotibialis

Vastus lateralis muscle

Patella

Figure 11.5 Right tensor fascia latae flap covering a right trochanteric pressure ulcer. Crista iliaca is the proximal border of the muscle. Often, it is unnecessary to free the flap all the way to this line. The tip of the flap is folded posteriorly and sutured to the adjacent posterior border of the flap.

Extensive, multiple and recurrent pressure ulcers

Extensive pressure ulcers are defined as pressure ulcers too large to heal secondarily or to be treated surgically by a single flap (Bergstrom et al 1994). Of these patients, 30–70% have more than one pressure ulcer at admission (Ch. 2; Thornhill-Joynes et al 1986, Garg et al 1992).

Extensive pressure ulcers are located in the pelvic region when reconstruction becomes an option. Large amounts of tissue are needed. A total thigh flap gives good soft tissue covering and can be folded to cover large defects on the ipsilateral pelvis, making wheelchair ambulation possible (Royer et al 1969). Since a hip disarticulation is necessary, only the presence of major pressure lesions justify the thigh flap. Modifications can be performed without amputation of the entire, or part of the extremity (Peters & Johnson 1990). A rectus abdominis myocutaneous flap is also a possibility (Kierney et al 1998). Spinal cord injured patients are the most common target group. To prevent spasms from tearing the flap, external fixation may be indicated for a few weeks. Ablative surgery with elimination of the whole region containing the pressure lesion sometimes may be indicated as the only possibility of controlling a pressure ulcer.

Multiple pressure ulcers should be treated in as few sessions as possible (Rubayi et al 1990). To treat one or a few pressure ulcers at separate sessions prolongs the course. Postoperatively, multiple flaps may call for special regimens and beds since positioning will often be a problem (see below; Ch. 7).

Recurrence is a special and all too common challenge with recurrence rates of 5–56% or even higher in special risk groups (Rubayi et al 1990, Evans et al 1994, Aggrawal et al 1996, Niazi & Salzberg 1997). The lack of tissue is pronounced in a recurrent ulcer, where the reconstructed or adjacent tissue has broken down.

There is no major difference in the treatment of primary and recurrent pressure ulcers. The design of the flap should preferably avoid hampering alternative local flaps, i.e. by cutting important blood vessels or scarifying future flaps. (A pressure ulcer can also recur after a second repair!) If a patient repeatedly develops pressure ulcers, the indication for continued surgery and the rehabilitation possibilities must be carefully considered.

The general technique for raising a myocutaneous flap is as follows:

1 After thorough debridement (Figs 11.6 and 11.7), the borders of the flap are drawn on the skin with the patient in a position that gives good access to the region. The skin and subcutaneous tissue is incised in sweeping cuts to the deep fascia.
2 The fascia is opened and is sutured to the skin and underlying muscle with a few sutures to prevent the skin island from being torn off the muscle.
3 The muscle is released from the surroundings, usually only leaving the vascular pedicle untouched (Fig. 11.8). Sometimes the muscle only needs to be partially released, and then the vessels do not need to be visualized.

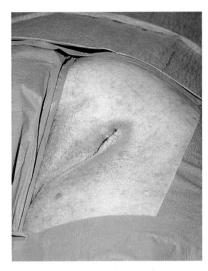

Figure 11.6　Right grade IV ischial pressure ulcer. Note the small skin defect. The skin could be closed without tension, but tissue is missing in the depth.

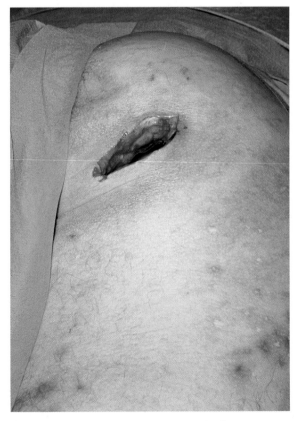

Figure 11.7　Right ischial pressure ulcer after debridement (same as Fig. 11.6).

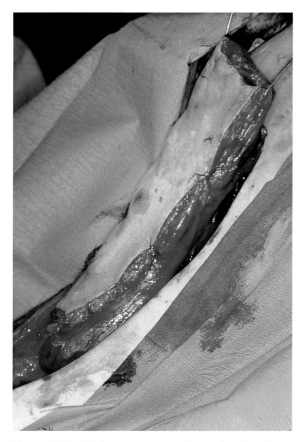

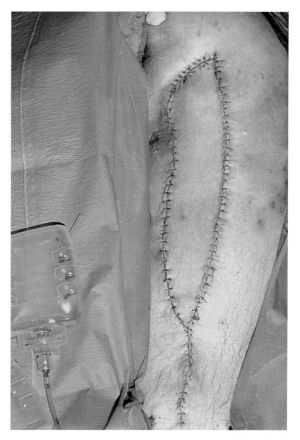

Figure 11.8 Right myocutaneous hamstring flap. Note mobilization of the flap across the ischial pressure ulcer defect (same as Figs 11.6 and 11.7).

Figure 11.9 Right myocutaneous V–Y hamstring flap covering a right ischial pressure ulcer (same as Figs 11.6–11.8).

4 The flap is now transpositioned into the pressure ulcer cavity and suturing is commenced (Fig. 11.9). Most frequently, myocutaneous flaps are needed in the pelvic region. The authors' favourites are shown in Table 11.1.

Closure of the surgical wound should be performed in layers to approximate the different tissue layers, keeping the whole area of sufficient and uniform thickness. Pull-out sutures can be used advantageously to place the deep muscle, to obliterate dead space and around bone. The number of sutures is a compromise between effective closure and a minimal amount of foreign material in the wound. Sutures should be removed when the wound is strong enough, usually after 2–3 weeks.

Table 11.1 Pressure ulcer location and surgical alternatives for reconstruction (authors' suggestions for repair). Notice the versatility of the gluteus maximus muscles in the treatment of sacral pressure ulcers

Pressure ulcer	First choice	Second choice
Sacral	Gluteus maximus	Gluteus maximus
Ischial	Hamstrings	Gluteus maximus
Trochanteric	Tensor fascia latae	Vastus lateralis

Drains are indispensable in flap surgery to reduce the risk of complications from haematoma. Suction drainage should be used. The drains should be left until drainage is limited to 10–20 cm^3. It has been suggested that suction prevents the formation of cavities beneath the flaps. If this effect is desired, drainage should be left for

2 weeks (Aggrawal et al 1996). However, the suction tube is a foreign body and a template for a tunnel from the surface to the obliterated space beneath the flap. If the tube is left too long, it can be a possible entrance for infective organisms. Foreign bodies also increase the risk of infection in a contaminated wound. The authors leave the drains in the former pressure ulcer cavity for 2 weeks and remove the drains in the donor site after a few days.

A thin, permeable bandage, for example a single layer of paper plaster, is found sufficient by us to cover the suture lines.

Antibiotics should always be administered in major reconstructive procedures for pressure ulcers (Garg et al 1992). In a wound without necrosis or infection a prophylactic dose given preoperatively is sufficient. If the operation is prolonged, the dose can be repeated, depending on the antibiotic used. If there has been bone involvement, or if the risk of infection is increased, administration of relevant antibiotics should be continued. In order to prevent postoperative infection it is advocated that antibiotics are used for 5 to 7 days (Garg et al 1992, Niazi & Salzberg 1997). Antibiotics against anaerobic organisms should be included for pressure ulcers in the pelvic region (Garg et al 1992). Since no consensus exists and no scientific proof has been published, both the length of the therapy and the choice of antibiotics vary. If no specific bacteria have been identified, the authors use a second-generation cephalosporin. This treatment can be given with metronidazole and possibly an aminoglycoside with increased risk of infection.

Prolonged administration of antibiotics is indicated in the treatment of osteomyelitis. Although no unequivocal recommendation exists, 2 weeks to 3 months are advocated (Thornhill-Joynes et al 1986, Anthony et al 1992, Deloach et al 1992). The authors prefer treatment for 3 months, but there is no evidence that extended antibiotic therapy reduces the risk of complications or recurrence (Thornhill-Joynes et al 1986). The antibiotics should only be stopped after leucocyte counts and erythrocyte sedimentation rate have been normalized. Initially, antibiotics are administered intravenously and after 2 weeks oral administra-

tion is commenced. Longer parenteral administration is often used (Deloach et al 1992).

Local administration of antibiotics is, in our opinion, not indicated in reconstructive procedures.

POSTOPERATIVE CARE

The surgical procedure is only one step in the successful surgical treatment of pressure ulcers. If sufficient measures are not taken postoperatively, the result will be recurrence.

Postoperative pressure ulcer prevention

After surgery, the operated area is still at risk. The region must be relieved of pressure to avoid impairment of the circulation in the flap and to avoid the development of a new pressure ulcer. The region can be relieved in two ways. The patient can be positioned to totally relieve the region, e.g. a hamstring flap can be relieved in the prone position. Tetraplegics, patients that are severely overweight and certain other patients might have respiratory problems if they are placed prone. Ulnar nerve compression and confusion have been described in a long-lasting prone position (Bergstrom et al 1994). Alternatively, the patient can be placed on a surface with sufficient pressure relief. Turning regimens must often be commenced. Patients are lifted into the new position (never slid). If possible, turning should be avoided to spare the flap from strain, but no new pressure ulcer caused by immobilization should be allowed to develop. The bed should be positioned to avoid visual isolation of the patient, e.g. turn the bed and remove the headboard to allow the patient a view other than the wall. Television, newspapers and conversation should be among the easily accessible entertainments.

A number of specialized beds and mattresses are available (Ch. 7). Air-fluidized beds and some of the low-air-loss beds are recommended for relieving pressure on flaps (Allen et al 1993, Niazi & Salzberg 1997). The time advocated for postoperative pressure relief is usually between 2 and 3 weeks, but up to 8 weeks has been advocated (Bergstrom et al 1994). A period of 3 weeks is the authors' choice.

After pressure relief the flap should be progressively loaded both according to pressure (from prone to supine and from supine to sitting) and time (from initially 15 min to the maximum of 2 h by doubling the time). A flap can usually be fully conditioned within 8–10 days. Some (Rubayi et al 1990) use a different schedule. In patients with normal mobility, usual behaviour can be resumed. In high-risk patients, pressure ulcer regions, operated or not, should never be loaded for more than 2 h. This has been shown experimentally as well as clinically to be a comparatively safe limit (Ch. 3; Bergstrom et al 1994). For practical reasons, wheelchair seating for several hours must often be accepted. A fixed plan for loading and mobilization should exist, but individual considerations should be acceptable. The patient should regularly, i.e. once per week, be assessed to evaluate the selected support surface.

Postoperative patient care

A convalescent should be offered an increased input of proteins and energy and a dietician should be a frequent guest in the department.

Contamination of the operation wound should be avoided in the first 3–5 days after surgery. In risk areas, an indwelling urine catheter and low-fibre or fluid diet in combination with constipating medicine can be helpful (Rubayi et al 1990, Bergstrom et al 1994, Niazi & Salzberg 1997). In patients with spinal cord lesions autonomic stimuli can provoke spasms or, if the spinal lesion is above the fifth thoracic segment, autonomic hyperreflexia.

Postoperative rehabilitation includes physical training to make the patient able to relieve pressure by moving; if possible, patients are mobilized. Spinal cord injured patients are taught to shift pressure intermittently by rocking or elevating the buttocks from the seat, etc. Caregivers should teach patients to take responsibility for themselves to a degree consistent with the patient's general condition and intellect. The patients must be instructed in daily visual control of the operated area and other pressure

risk areas and to take relevant action when signs of a pressure lesion are discovered.

Pressure ulcer prevention programmes with education and documentation of the action taken and follow up (US Department of Health and Human Services 1992, Bergstrom et al 1994) are important tools in reducing the recurrence rates and the prevention of new pressure ulcers. It should be noted that low compliance and carelessness of the patient are important reasons for recurrence (Maklebust & Magnan 1988).

THE NURSE'S ROLE

Without an educated and committed staff on all levels the surgical treatment of pressure ulcers is futile. The nurse's role in nursing and treating pressure ulcer patients cannot be overestimated. The Agency for Health Care Policy and Research's (1992) tenet 'surveillance, assessment, and intervention' embraces the nurse's work. A major goal is identification of the at-risk patient. The many problems with this are discussed in Chapter 6. Postoperatively, the patient is not necessarily in the same risk group as preoperatively, so assessment should not stop at the surgery. As with assessment, pressure ulcer prevention is a continuous process. Postoperatively, the demand for pressure ulcer prevention will change as the patient recovers.

General approach

When shall the nurse intervene? Always! And almost always in a multidisciplinary way. A pressure lesion must without exception be treated, and risk factors should always be detected and controlled.

A patient with a pressure ulcer has a high risk for developing another pressure ulcer in the peri- and postoperative period. Surveillance of the patient involves review of the whole body, with daily inspection of all pressure ulcer risk areas, control of correct function of the pressure-relieving device and attention to the patient's general condition. Different assessment scales exist (see Chs 6 and 8). Skin maintenance and ulcer cleansing is dealt with in Chapter 10 and pressure ulcer prevention and support surfaces in Chapter 7.

The nurse has a central role in the education of patients and relatives because of the frequent and close contact with the patients. This offers an opportunity for better contact, which is essential for effective instruction in prevention of pressure lesions and self-concern (Maklebust & Magnan 1988).

Postoperative care

The postoperative surveillance of a pressure ulcer patient does not deviate from the routines for other patients after comparable operations and conditions. In a few aspects the post pressure ulcer patient calls for special attention:

- The need for general pressure relieving is more pronounced than for most other patient groups.
- The operated area often needs total pressure relief (see 'Postoperative pressure ulcer prevention' in the previous section).

The reconstructed area should be observed intensively in the first postoperative period in case of flap failure. An adequate support surface and proper positioning takes these aspects into account. The flap is checked for underlying haematoma (the flap bulges and eventually changes colour; the area might become tense or fluctuate; blood may ooze from the suture lines). Insufficient circulation on the arterial side is indicated by a pale flap without capillary response. This can be caused by kinking of the flap or the vessels, external or internal pressure or stretching, or erroneous surgical method with insufficient arterial supply. In the case of venous insufficiency a cyanotic, congested flap develops from external or internal compressed venous outflow. This condition is as dangerous for flap survival as arterial insufficiency. Dehiscence is a symptom of spasms, too small a flap or incorrect positioning of the patient.

During rehabilitation, the flap should be inspected after each period of loading for signs of compromised circulation or mechanical overloading. The viability is assessed by inspecting the colour. Pallor will disappear a few seconds after removing the pressure. Reactive hyperaemia is a normal reaction to ischaemia, making redness of a flap after loading a physiological phenomenon,

but it should disappear within 30 min. A healthy flap looks like the normal skin on the donor site.

Measuring the surface temperature or blood flow in the flap is indicated under special circumstances, such as after free flap surgery. Simple clinical control is usually sufficient, but if temperature control is used, one should bear in mind that the temperature of the flap is influenced by the surroundings, thus obscuring the genuine flap temperature. Laser Doppler or transcutaneous oxygen measurements can also be used to monitor flap circulation.

The sutured incisional lines must be kept clean and dry to prevent infection. Crusts and contamination are carefully removed. Non-irritant liquids such as sterile saline are preferred. Manipulations should be kept to a minimum.

If complications arise, early action is mandatory and usually includes calling the surgeon.

Dealing with complications

Haematomas or seromas should be evacuated as soon as possible. If the patients are not in antibiotic therapy, they should be treated with a prophylactic in connection with evacuation of the accumulated fluid.

The treatment of insufficient circulation in the flap depends on the cause. Correction of positioning and support surfaces sometimes solve the problem. Removal of sutures can remove tension from the flap. If sutures are removed, the defect must be protected from contamination and infection. In other instances, the microcirculation can be improved by plasma expanders or other types of medication, thus bringing the local circulation to an acceptable level. Hyperbaric oxygen increases systemic oxygen supply and can make the flap survive until its own blood supply is improved (Deloach et al 1992). In some instances, surgery is necessary to regain sufficient circulation; if the circulation can only be secured by bringing the flap back to the donor side, this can be done. By delaying transposition of the flap about 1 week or more, circulation can adapt, allowing the flap to survive. In any flap failure it must be considered whether planning or surgery have been inadequate.

If the flap slowly develops necrosis, usually at the borders, an expectant attitude with deferment of surgery is assumed initially. When demarkation of the necrotic tissue is stable, revision of the flap can be performed.

Infection calls for immediate treatment. If the patient is not receiving antibiotics, this should be initiated. Administration of antibiotics is the treatment in cellulitis. If an abscess develops, acute surgery with incision and perhaps postoperative irrigation with antibiotics is indicated.

Spasms in spinal cord injured patients preferably should have been dealt with preoperatively; however, spasms might be provoked by surgery. Uncontrollable spasms and dehiscence call for a surgical 'wait-and-see' policy, since resuturing, in these cases, usually results in further rupture. Otherwise, resuturing can be performed according to usual surgical guidelines.

Recurrence calls for treatment and prophylaxis, as mentioned in the 'Extensive, multiple and recurrent pressure ulcers' section, earlier in this chapter.

CONCLUSION

The pressure ulcer patient's way through the system depends upon the local organization. In general, pressure ulcer patients are treated locally. Debridement can be performed by the local surgeons. Only in cases where interventions other than standard prophylaxis, wound care and debridement are expected, will the patient be examined by specialists. If surgical treatment is expected, the plastic surgeons who will perform the reconstructive procedures should be involved.

In the authors' area, obstinate pressure ulcers are evaluated by the Copenhagen Wound Healing Centre. If reconstructive or similar procedures are expected, the departments of plastic and reconstructive surgery are involved. The surgical treatment of pressure ulcers is a multidisciplinary task. Professional demands are high, courses complicated and problems frequent. Future progress is to be expected primarily in improved assessment and prophylaxis and, to a lesser degree, in technical developments in surgery.

SELF-ASSESSMENT QUESTIONS

1   (a)   Which grade of pressure ulcers are candidates for surgery?
    (b)   When is the most appropriate time for pressure ulcer surgery in a patient without sepsis:
          Emergency surgery?
          Electively, but as soon as possible?
          Postponed until the patient is stabilized?
          When the pressure ulcer starts to heal?
          How about a patient with sepsis?
    (c)   What type of flap is most appropriate in covering a pressure ulcer cavity with denuded bone after debrided osteomyelitis?
          And the same cavity, but without former osteomyelitis?
    (d)   How does a myocutaneous flap with normal circulation look?
          If the artery is obstructed?
          If the vein is clotted?
    (e)   When would you allow the patient to sit freely on a split-thickness skin graft or on a myocutaneous flap?
          For how long a time must the flap be loaded?

2   Make a plan for preoperative wound cleansing and pressure relief of a left-sided grade III ischial pressure ulcer without necrotic tissue on a 71-year-old woman.

    (a)   Would you change the regimens if the patient had an undislocated fracture of the right lateral malleolus (the fracture is treated with a plaster-of-Paris cast without loading on the foot)? Any special precautions?

    (b)   The patient develops necrotic tissue and soft bone in the pressure ulcer. New plan?

    (c)   The patient is a diabetic. She develops fever. No focus is found except odour and purulent secretion from the pressure ulcer. The diabetes is getting unstable, but is still well regulated with insulin. Make a priority of treatment of the diabetes, the fracture, the infection and the pressure ulcer.

REFERENCES

Agency for Health Care Policy and Research 1992 Pressure ulcers in adults: prediction and prevention. American Family Physician 46(3):787–794

Aggrawal A, Sangwan S S, Siwach R C, Batra K M 1996 Gluteus maximus island flap for repair of sacral pressure ulcers. Spinal Cord 34:346–350

Allen V, Ryan D W, Murray A 1993 Air-fluidized beds and their ability to distribute interface pressures generated between the subject and the bed surface. Physiological Measurement 14:359–364

Angrigiani C, Grill D, Siebert J, Thorne C 1995 A new musculocutaneous island flap from the distal thigh for recurrent ischial and perineal pressure sores. Plastic and Reconstructive Surgery 96(4):935–940

Anthony J P, Huntaman W T, Mathes S J 1992 Changing trends in the management of pelvic pressure ulcers: a review. Decubitus 5(3):44–51

Banwell P E 1999 Topical negative pressure therapy in wound care. Journal of Wound Care 8(2):79–84

Bergstrom N, Bennett M A, Carlson C E et al 1994 Treatment of pressure ulcers. Clinical practice guideline no. 15. Rockville, MD.

Deloach E D, DiBenedetto R J, Womble L, Gilley J D 1992 The treatment of osteomyelitis underlying pressure ulcers. Decubitus 5(6):32–41

Ercöcen A R, Apaydin I, Emiroglu M, Yilmas S, Adanah G, Tekdemir I, Yormuk E 1998 Island V–Y tensor fascia latae fasciocutaneous flap for coverage of trochanteric pressure sores. Plastic and Reconstructive Surgery 102(5):1524–1530

Espositio G E, Ziccardi P, Di Caprio G, Scuderi N 1991 Reconstruction of ischial pressure ulcers by skin expansion. Scandinavian Journal of Plastic and Reconstructive Surgery 27:133–136

Evans G R D, Dufresne C R, Manson P N 1994 Surgical correction of pressure ulcers in an urban centre: is it efficacious? Advances in Wound Care 7(1):40–45

Foster R D, Anthony J P, Mathes S J, Hoffman W Y 1997 Ischial pressure sore coverage: a rationale for flap selection. British Journal of Plastic Surgery 50:374–379

Frantz R A, Bergquist S, Sprecht J 1995 The cost of treating pressure ulcers following implementation of a research-based skin care protocol in a long-term facility. Advances in Wound Care 8(1):36–45

Garg M, Rubayi S, Montgomerie J Z 1992 Postoperative wound infection following myocutaneous flap surgery in spinal cord injury patients. Paraplegia 30:734–739

Gray B C, Salzberg C A, Petro J A, Salisbury R E 1990 The expanded myocutaneous flap for reconstruction of the difficult pressure sore. Decubitus 3(2):17–20

Hagerty R C, Gould W L 1995 The split gluteus maximus muscle turnover flap. Plastic and Reconstructive Surgery 96(6):1459–1462

Jørgensen L N, Kallehave F, Christensen E, Siana J E, Gottrup F 1998 Less collagen production in smokers. Surgery 123:450–455

Kierney P C, Cardenas D D, Engrav L H, Grant J H, Rand R P 1998 Limb-salvage in reconstruction of recalcitrant pressure sores using the inferiorly based rectus abdominus myocutaneous flap. Plastic and Reconstructive Surgery 102(1):111–116

Kroll S S, Hamilton S 1989 Multiple and repetitive uses of the extended hamstring V–Y myocutaneous flap. Plastic and Reconstructive Surgery 84(2):296–302

Kuhn B A, Coulter S J 1992 Balancing the pressure ulcer cost and quality equation. Nursing Economics 10(5):353–359

Lewis V L, Bailey M H, Pulawski G, Kind G, Basikioum R W, Hendri W H 1988 The diagnosis of osteomyelitis in patients with pressure sores. Plastic and Reconstructive Surgery 81(2):229–232

Linder R M, Morris D 1990 The surgical management of pressure ulcers: a systematic approach based on staging. Decubitus 1(2):32–38

Maklebust H A, Magnan M A 1988 Approaches to patient and family education for pressure ulcer management. Decubitus 5(7):18–28

Minns R M, Sutton R A 1991 Carbon fibre pad insertion as a method of achieving soft tissue augmentation in order to reduce the liability to pressure sore developement in the spinal injury patient. British Journal of Plastic Surgery 44:615–618

Naito M, Ogata K 1994 Vulnerability of the skin circulation without underlying muscle. An experimental study. 33rd Annual Scientific Meeting of the ISOP, Kobe p. MT V-1

National Pressure Ulcer Advisory Panel (NPUAP) 1989 Pressure ulcer prevalence, costs, and risk assessment: consensus development conference statement. Decubitus 2(2):27–28

Niazi Z B M, Salzberg C A 1997 Surgical management of pressure ulcers. Ostomy/Wound Management 43(8):44–52

Park S, Koh K S 1998 Superior gluteal vessel as a recipient for free flap reconstruction of lumbosacral defect. Plastic and Reconstructive Surgery 101(7):1842–1849

Peters J W, Johnson G E 1990 Proximal femurectomy for decubitus ulceration in the spinal cord injury patient. Paraplegia 28:55–61

Pressure Ulcer Guideline Panel 1995 Pressure ulcer treatment. American Family Physician 51(5):1207–1222

Regan M B, Byors P H, Mayrovitz H N 1995 Efficacy and comprehensive pressure ulcer prevention program in an extended care facility. Advances in Wound Care 8(3):49–55

Rodriques G P, Garber S L 1994 Prospective study of pressure ulcer risk in spinal cord injury patients. Paraplegia 32:150–158

Royer J, Pickrell K, Georgiade N, Madick R, Thorne F 1969 Total thigh flap for extensive decubitus ulcers. Plastic and Reconstructive Surgery 44(2):109–118

Rubayi S R, Cousins S, Valentine W A 1990 Myocutaneous flap. Surgical treatment of severe pressure ulcers. AORN Journal 52(1):40–55

Rudensky B, Lipschitz M, Isaacsohn M, Sonnenblick M 1992 Infected pressure sores: comparison of methods for bacterial identification. Southern Medical Journal 85(9):901–903

Sapico F L, Ginunas V J, Thornhill-Joynes M et al 1986 Quantitative microbiology of pressure sores in different stages of healing. Diagnostic Microbiology and Infectious Disease 5:31–38

Siddique A, Wiedrich T, Lewis V L 1993 Tensor fascia latae V–Y retroposition myocutaneous flap: clinical experience. Annals of Plastic Surgery 31:313–317

Siegler E L, Lavaizzo-Mourey R 1991 Management of stage III pressure ulcers in moderate demented nursing home residents. Journal of Geriatric Internal Medicine 6(6):507–513

Smith J W, Aston S J (eds) 1991 Grabb and Smith's plastic surgery. Little, Brown and Company, London, pp 3–90 1259–1297

Strauch B, Vasconez L O, Hall-Findlay E J (eds) 1990 Grabb's encyclopedia of flaps. Little, Brown and Company, London, pp. 1529–1800

Thornhill-Joynes M, Gonzales F, Steward C A, Kanel G C, Lee G C, Capen D A, Sapico F L 1986 Osteomyelitis associated with pressure ulcers. Archives of Physical Medicine and Rehabilitation 57:314–318

US Department of Health and Human Services 1992 Preventing pressure ulcers. A patient's guide. Decubitus 5(3):34–40

Wingate G F, Lewis V L, Green D, Wiedrich T A, Koenig W J 1992 Desmopressin decreases operative blood flow loss in spinal cord injured patients having flap reconstruction of pelvic pressure sores. Plastic and Reconstructive Surgery 89(2):279–282

12 *Mary Dyson and Courtney Lyder*

Wound management: physical modalities

INTRODUCTION

The aim of wound treatment should be to replace wound management by wound healing. Physical modalities can be used, together with best clinical practice in wound management, as a means of progression from management to healing.

The physical modalities currently used in wound healing include the following (McCulloch et al 1995):

- Ultrasound
- Low-intensity laser therapy (LILT)
- Electrical stimulation.

When used correctly, they can accelerate the healing of acute wounds, provided that these are not already healing optimally. They can also initiate and/or accelerate the healing of chronic wounds provided that the metabolic status of the patient is such that healing is possible; for example, there must be an adequate blood supply to each injured region. Following transduction within the tissues, these physical modalities can accelerate the acute inflammatory phase of healing and do so, in part, by stimulating the activity of the cells involved in growth factor production. This leads to more rapid entry of the wound into the proliferative phase of repair, and in some instances to the development of stronger reparative tissue.

Selection of an appropriate physical treatment should be based on an understanding of the process of wound healing and of the mode of action of the modalities; the latter is addressed in this chapter.

Regular assessment of the wound, ideally using a non-invasive objective technique such as high frequency (20 MHz) ultrasound imaging (Sussman & Dyson 1998), is recommended so that the effectiveness of treatment can be monitored and changes made in the treatment protocol if this is in the best interests of the patient. The chapter ends with a description of this technique; its role in the assessment of the development and healing of pressure ulcers is emphasized.

ULTRASOUND

What is ultrasound?

Ultrasound (US) is a mechanical vibration transmitted at a frequency above the upper limit of human hearing (i.e. higher than 20 kHz) – 1 hertz (Hz) is 1 cycle per second, 1 kilohertz (kHz) is 1000 cycles per second and 1 megahertz (MHz) is 1 000 000 cycles per second. Megahertz frequencies of US, typically 0.75–3 MHz, have been used to treat damaged skin and other tissues for over 40 years (Dyson 1995). In the last decade kilohertz frequencies of US, typically 30–50 kHz, have also been found to have therapeutic efficacy (Peschen et al 1997). Frequency and wavelength are inversely related; the lower the frequency the longer the wavelength. Kilohertz US is therefore also known as long wave US; this form of US is more penetrative than MHz US. Both kilohertz and megahertz US are transmitted readily through water and fat, and are absorbed by proteins. Kilohertz US, unlike megahertz US, is also transmitted readily through bone and metal. US is reflected from the interfaces between substances which differ acoustically, e.g. protein and water, soft tissues and bone, air and skin, etc., a property that is made use of when US is used diagnostically.

The energy of a beam of US transmitted through tissue gradually decreases in intensity as a result of absorption, scattering and reflection. The intensity (measured in W/cm^2) available at any depth within the tissue is inversely proportional to that depth, i.e., the greater the depth the less the amount of energy remaining in the beam. The rate of loss of energy from the beam depends on the wavelength, which is inversely proportional to the frequency of the US. The higher the frequency the shorter the wavelength and the more rapid the energy loss from the beam. A frequency of 3 MHz is therefore suitable for treating skin and superficial subcutaneous soft tissues, but not sufficiently penetrative for treating deep wounds in muscle or bone. Some of the energy in a 1 MHz beam will be absorbed in the skin, but proportionally less than in a higher MHz beam. Similarly, some energy from a kHz beam will be absorbed superficially, but proportionally less than in a MHz beam. Conversely, the lower the frequency of the US beam, the greater the depth to which it can penetrate.

US beams are non-uniform in terms of intensity, and can be delivered in either continuous or pulsed fashion. Because of this, the type of intensity should be specified when US is applied therapeutically. The intensity averaged across the face of the treatment head is the spatial average (SA); the intensity averaged in time is the temporal average (TA). When pulsed US is used it is important to distinguish between the pulse average (PA), i.e. the average intensity during the pulse, and the temporal average (TA), i.e. the average intensity during the pulse repetition cycle, which takes into account the absence of energy in the gaps or spaces between the pulses. The term temporal peak (TP) is also used to describe the intensity during the pulse. When US is used continuously, without pulsing, the intensity is described as I(SATA); when it is used in pulsed fashion the intensity should be described

as both I(SATA) and either I(SAPA) or I(SATP). Note that I(TP) and I(PA) are identical values.

Therapeutic ultrasound equipment

This typically consists of a microcomputer-controlled high-frequency generator linked by a coaxial cable to an applicator or treatment head. The treatment head contains a transducer (a component that changes one form of energy into another, in this case electrical energy to US).

Examples of therapeutic devices producing MHz US, kHz US and both kHz and MHz US are shown in Figures 12.1, 12.2, and 12.3 respectively. There is evidence that both MHz and kHz US can stimulate wound healing, as described below. An advantage of MHz US is that its mode of action is better understood and that more of its energy is absorbed in the superficial tissues; 3 MHz is absorbed more superficially than 1 MHz. In contrast, since less of the energy of kHz US is absorbed in the superficial tissues, more is available for absorption by the deeper tissues.

KEY POINTS

◆ Use whatever therapeutic US device is available, since some energy will be absorbed in the injured tissue whatever the frequency of the US

◆ If you have a choice, select a higher frequency for superficial injuries and a lower frequency for deeper injuries.

Application of ultrasound to a wound

Since US is reflected from air/soft tissue interfaces, it has to be transmitted into the tissues via either a coupling gel or water. If the skin is broken, the cavity of the wound should be filled with warm sterile saline and covered by either a film dressing such as OpSite (Smith & Nephew) or a hydrocolloid dressing such as Granuflex (ConvaTec) or Geliperm (Geistleich Pharmaceuticals), all of which transmit US readily into the tissues to be treated.

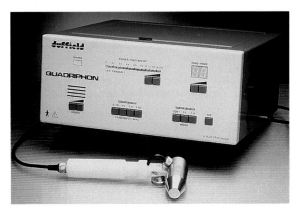

Figure 12.1 Ultrasound therapy device producing MHz ultrasound.

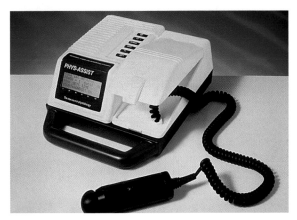

Figure 12.2 Ultrasound therapy device producing kHz ultrasound.

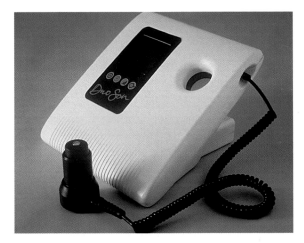

Figure 12.3 Ultrasound therapy device producing kHz and MHz ultrasound either separately or simultaneously.

Treatment parameters

When using ultrasound to treat a patient the following parameters should be recorded:

- Frequency (in Hz)
- Duration of treatment (in min)
- Continuous or pulsed application
- If pulsed, pulse duration (in ms) and space duration (also in ms)
- Intensity (in W/cm^2):
  - as I(SATA) for both continuous and pulsed applications
  - and either I(SAPA) or I(SATP) if pulsed.

A typical treatment for a pressure ulcer is as follows:

- F = 3 MHz
- Duration of treatment: 5 min
- Pulsed
- Pulse duration, 2 ms; space duration, 8 ms (also referred to as a 20% duty cycle, since the US is on for 20% of the treatment time)
- I(SATA) = $0.2 \, W/cm^2$
- I(SAPA) = I(SATP) = $1.0 \, W/cm^2$.

Ultrasound bioeffects relevant to therapy

US can be used to heat tissues. If the tissue temperature does not exceed 45°C this can be beneficial, provided that the tissue treated has an adequate blood supply. Temperature increases of less than 1°C are not considered to be clinically significant, since they are within the range of normal diurnal variation. US also produces predominantly non-thermal effects, some advantageous and others potentially damaging; the former are responsible for the cellular changes which initiate and/or accelerate healing, while the latter are readily avoided.

Thermal effects of ultrasound

The application of US in the I(SATP) range of between 1.0 and $2.0 \, W/cm^2$ increases the temperature of vascularized tissue to a therapeutically beneficial level. Care must be taken to ensure that the temperature reached does not

179

exceed 45°C, above which the tissue will be damaged and may become necrotic. Within the I(SATP) range noted above, both 1 and 3 MHz US equipment produce clinically significant therapeutic heating; kHz equipment does not. It is found that 1 MHz US produces clinically significant heating to a depth of approximately 5 cm whereas 3 MHz only does so to a depth of approximately 2 cm. Thermal effects can be reduced by pulsing, since this reduces the I(TA) and thus the total amount of energy available for absorption.

To produce a therapeutic effect the US has to be absorbed by the injured tissues. Absorption involves transduction of the US into another form of energy (ultimately into heat). As indicated above, high frequencies are more readily absorbed than lower frequencies and produce a greater heating effect in tissues. The greatest absorption, and therefore heating, is produced in the proteinaceous components of tissues.

Do not attempt to heat damaged tissue by ultrasonic or any other means if the blood supply to the region is impaired, because there is reduced ability to dissipate the applied heat and burning could occur. In such regions, the predominantly non-thermal effects of US produced by lower intensities, e.g. I(SATA) = 0.1 W/cm², I(SAPA) = 0.5 W/cm², pulsed 2 ms on, 8 ms off, F = 1–3 MHz, can be used safely and effectively. kHz US can be used in continuous mode, again for its non-thermal effects.

Non-thermal effects of ultrasound

These occur at lower spatial average, temporal average intensities than are required for thermal effects. With MHz US, these intensities are usually achieved by pulsing. The main predominantly non-thermal mechanisms by which US can stimulate tissue repair are cavitation and acoustic streaming

Cavitation is the production of micrometre-sized bubbles in the coupling medium used to transmit US into the body and in the fluids within the tissues. These bubbles oscillate in the US field, alternately expanding and contracting as they are subjected to the mechanical vibrations which comprise the US wave. At low (therapeutic) intensities the bubbles do not change greatly in size; this is termed stable cavitation and is beneficial. Acoustic streaming, the unidirectional flow of fluid, occurs around the stable bubbles and around cells within the tissues. This reversibly increases the permeability of the cell membranes to ions such as calcium, which stimulates cell activity. If the intensity of the US is too high then the bubbles change in size dramatically and can implode, producing highly localized tissue damage. This is termed transient cavitation. It is most likely to occur if the device is used at maximum power and if the applicator or treatment head is kept still during irradiation. The US can then be reflected to and fro between the applicator and a reflective interface such as that between soft tissue and bone, producing a standing wave in which energy can accumulate to a damaging level.

For effective and safe treatment of injured tissue:

- Use the lowest intensity that produces the required stimulatory effect
- Move the applicator during treatment, to avoid the formation of harmful standing waves.

How ultrasound stimulates wound healing

Basic mechanism

Non-thermal levels of US can induce stable cavitation and bubble-associated streaming, which reversibly increase the permeability to calcium ions of the plasma membranes of cells subjected to this fluid flow (Dyson 1995). Entry of calcium ions into the cell is a stimulus to cell activity. Cells in the path of the beam migrate, grow, proliferate, differentiate, phagocytose, synthesize and secrete matrix components and growth factors, according to their capabilities. These activities are all required for effective wound healing. US acts as a stimulus which the cells transduce into electrical and thermal energy. An amplified response then occurs, the nature of which depends on the type of cell involved; thus macrophages phagocytose debris and release growth factors which stimulate cell activity further, and can move the wound from acute inflammation to the proliferative phase of healing.

Effect of ultrasound on acute wounds

Used at low intensity during the acute inflammatory phase of healing, US can shorten inflammation, so that the wound enters the proliferative phase of repair more rapidly (Dyson 1995). Ultrasound is not anti-inflammatory; it does not inhibit inflammation but does shorten its duration. The production by immuno-inflammatory cells of the growth factors needed for progress into the proliferative phase of healing is stimulated by US and not inhibited, as would occur if the treatment was anti-inflammatory. US therapy therefore assists the body to heal itself. If healing is already progressing optimally, then US treatment cannot accelerate it. If, however, as is generally the case, there is scope for acceleration, then this can be achieved.

It has also been found that acute injuries treated with US in the inflammatory phase develop stronger tissue than control, sham-irradiated wounds (Hart 1993).

 KEY POINT

- ◆ Use US as soon as possible after injury, so that acute inflammation is accelerated and entry into the proliferative phase of healing occurs as rapidly as possible.

Effect of ultrasound on chronic wounds

For US to assist the healing of chronic wounds, these must first be treated so that at least part of the wound is in the acute inflammatory phase of repair. This can be achieved most readily by debriding the wound, either surgically or ultrasonically. The application of a single thermal-level treatment of MHz US can generally achieve this, as can kHz US, applied via a water bath in which acoustic streaming removes superficial necrotic tissue and occasionally produces tingling and pinhead-sized bleeding (Peschen et al 1997).

In leg ulcers, once acute inflammation begins, the application of 3 MHz US at an I(SATP) of 1.0 W/cm², I(SATA) of 0.2 W/cm², pulsed 2 ms on, 8 ms off, for between 5 and 10 min three times weekly has been shown to accelerate healing significantly more than in sham-irradiated controls (Dyson 1995). The application of kHz US via a water bath similar to the podiatry bath shown in Figure 12.4 has also been shown to stimulate the healing of chronic venous ulcers significantly. Peschen et al (1997) treated such wounds with continuous 30 kHz US at an I(SATA) of 0.1 W/cm²

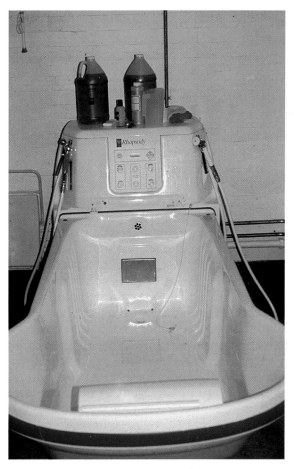

Figure 12.4 Podiatry bath incorporating a kHz ultrasound therapy transducer.

for 10 min three times a week and compared their healing with a control group. Both the experimental and the control wounds were treated conventionally in that they were covered with hydrocolloid dressings and compression therapy was applied. After 12 weeks, the experimental group, i.e. the group treated with US, showed an average decrease in ulcer area of 55.4% compared with only 16.5% in the control group – a highly significant difference ($P < 0.007$; $n = 24$).

No reports are available on the effect of kHz US on the healing of pressure ulcers, but 1 MHz has been used successfully, producing reduction in wound area, depth and undermining (reported by Sussman & Dyson 1998). Pulsed 1 MHz US at an I(SATP) of 0.5 W/cm^2, an I(SATA) of 0.1 W/cm^2 and a 20% duty cycle was applied to the periwound area for 5 min daily following the initiation of acute inflammation without adverse reaction.

The use of ultrasound to relieve pain and oedema

Reduction in pain, frequently associated with oedema, is an important part of wound healing. It results in reduced muscle guarding and increased activity, which aids circulation in the injured region and thus improves the local environment so that healing is encouraged. The reduction in oedema and in pain is indicative of progress through acute inflammation toward the proliferative phase of wound healing. The application of non-thermal levels of US over hydrogel or transparent film dressings to painful skin tears has been found to reduce pain 'after one or two treatments and to disperse ecchymosis within 6 to 10 sessions, depending on the size of the area involved' (reported by Sussman & Dyson 1998). Pulsed 1 MHz US was used at an I(SATP) of 0.5 W/cm^2, an I(SATA) of 0.1 W/cm^2 and a 20% duty cycle for 5 min daily to the periwound area. Had a 3 MHz applicator been available this would have been selected because of the superficial nature of the wounds being treated. An advantage of this method of application is that the dressing can remain on the wound during and between treatments.

Treatment of stage I pressure ulcers with ultrasound

Treatment with non-thermal levels of US increases the dispersal of haematoma, such as are found in stage I pressure ulcers, possibly by increasing the efficiency of phagocytosis of extravasated blood (McDiarmid et al 1985). Patients with deeper partial-thickness ulcers tended to heal more quickly than sham-irradiated controls but the results of a pilot study involving 40 patients were not statistically significant. According to McDiarmid & Burns (1987), infected ulcers responded better than clean ulcers, the stimulation of healing being statistically significant in the former but not in the latter. It is suggested that this may be because the infected wounds had been activated by the infection and were in the acute inflammatory phase which ultrasound and other forms of electrotherapy have been shown to accelerate (Young & Dyson 1993).

BOX 12.1   RECOMMENDATION

An effective protocol for treating pressure ulcers with US is as follows: pulsed 1 Mz US at an I(SATP) of 0.5 W/cm^2, an I(SATA) of 0.1 W/cm^2, and a 20% duty cycle for 5–10 min, according to the size of the ulcer, for 5–7 times a week for 1–2 weeks, or until the colour of the affected skin returns to that of the adjacent uninjured skin (Sussman 1993).

LOW-INTENSITY LASER THERAPY (LILT)

What is LILT?

Laser is an acronym for light amplification by the stimulated emission of radiation. Unlike US, light and other forms of electromagnetic radiation, such as radio waves and X-rays, do not require a transmission medium. All that light requires to reach a wound is that the wound be either exposed or covered by a transparent dressing.

Light consists of a range of wavelengths visible to the human eye, from violet, the shortest wavelength to red, the longest wavelength. Exposure to red light and/or infrared, which is just beyond our range of vision, has been found to stimulate wound healing (Mester et al 1985; Dyson & Young 1986). Light, as produced by the sun or a light bulb, is a spontaneous emission of electromagnetic radiation. The energy of the emitter is absorbed by atoms causing their electrons to move to higher-energy orbits where they are unstable and fall spontaneously to lower-energy orbits, releasing the energy they acquired as photons. The wavelength, and therefore the perceived colour, of the emitted light is determined by the difference in energy between the higher and lower orbits. So-called white light contains a mixture of all visible wavelengths.

The stimulated emission of radiation occurs when a photon interacts with an energized atom, where an electron is already in a higher orbit. If the energy of the incident photon equals the energy difference between the electron's excited and resting states, the photon emitted from the atom when its energized electron returns to its resting state has the same properties as that of the incident photon, which is also emitted. This process is repeated in the adjacent atoms, producing laser. Unlike light from non-laser sources, it is:

- monochromatic, i.e. of a single wavelength
- collimated, i.e. the rays are virtually parallel
- coherent, i.e. in phase, the troughs and peaks of the waves coinciding in time and space.

Of these characteristics, monochromaticity is of particular importance in the production of lasers' effects on tissues. This is probably because absorption, which is essential for the production of any effect on tissues, is wavelength-specific, substances of different colours absorbing light of different wavelengths. Lasers allow light energy of a specific wavelength to be delivered efficiently to the tissue components that benefit from modulation by it.

LILT is an acronym for low-intensity laser therapy (Baxter 1994). The first lasing devices used medically were of high intensity and were used to thermally coagulate and cut tissue. In contrast, LILT involves the use of lasing devices which operate at intensities which are too low to do this.

LILT equipment

This equipment has three essential components.

- A *lasing medium*, capable of being energized sufficiently for lasing to take place. Different media produce different wavelengths of radiation. For example, a mixture of helium and neon gases, termed HeNe, produces monochromatic red light with a wavelength of precisely 632.8 nm. In contrast, gallium–aluminium–arsenide (GaAlAs) semiconductor diodes also produce monochromatic light, but with a wavelength typically within the red–infrared range of 630–950 nm.
- A *resonating cavity* which contains the lasing medium and has two parallel surfaces, one totally reflecting and the other partially reflecting. The photons of light produced during lasing are reflected to and fro between these surfaces, and leave as a laser beam through the partly reflecting surface. The cavity of an HeNe laser is many centimetres long but that of a GaAlAs semiconductor diode is tiny, the diode itself being the lasing material and its polished ends the reflecting surfaces. Because of their small size and ease of use, most LILT devices are currently of the GaAlAs type (Fig. 12.5). Their treatment heads contain either one or many diodes. Those with a single diode resemble laser pens or pointers and are designed to treat trigger and acupuncture points but can also be used to treat points around and within wounds. Those with many diodes are termed cluster probes and allow large areas, such as the surface of pressure ulcers, to be treated rapidly. Cluster probes house up to 50 diodes, groups of which produce light of different wavelengths in the red and infrared range, allowing different cellular components and cell types to be targeted simultaneously.

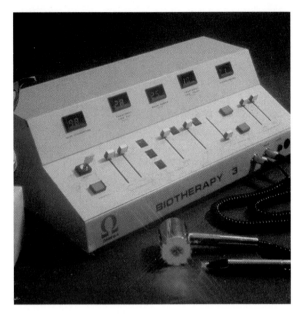

Figure 12.5 A LILT device showing single diode and multidiode cluster probes.

- *A power source*. The power source, either mains electricity or battery, is used to pump energy into the lasing medium via a transformer and control unit housed in a base unit.

Application of LILT to a wound

LILT can be applied to pressure ulcers by direct contact to the periwound area and to the wound area if the skin is unbroken, and/or using a non-contact method via a transparent dressing if the skin is damaged.

Baxter (1996) recommends the use of a single diode probe to treat the intact skin around the wound at about 1–2 cm from its edge by direct contact, the points being 2–3 cm apart. The probe should be pressed firmly onto the skin to reduce attenuation (i.e. energy loss) by temporarily displacing from the region erythrocytes which would absorb some of the incident energy. It is recommended that the energy density applied be no more than 10 J/cm², joules being calculated by multiplying the power density (in W/cm²) by the irradiation time in seconds.

Areas lacking a protective covering of skin should be covered with a transparent dressing

and are most conveniently treated with a cluster probe which can either be placed in contact with the dressing or held a few millimetres above it. Mester et al (1985) recommended the use of 4 J/cm² for the treatment of the wound bed.

Treatment parameters

When LILT is used to treat a patient the following treatment parameters should be recorded:

- Wavelength (in nm)
- Duration of treatment (in min)
- Power output of the device (in mW)
- Power density (in mW/cm²), calculated by dividing the power output by the spot size (irradiating area) of the laser. Semiconductor diodes typically have a spot size of 0.1–0.125 cm². For cluster probes this must be multiplied by the number of diodes
- Energy density (in J/cm²); see text above for method of calculation
- Pulse repetition rate (in Hz, i.e. number of pulses per second), if used in pulsed mode.

LILT bioeffects relevant to therapy

Like ultrasound, light must be absorbed by the components of tissue if it is to have a therapeutic effect. Research on mammalian keratinocytes, macrophages, fibroblasts and endothelial cells, all of which are of importance in wound healing, has generally demonstrated stimulation of cell activity, provided that appropriate wavelengths and energy densities are used. Much of this work has been critically reviewed by Baxter (1994). The wavelength of the light must be such that components within the cell can absorb it. Red light is absorbed by cytochromes in the mitochondria, while certain wavelengths of infrared light are thought to be absorbed by proteins of the cell membrane. A temporary increase in permeability of the cell membrane to calcium ions has been demonstrated (Young et al 1990). It is suggested that this may be the mechanism by which LILT at these wavelengths of light can act as a stimulus to cell activity, as has been shown to occur with ultrasound therapy.

How LILT stimulates wound healing

Basic mechanism

It is suggested that the triggering of cell activity by reversible changes in membrane permeability following absorption of light is the basic mechanism by which light, and other electrotherapeutic modalities, used at levels too low to produce clinically significant tissue heating, stimulate tissue repair (Young & Dyson 1993). Studies of macrophages exposed *in vitro* to light produced by laser diodes and superluminous diodes have shown that an increase in calcium uptake can occur. This is dependent upon energy density and wavelength (Young et al 1990). Energy densities of 4 and 8 J/cm^2 were found to be significantly effective, whereas 2 and 16 J/cm^2 were not. Of the wavelengths tested, 660, 820 and 870 nm were significantly effective, whereas 880 nm was not. Light at 660 nm is red and would be expected to be absorbed within the mitochondria, where it has been shown to stimulate ATP production and cytoplasmic H$^+$ concentration, which can affect plasma membrane permeability (Karu 1988). At wavelengths of 820, 870 and 880 nm light lies in the infrared range, and it has been suggested that this is absorbed by proteins in the plasma membrane of the cells. Since some of these proteins vary in different cell types, this may, at least in part, explain why different wavelengths of infrared light selectively affect different cell types involved in the healing process. Thus, 870 and 880 nm light was found to affect the activity of macrophages significantly, but not that of mast cells (El Sayed & Dyson 1990); in contrast, 820 nm light affected both cell types significantly. Appropriate selection of wavelength could, therefore, allow specific cell types to be targeted. The use, for example, of 870 or 880 nm light would be expected to stimulate the release of growth factors from macrophages, thus stimulating repair but not the degranulation of mast cells, which would be expected to be pro-inflammatory. More research is needed to discover which infrared wavelengths selectively affect other cells involved in the wound healing process.

Stimulation of the plasma membrane of a cell leads to its activation. Stimulation of the cells involved in wound healing would be expected to produce accelerated wound healing, as has been found. Unlike ultrasound, which does not affect particular cell types selectively, some wavelengths of infrared 'light' are selective in their action. Different wavelengths are absorbed by different cell types, and only those wavelengths which can be absorbed are effective.

KEY POINTS

- Use red light if you wish to affect all the cells involved in the healing process
- Use infrared radiation of 870 or 880 nm wavelength if you want to avoid stimulating mast cells.

Effect of LILT on acute wounds

As with ultrasound or any other modality, the stimulation of healing of acute wounds by LILT is only possible if they are healing suboptimally; for example, if they are in a dry environment. In such wounds, the production of granulation tissue can be stimulated (Haina et al 1982), as can wound contraction (Dyson & Young 1986) and the tensile strength of acute wounds (Abergel et al 1987). The most effective energy density of those tested was generally found to be 4 J/cm^2.

Effect of LILT on chronic wounds

A questionnaire survey of physiotherapy departments in Northern Ireland by Baxter et al in 1991 showed that, of the physical modalities available in these departments, LILT was the most popular for the treatment of wounds. Baxter (1994) states that 'laser therapy is often the physiotherapeutic modality of choice in a variety of conditions including trophic, diabetic and decubitus ulcers, particularly if these have become chronic and/or unresponsive to other treatment approaches'. Work on the effect of LILT on chronic ulcers extends back to that of Mester in the 1960s. In 1985, Mester et al surveyed the treatment of over 1000 ulcer patients with LILT at an energy density of $4 J/cm^2$; they showed 50–100% healing, the variation being related to the type of lesion. It is suggested that the induction of acute inflammation in chronic wounds should precede treatment with LILT, since it has been shown that LILT can accelerate this (Young & Dyson 1993).

The use of LILT to relieve pain and oedema

Zhukov et al (1979), using a HeNe laser producing red light, found that post-thrombophlebitic oedema and leg ulceration could be reduced by treatments with energy densities as low at $0.1 J/cm^2$. Reduction of oedema would be expected to reduce ulcer-associated pain. LILT has also been used to relieve postoperative pain associated with mastectomy (Martino et al 1987).

ELECTRICAL STIMULATION

What is electrical stimulation as applied to wound healing?

According to Sussman & Byl (1998) 'electrical stimulation for wound healing is defined as the use of a capacitive coupled electric current to transfer energy to a wound'. Although there are other methods of transferring electricity to tissue, e.g. via implanted electrodes (reported by Becker & Selden 1985), capacitive coupling is the most widely available and has the advantage of being non-invasive.

Capacitively coupled electrical stimulation of wound healing involves the transference of electric current through an electrode pad applied to the moistened skin or wound bed which form a wet conductive medium. At least two electrodes are needed to complete the circuit.

- In the monopolar technique the electrodes are placed either
  - within the wound or
  - on the intact skin some distance from the wound.
- In the bipolar technique the electrodes are placed on either side of the wound, straddling it.

The polarity of the electrodes can be varied, since this affects their bioeffects (see below). Polarity determines the direction of current flow, since electrons move from the negative pole (the cathode) to the positive pole (the anode). Current flow can be unidirectional or bidirectional.

Electrical stimulation can be delivered in a wide variety of waveforms as follows:

1. Continuous unidirectional direct current (also termed galvanic).
2. Monophasic pulsed direct current, the pulses or phases being either:
   (a) square wave or
   (b) containing two peaks.
3. Continuous alternating current, also termed biphasic or bipolar. It can be:
   (a) either balanced or unbalanced and
   (b) either symmetrical or asymmetrical.

These waveforms are illustrated in Figure 12.6.

Electrical stimulation equipment

Electrical stimulators consist of a power source, an oscillator circuit, an output amplifier and electrodes. Portable stimulators are battery powered. Many electrical stimulators use microprocessors which provide the user with a choice of waveforms and protocols for wound treatment, which should always be able to be altered according to the response of the patient to treatment. Electrical stimulators should be calibrated regularly and their output checked between calibration using a multimeter.

The electrodes complete the circuit between the stimulator and the body. They must be good conductors. Aluminium foil is recommended by Sussman & Byl (1998) because it is non-toxic, inexpensive, disposable, conformable and can be cut to the size required. The surface area of the electrode affects current density; the smaller the surface area the greater the current density and the deeper its penetration, and therefore its effect. The further apart the electrodes are the deeper the current penetrates; the greater the amplitude, the deeper the penetration. Typically, one small and one larger electrode are used: the smaller, termed the active electrode, has the greater current density; the larger is termed the dispersive electrode.

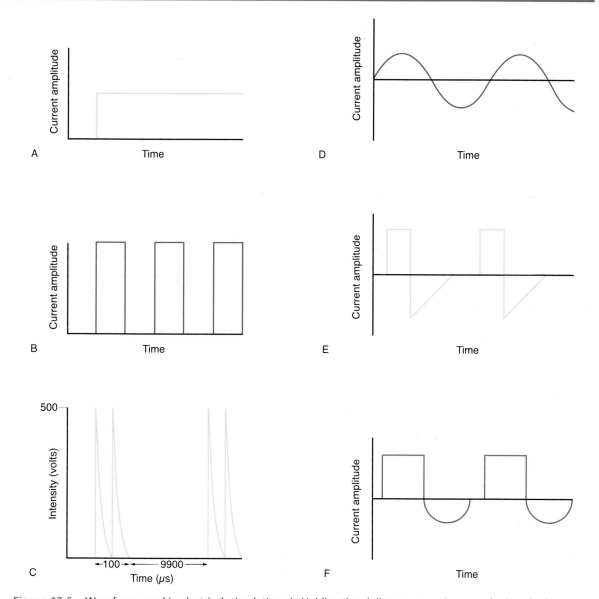

Figure 12.6 Waveforms used in electrical stimulation: A, Unidirectional direct current; B, monophasic pulsed current; C, high-voltage pulsed current showing twin-peaked monophasic waveform; D, balanced symmetrical alternating (biphasic) current; E, balanced asymmetrical alternating (biphasic) current; F, unbalanced asymmetrical biphasic current (modified from Sussman & Byl, 1998).

There are two types of direct current devices which have been used to stimulate healing:

- low voltage, typically 60–100 V
- high voltage, typically 100–500 V.

A high-voltage electrical stimulator (HVES) has a maximum electrical charge of only 10–15 micro-coulombs (μC), which is considered to be very safe (Alon & De Domenico 1987).

The amplitude of the voltage can be varied; by doing this, the current, measured in microamps (μA) is also varied, since according to Ohm's law $V = IR$, where V is voltage, I is current and R is resistance. Some electrical stimulators give a readout of the voltage and others of the current when the amplitude is changed.

Alternating current devices, which resemble transcutaneous neural stimulators (TENS devices) but have a different waveform, have also been used to stimulate healing.

Application of electrical stimulation to a wound

The wound must be covered by a dressing that permits the conduction of current into the wound, which must be kept moist since fluid is essential for transmission of the current. A study by Bourguignon et al in 1991 found that:

● occlusive film dressings are poor conductors
● both fully hydrated hydrocolloid dressings and hydrogels are good conductors.

In addition to conducting electrical current from electrodes the last of these also promote healing by:

● maintaining a moist environment
● promoting an injury current via this moisture
● retaining growth factors which stimulate healing.

Treatment parameters

Direct current

High-voltage pulsed current usually has a monophasic twin-peak waveform. When used to stimulate wound healing the parameters selected are usually as follows:

● Voltage = 80–200 V
● Pulse rate = 50–120 pulses/s
● Peak duration = 5–20 μs
● Polarity, variable.

Monophasic low-voltage microcurrent electrical stimulation (MENS) is typically applied using the following parameters to stimulate the healing of soft tissue (Gersh 1989):

● Voltage < 100 V
● Amperage = 200–300 μA

When used to stimulate bone repair, 20 μA has been shown to be effective (Friedenberg et al

1970). The pulse duration is greater than that of high-voltage devices.

Alternating current

Alternating current is used without pulsing. Its most effective waveform for stimulating wound healing is unbalanced (i.e. with the polarity of one pole predominating) and asymmetrical, in contrast to the balanced asymmetrical waveform used in TENS devices to reduce pain (Sussman & Byl 1998).

Selection of treatment

In selecting protocols for the electrical stimulation of wound healing it should be appreciated that the wound has different requirements at different stages of the healing process. The effects of polarity, biphasic currents, frequency and amplitude should all be considered.

1. Polarity: this is important when using direct current and monophasic pulsed current. The negative pole is generally used as the active electrode during acute inflammation or when the wound is overtly infected. The polarity is then varied, with the aim of matching electrode polarity with changes in the injury potential polarity (Kloth & Feedar 1988). This is an area where more research in required.
2. Biphasic current: Baker et al (1996) found that the best outcome of the treatments they tested on pressure ulcers in patients with spinal cord injuries was obtained with an asymmetrical waveform biased toward the negative pole.
3. Frequency: this has been varied widely for high-voltage pulsed currents. A proposed reason for this is its effects on blood flow; lower pulsing frequencies produce higher mean blood flow velocity in animal experiments (Mohr et al 1987).
4. Amplitude: this is usually kept constant and is reported as either voltage (100–200 V for high-voltage pulsed currents) or in milliamperes (35 mA for low-voltage direct current). When using high voltage this should be adjusted so that the patient

remains comfortable. If the patient has intact sensation then 100 V may be the maximum tolerable level.

The optimum pattern of treatments using electrical stimulation is still not known. The main variable tested has been polarity. For high-voltage pulsed currents Sussman & Byl (1998) recommend that the active electrode be negative during the acute inflammatory phase and to treat oedematous areas, should alternate between negative and positive every 3 days during granulation tissue development and should alternate daily during re-epithelialization and remodelling.

Electrical bioeffects relevant to therapy

Interactions between the living cells of the tissues of the body create a bioelectrical environment which is modified by injury. The aim of electrical stimulation is to increase the speed at which this is normalized, increasing the rate of repair.

The superficial aspect of the intact epidermis has an electronegative charge of about −23 mV compared with its deep aspect (i.e. adjacent to the dermis). This charge difference is maintained by the sodium pump which moves positively charged sodium ions to the deep aspect of the epidermis, leaving an excess of negatively charged chloride ions on its superficial aspect. The epidermis thus has an electrical potential across it and acts as a battery which maintains this potential. When the epidermis is disrupted by injury, current can flow as ions are transmitted through the tissue fluid between the damaged regions of the epidermis. This unidirectional current flow attracts cells involved in repair into the wound bed by a process termed galvanotaxis. When healing is either completed or arrested, this current, referred to as an injury current, disappears.

How electricity stimulates wound healing

Electrical stimulation mimics the injury current and has been described as being able to jump-start or accelerate the healing process (Gentzkow et al 1991).

Effect of electrical stimulation on acute wounds

Used correctly electrical stimulation accelerates acute inflammation and proliferation.

Effect of electrical stimulation on chronic wounds

The restoration of an injury current by electrical stimulation may have the effect of initiating healing by inducing local acute inflammation, as can the other physical modalities described in this chapter.

The use of electrical stimulation to relieve pain and oedema

This can be done by the application of high-voltage pulsed current and TENS using portable units. The procedures involved can often be carried out by the patient after appropriate training, but the clinician should monitor treatment outcome and intervene where appropriate.

Treatment of pressure ulcers with electrical stimulation

In a case study described by Kloth (1995) the treatment of a pressure ulcer on the right ischial tuberosity of a 24-year-old paraplegic man is described. High-voltage pulsed current stimulation is recommended to accelerate wound healing, with the electrode being placed over saline-moistened gauze which was used to pack the wound. The voltage should be set between 75 and 200 V to provide a tingling paraesthesia at a frequency of 100 pulses/s. If healing ceases, then the polarity should be reversed daily. Regular monitoring of the healing process is essential.

THE NEED FOR NON-INVASIVE ASSESSMENT OF PRESSURE ULCER DEVELOPMENT AND THE EFFECTIVENESS OF TREATMENT

The effectiveness of physical modalities and other methods of wound treatment should be monitored in every pressure ulcer so that the treatments can be adjusted to produce the optimal outcome, the healed wound. Photography of the wound site is of value, but only shows the wound surface. Non-invasive, and therefore non-damaging, objective assessment of structural changes deep within the wound and in the adjacent intact soft tissues, can be achieved by the use of high-resolution diagnostic ultrasound operating at a frequency of 20 MHz and higher.

Ultrasound can be used to detect the early stages of pressure ulcer development (Miller & Dyson 1996) and healing in skin and underlying tissues (Dyson et al 1999) regardless of level of pigmentation. Concerns about the inability of clinicians to accurately detect stage I pressure ulcers in people with darkly pigmented skin have been raised (Graves 1990, Bennett 1995, Lyder 1996, Henderson et al 1997). This is due to reliance on the assessment parameter of colour change, specifically redness, for all patients, rather than considering the different colour change hues of blue–purple in people with darkly pigmented skin. Since the assessment of colour is affected by the quality and quantity of the light source used, its value as the only indicator of stage I pressure ulcers is questionable. Inclusion of other characteristics such as skin temperature, stiffness and sensation has therefore been proposed (Henderson et al 1997), together with the use of high-resolution ultrasound B-scans (Miller & Dyson, 1996).

A portable, user-friendly, digital high-resolution ultrasound scanner (Fig. 12.7) has recently been developed which allows skin and subcutaneous tissues (Fig. 12.8) and connective tissue distortion caused by oedema and associated with stage I pressure ulcers to be visualized (Fig. 12.9) and digitally analysed. The ultrasound scanner (*http:\\www.longportinc.com*), which operates at a centre frequency of 20 MHz, provides a resolution of the order of 65 μm, clear discrimination between acoustically different materials, linear measurement and image analysis. Collectively, these features allow assessment of the development of a pressure ulcer and the progress of healing in a rapid and reproducible manner. The device's portability and ease of use

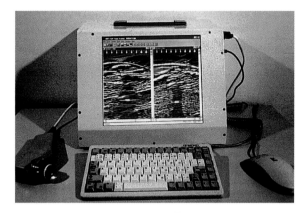

Figure 12.7 A high-resolution (20 MHz) diagnostic ultrasound digital scanner. Showing on the screen of the scanner are B-scans of an acute wound 3 days (left) and 7 days (right) after injury. The dark areas of the scans represent the healing wound.

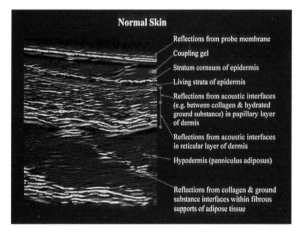

Figure 12.8 20 MHz ultrasound B-scan of intact thin skin, labelled to identify those components of the skin that can be distinguished ultrasonically.

by the nurse allows it to be taken to patients wherever they are located, be this at home, in a clinic, hospital, hospice or even in an ambulance. The B-scans of pressure ulcers, or of the skin and subcutaneous soft tissue at each pressure point, take only a few seconds to produce; they are stored electronically and can be either interpreted on the spot, or transmitted elsewhere via the internet for detailed analysis and comparison.

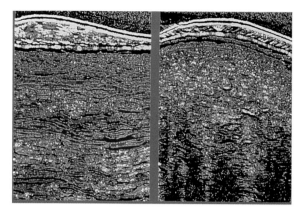

Figure 12.9 Two 20 MHz ultrasound B-scans. On the left is the normal skin of the heel of a geriatric patient at risk of pressure ulcer development. The scan shows intact epidermis, dermis and subcutaneous tissue. On the right is damaged skin and subcutaneous tissue of the other heel of the same patient, indicative of the development of a pressure ulcer. Note that although the appearance of the epidermis and papillary layer of the dermis is similar to that in the scan on the left, distortion indicative of oedema is present in the reticular layer of the dermis and in the subcutaneous tissue. Oedematous regions appear dark in the B-scan.

While the specific characteristics of early pressure-related injury are yet to be defined, awareness of the need to educate clinicians in culturally sensitive assessment techniques is growing (Bennett 1995). Use of the ultrasound scanner described above greatly increases both the sensitivity and specificity of correctly identifying stage I pressure ulcers, particularly in darkly pigmented skin. Dependence on less accurate measures to identify stage I pressure ulcers in skin regardless of its level of pigmentation could be eradicated by the use of this equipment. The implementation of appropriate preventative measurements (Ch. 7) and treatments, such as the use of the physical modalities described above, could significantly decrease the incidence of pressure ulcers in those at risk, leading to improvement in the quality of life and savings in the cost of health care. The effectiveness of these measures can now be assessed readily, objectively and without damage or discomfort to the patient.

CASE STUDY 12.1

Pressure ulcer treated with ultrasound therapy

The patient is an 88-year-old female admitted to the geriatric ward of a city hospital 2 weeks ago.

There is a stage III pressure ulcer on her left elbow. This was described as a stage II ulcer on her admission to hospital. Necrotic tissue is present. The wound is being kept moist, there is no overt bleeding and the ulcer is clean. Healing is impaired.

She has a history of systemic arteriosclerotic disease and has had several strokes, as a result of which she cannot change her position when in bed. She has reduced sensation and cannot communicate verbally. The mobility of her elbow, hip and knee joints is limited by the development of contractures.

Her skin is darkly pigmented. No redness is visible around the pressure ulcer; however, parts of the wound margin appear purplish and swollen. The skin over her pressure points is being inspected twice daily for signs of reddening.

Treatment consists of debridement, removal of pressure trauma by regular repositioning and the use of a pressure-relieving mattress, passive movement of the joints of the extremities in an attempt to improve the local circulation, use of a hydrocolloid dressing and daily ultrasound therapy.

Assessment is by daily visual inspection and photography and daily ultrasound B-scan immediately after ultrasound therapy.

Granulation tissue was detectable ultrasonically within 7 days of the commencement of treatment, when contraction deep within the bed of the wound became measurable. During the second week the surface began to decrease in size as re-epithelialization commenced. Ultrasound reflections from within the granulation tissue gradually increased as more collagen bundles were produced. More contraction was seen deep within the wound than at the surface. The ulcer took 12 weeks to close. By this time, the ultrasound reflections were those to be expected in scar tissue and remained fewer and of a different pattern to those of the adjacent uninjured skin.

1 State two methods, one involving ultrasound, which could be used to initiate acute inflammation in this patient's pressure ulcer. Why is the initiation of acute inflammation required?

2 List the treatment parameters appropriate for the treatment of this patient's pressure ulcer with ultrasound therapy after the initiation of acute inflammation. What dressings should be used over open wounds to be treated and/or examined with ultrasound? Is it necessary to remove these dressings prior to exposure to ultrasound?

CASE STUDY 12.1 (*contd.*)

3 Is the visual detection of redness in the skin an appropriate method of detecting the onset of pressure ulcers in patients, who, like this lady, have dark skins? What additional techniques are appropriate?

4 Can ultrasound be used to detect oedema in the early stages of pressure ulcer formation? What frequency of ultrasound is appropriate? Does oedematous soft tissue transmit ultrasound to a greater or to a lesser degree than does non-oedematous soft tissue?

SELF-ASSESSMENT QUESTIONS

1 What effects do acoustic microstreaming have on injured tissue?
2 Where within a living cell is red light absorbed? What effects do this absorption have on cell activity? How does this affect wounds in which healing is delayed?
3 What is an injury current? When and how is it produced?
4 Is ultrasound anti-inflammatory? How does it accelerate acute inflammation?

REFERENCES

Abergel R P, Lyons R F, Castel J C 1987 Biostimulation of wound healing by lasers; experimental approaches in animal models and fibroblast cultures. Journal of Dermatology and Surgical Oncology 13:127–133

Alon G, De Domenico G 1987 High voltage stimulation: an integrated approach to clinical electrotherapy. The Chattanooga Group, Hixson

Baker L L, Rubayi S et al 1996 Effect of electrical stimulation waveform on healing of ulcers in human beings with spinal cord injury. Wound Repair and Regeneration 4:21–28

Baxter G D 1994 Therapeutic lasers: theory and practice. Churchill Livingstone, Edinburgh

Baxter D 1996 Low intensity laser therapy. In: Kitchen S, Bazin S (eds) Clayton's electrotherapy, 10E. WB Saunders, London, pp. 197–217

Becker R O, Selden G 1985 The body electric: electromagnetism and the foundation of life. Morrow, New York

Bennett M 1995 Report of the task force on the implications for darkly pigmented intact skin in the prediction and prevention of pressure ulcers. Advances in Wound Care 8:34–35

Bourguignon G L et al 1991 Occlusive dressings unsuitable for use with electrical stimulation. Wounds 3(3):127

Dyson M 1995 Role of ultrasound in wound healing. In: McCulloch J M, Kloth L C, Feedar J A (eds) Wound healing: alternatives in management, 2nd edn. Davis, Philadelphia, pp. 318–346

Dyson M, Young S 1986 The effects of laser therapy on wound contraction and cellularity. Lasers Med Sci 1:125–130

Dyson M, Moodley S, Verjee L, Verling W, Weinman J, Wilson P 1999 Wound healing assessment using 20 MHz ultrasound. Skin Res Technol 5(2):131

El Sayed S O, Dyson M 1990 Comparison of the effect of multiwavelength light produced by a cluster of semiconductor diodes and of each individual diode on mast cell number and degranulation in intact and injured skin. Lasers Surg Med 10:559–568

Friedenberg Z B, Andrews E T, Smolenski B I, Pearle B W, Brighton C T 1970 Bone reaction to varying amounts of direct current. Surg Gynecol Obstet 131:894–899

Gentzkow G D, Pollack S V et al 1991 Improved healing of pressure ulcers using Dermapulse, a new electrical stimulation device. Wounds 3:158–160

Gersh M 1989 Microcurrent stimulation: putting it into perspective. Clin Manag 9(4):51–54

Graves D 1990 Stage I pressure ulcer in ebony complexion. Decubitus 3:4

Haina D, Brunner R, Lanthaler M et al 1982 Animal experiments in light induced wound healing. Laser Basic Biomed Res 22:1

Hart J 1993 The effect of therapeutic ultrasound on dermal repair with emphasis on fibroblast activity. London: University of London (PhD thesis)

Henderson C, Ayello E, Sussman C et al 1997 Draft definition of stage I pressure ulcers: inclusion of persons with darkly pigmented skin. Advances in Wound Care 10:34–35

Karu TI 1988 Molecular mechanisms of the therapeutic effect of low-intensity laser irradiation. Lasers Life Sci 2(1):53–74

Kloth L C 1995 Electrical stimulation in tissue repair. In: McCulloch J M, Kloth J C, Feedar J A (eds) Wound healing: alternatives in management, 2nd edn. Davis, Philadelphia, pp. 275–310

Kloth L C, Feedar J 1988 Acceleration of wound healing with high voltage, monophasic, pulsed current. Phys Ther 68:503–508

Lyder C 1996 Examining the inclusion of ethnic minorities in pressure ulcer prediction studies. JWOCN 23:257–260

McCulloch J M, Kloth L C, Feedar J A 1995 Wound healing: alternatives in management, 2nd edn. Davis, Philadelphia

McDiarmid T, Burns P N 1987 Clinical applications of therapeutic ultrasound. Physiotherapy 73(4):155–162

McDiarmid T, Burns P N, Lewin G T, Mackin D 1985 Ultrasound and the treatment of pressure sores. Physiotherapy 71(2):66–70

Martino G, Fava G, Galperti G et al 1987 CO_2 laser therapy for women with mastalgia. Lasers Surg Med 7:78

Mester E, Mester A F, Mester A 1985 The biomedical effects of laser application. Lasers Surg Med 5:31–39

Miller M, Dyson M 1996 Principles of wound care: a professional nurse publication. Macmillan Magazines, London

Mohr T, Akers T, Wessman H C. 1987 Effect of high voltage stimulation on blood flow in the rat hind limb. Phys Ther 67:526–533

Peschen M, Weichenthal M, Schopf E, Vanscheidt W 1997 Low-frequency ultrasound treatment of chronic venous leg ulcers in an outpatient therapy. Acta Dermatol Venereologica 77:311–314

Sussman C 1993 Ultrasound for wound healing. The Chattanooga Group, Hixson

Sussman C, Byl N 1998 Electrical stimulation for wound healing. In: Sussman C, Bates-Jensen B M (eds) Wound care: a collaborative manual for physical therapists and nurses. Aspen Publishers, Gaithersburg, pp. 357–388

Sussman C, Dyson M 1998 Therapeutic and diagnostic ultrasound. In: Sussman C, Bates-Jensen B M (eds) Wound care: a collaborative manual for physical therapists and nurses. Aspen Publishers, Gaithersburg, pp. 427–445

Young S R, Dyson M 1993 The effect of ultrasound and light therapy on tissue repair. In: Macleod D A D, Maughan C, Williams C R, Sharo J C M, Nutton R (eds) Intermittent high intensity exercise. Chapman and Hall, London, pp. 321–328

Young S R, Dyson M, Bolton P 1990 Effect of light on calcium uptake by macrophages. Laser Therapy 2:53–57

Zhukov B N, Zolotariova A I, Musienko S M et al 1979 Use of laser therapy in some forms of post-thrombophlebitic disease of the lower extremities. Klinicheskaia Khirurgiia 7:46–47

13 *Susan McLaren and Sue Green*

Nutritional factors in the aetiology, development and healing of pressure ulcers

INTRODUCTION

Nutrients provide essential substrates for body tissue metabolism, also influencing its rate and direction via hormonal signalling and enzyme activity (McLaren 1997). In a healing wound, nutrients provide the metabolic fuel for a variety of cell species, including leucocytes, lymphocytes, macrophages and fibroblasts which play a vital role in orchestrating cellular and biochemical events intrinsic to different stages of the healing process. Nutrients also provide the fundamental components from which new cellular structures and their supporting extracellular matrix of collagen, elastin, proteoglycans, fibronectins and integrins are synthesized (Meyer et al 1994, McLaren 1997). A dispassionate consideration of these facts suggests that nutrients can potentially influence all stages of healing in acute and chronic wounds and, indeed, affect aspects of recovery, but what is the evidence that they do? Recent systematic reviews of the clinical research literature, notably by Klein et al (1997), Green (1999) and Stratton & Elia (1999), have provided evidence supporting the vital role of effective nutritional support during recovery in patients suffering from a wide range of medical disorders. General conclusions are that malnourished states are common in hospitalized populations and that severe protein energy malnutrition can lead to an increased morbidity and mortality. Adverse outcomes frequently cited include increased lengths of hospital stay and institutional costs, decreased functional capacity, depressed immune function, increased vulner-ability to drug side effects, impaired wound healing and pressure ulcers (Green 1999). In many studies covering a range of diagnostic groups, the provision of rapid, effective nutritional support either oral, enteral or parenteral can lead to improved clinical outcomes (Klein et al 1997, Green 1999, Stratton & Elia 1999).

However, scrutiny of the research evidence suggests that there are problems inherent in demonstrating that nutritional factors affect the aetiology and healing of pressure ulcers or other types of chronic wounds. In clinical studies, many variables, notably age, medical diagnosis, drug treatment, social, psychological and nutritional status, can all influence outcomes such as pressure ulcer healing, which pose a challenge for research study design. Authors of the reviews cited above have emphasized the need for rigour in constructing scientifically robust, ethical study designs with clearly defined outcome measures and end points which attempt to overcome some of the problems posed by confounding variables. Other issues, raised by Albina (1994), are the need for caution in extrapolating findings from research work using in-vivo animal models to wound healing in humans. Anatomical, functional and metabolic differences exist between animals and humans which can impact on healing. For example, wound collagen deposition occurs more rapidly in rodents, and tolerance of fasting is poorer owing to a higher basal metabolic rate – both important points to bear in mind when interpreting findings of research studies.

The importance of using clearly defined, reliable, valid, specific outcome measures to evaluate healing in research investigations is also vital. For example, a finding that pressure ulcer sepsis was significantly associated with poor nutritional status solely based on the presence of microorganisms cultured from wound swabs could be challenged, since all chronic wounds contain bacteria, and those found may represent secondary colonization or contamination (Gilchrist & Morison 1997). Similarly, 'delayed healing' may be cited as an outcome measure in nutrition research studies. In interpreting this, Albina (1994) emphasized the importance of making distinctions between adequate or poor outcomes which follow delayed healing and impaired healing, which uniformly results in poor wound outcome.

In this chapter, an emphasis has been placed on evidence gained from clinical research wherever possible. Readers should note that the volume of material available relating to the influence of nutritional factors on the aetiology, development and healing of pressure ulcers is not abundant, and the influence of malnutrition is a recurring theme. Further research is urgently needed to evaluate the impact of obesity on the development and healing of pressure ulcers.

CLINICAL POPULATION STUDIES

A number of investigations have examined the role of nutrition in the development and subsequent rate of healing of pressure ulcers. Cross-sectional studies have suggested that a low protein and energy intake, low body weight and triceps skin-fold thickness, low serum albumin and low haemoglobin levels can be associated with the presence of pressure ulcers (Breslow & Bergstrom 1994). Prospective studies have also identified poor dietary intakes and poor nutritional status as possible risk factors for the development of a pressure ulcer. More specifically, Moolten (1972), Allman et al (1986), Pinchcofsky-Devin & Kaminski (1986), Sitton-Kent & Gilchrist (1993), Meaume et al (1994) and Gilmore et al (1995) found that poor nutritional status indicated by hypoalbuminaemia, and poor food intake was associated with pressure ulcer presence (Berlowitz & Wilking 1989, Gilmore

et al 1995). Furthermore, the severity of pressure ulcers has been associated with severity of malnutrition, as indicated by a low serum albumin level and total lymphocyte count (Pinchcofsky-Devin & Kaminsky 1986).

However, the association of poor nutritional status and dietary intake with pressure ulcers needs closer examination since the presence of pressure ulcers could potentially lead to poor nutritional status through loss of protein from the wound or due to infection. Similarly, poor dietary intake could be associated with increased physical dependence, which could be the causal factor associated with pressure ulcer development. However, prospective studies suggest that poor nutritional status may predispose to the development of pressure ulcers. Several studies have shown that individuals with low serum albumin levels (Allman et al 1986, Ek 1987, Ek et al 1991) and/or a poor dietary intake (Berlowitz & Wilking 1989, Ek et al 1991, Bergstrom & Braden 1992) are more likely to develop pressure ulcers.

Ek (1987) examined 515 consecutive admissions to a long-term medical ward. Each patient was assessed on admission and followed up weekly for 26 weeks or until discharge. A modified Norton Scale, serum albumin and skin test reactivity was used to assess nutritional status. Findings demonstrated that low serum albumin level and skin anergy was associated with the development of pressure ulcers. In a subsequent study, Ek and colleagues (1991) replicated their previous findings that pressure ulcer development was associated with low serum albumin levels. Bergstrom & Braden (1992) studied 200 newly admitted residents to a skilled nursing facility. Dietary intake and serum albumin levels were assessed weekly and found to be lower in subjects that developed pressure ulcers, but other biochemical measures were unaffected.

Guralnik et al (1988) examined the occurrence of pressure ulcers over 10 years in a large cohort of 5193 older adults and found anaemia was associated with the development of pressure ulcers.

One large study of 2373 patients in a large hospital identified reduced appetite as a risk factor for the development of pressure ulcers (Perneger et al 1998). Interestingly, in this study the presence of a nasogastric tube or intravenous nutrition was also associated with the development of pressure ulcers.

Nutritional factors have been shown to have some value when used in pressure ulcer risk assessment. The nutritional component of the Braden Scale has been found to contribute significantly to risk for pressure ulcer development (Schue & Langemo 1998). Nutritional status markers have also been shown to be predictive of pressure ulcer development when included as a component of functional assessment (Zulkowski 1998).

Conclusions from the studies mentioned above suggest that malnutrition can be considered a risk factor for the development of pressure ulcers, and a risk factor that is potentially reversible (Thomas 1997). However, some investigations have failed to show associations between poor dietary intakes and the subsequent development of pressure ulcers (Lewis 1998). Kemp et al (1990) examined 125 surgical patients and found no association between those who developed pressure ulcers and declining serum albumin levels. Similarly, poor nutritional intake has not been associated with pressure ulcer outcome in some studies (Myers et al 1990). Finucane (1995) summarized much of the research in this area and concluded that although some studies show low serum albumin and poor nutritional intake is associated with the presence and development of pressure ulcers, some do not. The impact of confounding variables on nutritional outcome measures in some clinical conditions should be borne in mind here, notably on serum albumin levels which in some diagnostic groups may be more indicative of disease severity than nutritional status.

Few studies have examined the effect of nutritional supplementation on the healing of pressure ulcers. For many years the ingestion of a high-protein diet has been suggested to increase pressure ulcer healing (Mulholland et al 1943). Myers et al (1990) examined the effect of nutritional support on the healing of pressure ulcers over 7 days and found no differences in the rate of healing in the supplemented patients, although the authors reported that a normal transferrin level was correlated with improvement in stage and size of ulcers, suggesting a nutritional role in the development of pressure ulcers. Ek et al (1991) suggested that patients who received an extra dietary supplement developed fewer pressure ulcers; and that healing was also improved. Breslow et al (1993) demonstrated that patients receiving a high-protein supplement showed improved healing of pressure ulcers compared with those receiving a lower protein supplement. Finucane (1995) concluded that pressure ulcer healing has been shown to be improved with nutritional supplementation in some studies but not others and that this warrants further investigation. In summary, many studies demonstrate that the presence and development of pressure ulcers is more likely to occur in malnourished individuals (Breslow 1991); however, some studies do not support this. Poor nutritional status may therefore be a contributory factor to the development of pressure ulcers, but may not be a major causal factor.

MALNUTRITION AND OBESITY: DEFINITIONS

Keller (1993) defined malnutrition as a general term that encompasses undernutrition associated with inadequate food intake, overnutrition caused by excessive food consumption, which can lead to obesity, and imbalances and deficiencies in the intake of specific nutrients. Undernutrition is most commonly found in patients with pressure ulcers, and is defined as 'a continuum that originates with an inadequate nutrient intake and is followed by a progressive series of metabolic, functional and body composition changes' (Klein et al 1997). In contrast, obesity, which may mask specific nutrient deficiencies, can be defined as an increased body fat content, which frequently results in increased morbidity, mortality or a reduction in performance capacity (Stordy 1988).

Body mass index

Body mass index (BMI) can be used to assess malnutrition and obesity in adults and is a computation of weight in proportion to height. It is calculated using the formula: weight (kg)/height^2 (m). In adults, BMI is used extensively to define underweight (BMI less than 19), normal weight (BMI 19–25), overweight (BMI 26–30) and obesity (BMI greater than 30). A BMI of 19–25 is seen as most desirable in health terms. However, BMI in an older person should be interpreted more cautiously for several reasons: first, body composition changes as the body ages (De Groot et al 1996); secondly, people with a BMI of greater than 26, who appear well nourished, may have lost a considerable amount of weight in the months before measurement (McWhirter & Pennington 1994); and thirdly, BMI and health risks may not show the same associations in the elderly as they do in younger adults.

In younger adults, mortality increases with increasing BMI (Kushner 1993). The elderly population may, however, show a different pattern. A BMI of 26–30 in younger adults suggests that a person is overweight and should consider losing weight for health reasons. In the elderly, especially the older elderly, BMI associated with low mortality increases with age and may be greater than 26 (Rissanen et al 1989, 1991). A BMI of over 30 in younger adults indicates obesity and this is associated with increased mortality. In contrast, in the older person there is some debate as to whether increased mortality is associated with obesity (Kushner 1993). Low weight (BMI less than 19) has been shown in a number of studies to be associated with high mortality (Tayback et al 1990). In the hospital environment, decreased BMI is linked with increased mortality in the elderly.

In summary, an elderly person with a BMI of less than 19 is at risk of malnutrition. There is little evidence to suggest that the elderly person with a BMI of 26–30, especially the older elderly person, would gain any health benefits from losing weight. However, some medical conditions do make weight loss advisable. If an older adult is obese it may or may not be appropriate for a reducing diet to be recommended; this will depend on the decision of the multidisciplinary team.

Vulnerable groups

On admission to hospital 10–40% of older adults show evidence of undernutrition which can increase by the time of discharge (McWhirter & Pennington 1994; Muhlethaler et al 1995; Potter et al 1995). Increased age is also an established contributory factor in the development of pressure ulcers, since 60–70% of all patients affected are elderly (Barbenel et al 1977, Melcher et al 1988). Significant relationships between increased age, poor nutritional status, inadequate dietary intakes and development of pressure ulcers have been found in several of the studies cited earlier in this chapter, notably by Pinchcofsky-Devin & Kaminsky (1986), Bergstrom et al (1987), Berlowitz & Wilking (1989), Bergstrom & Braden (1992), Meaume et al (1994) and Finucane (1995).

Reasons why older adults are vulnerable in relation to undernutrition are wide ranging and include concurrent illness factors which can lead to reduced food intake (Table 13.1) and factors associated with the care setting. In particular:

- Ageing is variably marked by lower levels of hunger, increased satiety, diminished acuity for taste and smell which can diminish appetite and food intake (Morley 1995).
- Inadequate income can reduce the range and quality of nutrients purchased, leading to consumption of a monotonous, imbalanced diet.
- Social and psychological factors, including living alone, bereavement, social isolation and depression, can exert adverse effects on food intake in older adults. Physical disability and immobility can exacerbate these effects (Morley 1995).
- Drug side effects can negatively affect food intake, notably by causing anorexia, nausea and vomiting. These can result from treatment with aspirin, digoxin, hydralazine, warfarin or mineral oil laxatives used in medical conditions common in older adults. Antineoplastic drugs and corticosteroids can directly inhibit wound healing (Telfer & Moy 1993).
- Lack of organization of nutritional services in hospitals, inadequate resource management

Table 13.1 Diseases that may result in protein-energy malnutrition (reproduced from 'Eating Matters' by kind permission of the Centre for Health Services Research, University of Newcastle-upon-Tyne)

Reduced nutrient intake

Reduced mobility and/or cognition, sensation, perception impairing food purchase and/or preparation (e.g. stroke, Parkinson's disease, dementia, cardiac failure, pulmonary disease, musculoskeletal trauma, osteo/rheumatoid arthritis)

Loss of functional independence in eating, motor skills (e.g. stroke, Parkinson's disease, osteo/rheumatoid arthritis, dementia, musculoskeletal trauma)

Loss of appetite (e.g. depression, anxiety, cancer, infection (any cause), pain (any cause), renal and liver diseases)

Nausea and vomiting (e.g. some types of cancer, renal, liver disease)

Impaired oral food retention/ingestion, chewing, swallowing (e.g. dementia, stroke, cancer of the oesophagus, pharynx, oral cavity)

Decreased nutrient digestion/absorption

Chronic gut inflammation (e.g. ulcerative colitis, Crohn's disease, enteropathies, malabsorption syndromes, gastrointestinal infection, cancer)

Liver disease

Pernicious anaemia (reduced vitamin B_{12} absorption)

Increased metabolic utilization of nutrients/disposal

Metabolic responses to injury (e.g. burns, sepsis, orthopaedic trauma, grade IV pressure ulcers complicated by sepsis)

Cancer cachexia syndrome

Hyperthyroidism

Chronic obstructive pulmonary disease (COPD) associated with hyperventilation

---

policies, lack of training and knowledge of nursing and medical staff in nutrition support, and a lack of practice guidelines and nationally agreed standards for nutrition support can contribute to the development of disease-related malnutrition (Green 1999).

In conclusion, older adults constitute a highly vulnerable group for the development of undernutrition and pressure ulcers; some common contributory factors are evident in the genesis of both.

Relationship between nutritional risk, wound healing and pressure ulcers

Figure 13.1 shows potential links between factors which can lead to impaired nutritional status, and an increased risk of pressure ulcer development. Protein-energy malnutrition, once established, can adversely affect all body systems, resulting in altered body composition, and an array of functional tissue and organ deficits. The relationships between selected key deficits and wound healing are summarized in Figure 13.2. It is vital that individuals who are at high nutritional risk are identified at an early stage, through effective screening processes following hospital admission. Appropriate nutritional support can then be given to minimize the risk of pressure ulcer development and improve other clinical outcomes.

MACRONUTRIENTS

Energy for tissue metabolism and healing is provided principally by glucose and fatty acids; proteins provide amino acids for the synthesis of new structural components of tissue and in injury, the synthesis of acute-phase reactants. These are proteins synthesized by the liver during the metabolic response to stress and injury, which are systemic mediators of inflammatory responses. Specific amino acids, e.g. glutamine, are used as a metabolic fuel by macrophages during the process of healing. The roles of specific macronutrients are described below.

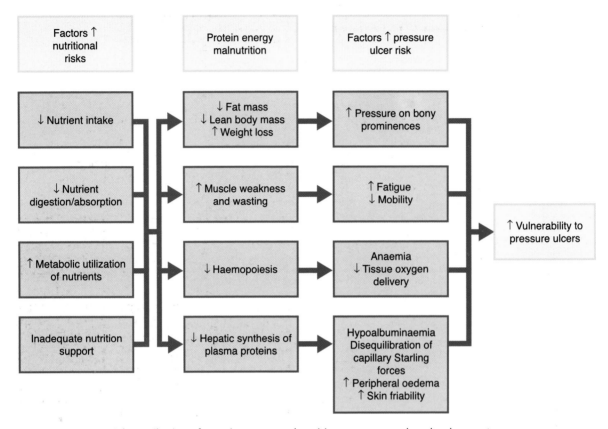

Figure 13.1 Potential contribution of protein-energy malnutrition to pressure ulcer development.

Glucose

During the early stages of healing (inflammatory response and destructive phase), factors released by damaged cells and platelets chemically attract neutrophils to the wound site, followed by monocytes and macrophages. Collectively these cells comprise the 'cellular infiltrate' which functions to remove devitalized tissue and bacteria. Leucocytes and macrophages release cytokines and growth factors which stimulate fibroblast production and thereby, collagen synthesis (Edwards & Moldawer 1998). Fibroblasts also synthesize other components of the new extra-cellular matrix, notably hexosamine sugars and proteoglycan polymers. Glucose is a vital energy substrate for leucocytes and macrophages, which have an increased capacity for aerobic glycolysis linked to pyruvate oxidation. The metabolic benefits are that the concentrations of intermediate

metabolites required for the synthesis of macro-molecules intrinsic to healing are raised (Falcone & Caldwell 1990). Wound angiogenesis, haematocrit and tissue perfusion factors which support aerobic metabolism are also necessary for efficient energy production from glucose. It is vital that dietary intakes of carbohydrate are adequate to meet energy requirements during healing. The determination of energy requirements, which includes a consideration of wound metabolism and injury, is discussed later in this chapter.

Protein

Evidence substantiating a vital role for protein in the healing of acute and chronic wounds has emerged largely from animal studies of dietary deficiency. Early work, reviewed by Hunt & Zelderfeldt (1969) and Ruberg (1984), found that effects of dietary protein depletion were an exten-

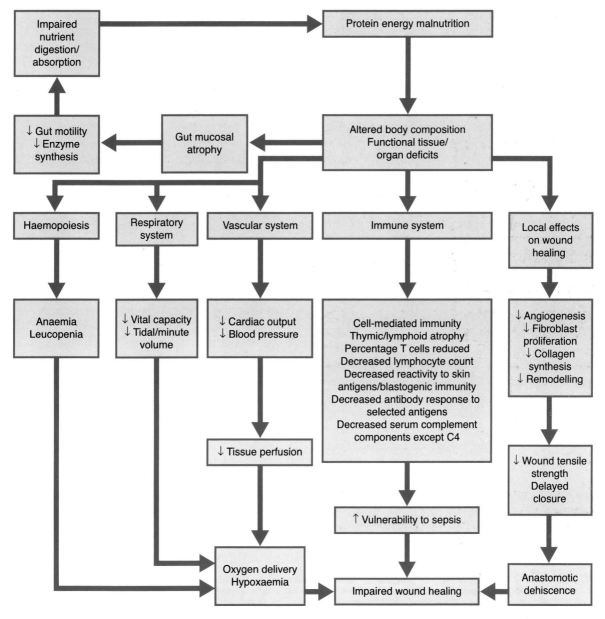

Figure 13.2 Effects of malnutrition on wound healing. Reproduced with permission from Macmillan Magazines Ltd. From McLaren S 1992 Proceedings of the 1st European Conference on Advances in Wound Management.

sion of the 'lag' phase of healing, decreased fibroblast proliferation, collagen and proteogly-can synthesis, decreased formation of new capillary vessels and adverse effects on the final stages of wound remodelling. Hypoalbuminaemia was acknowledged to impair healing because of the secondary development of oedema, which can increase the diffusion distance for nutrients from capillaries to tissues. Subsequent studies in rodents found that preoperative dietary protein depletion could decrease the bursting strength in colonic anastomoses – effects which were reversed by postoperative feeding which combined balanced amounts of amino acids and dextrose (Ward 1982).

Clinical research in patients with pressure ulcers has confirmed an association with hypoalbuminaemia, negative nitrogen balance and inadequate intakes of dietary protein, and improvements in dietary intakes has been associated with the development of fewer pressure ulcers. Studies by Allman et al (1986) found lower serum albumin concentrations in patients with established ulcers compared with those judged 'at risk' of developing pressure ulcers.

A community dietary survey by Green et al (1999) found that patients with pressure ulcers had lower dietary intakes of protein than a control group. Ek et al (1991) found that fewer pressure ulcers developed in an experimental group provided with a liquid nutrient supplement containing 8 g protein and 200 kcal per 24 h (in addition to a hospital diet of circa 2200 kcal in 24 h) in comparison with an unsupplemented control group. Multivariate analysis confirmed that low serum albumin levels and low food intakes were predictors of pressure ulcer development.

The assumptions underpinning these findings are that a low dietary protein intake can result in a decline in serum albumin concentrations, increasing the risk of pressure ulcer development. However, interpretation should consider the following:

- Plasma proteins can be lost in exudate from ulcers of any severity, but particularly from a grade IV ulcer.
- The serum albumin concentration declines markedly during metabolic responses to injury, sepsis and trauma, liver disease, nephrotic syndrome and enteropathies. Albumin also has a relatively long half-life of 18–20 days and a large body pool size of 5 g/kg body weight. Changes in serum albumin levels do not therefore provide a reliable index of short-term changes in nutritional status caused by altered food intakes in these conditions; research findings in patients with pressure ulcers should therefore be judged in the context of medical

diagnosis and dietary data (McLaren 1992). Similarly, effects of supplements should be judged in the context of their total macronutrient/micronutrient and energy content; not one nutrient alone, e.g. protein.

Amino acids

In a healing wound all essential and selected non-essential amino acids (i.e. glutamine, arginine) are used for:

- the synthesis of purines and pyrimidine components of nucleic acids
- the formation of structural proteins for cytoskeletons, i.e. actin, myosin, elastin, keratin
- the synthesis of procollagen (proline, lysine), collagen (methionine, cysteine), hexosamines and proteoglycans of the new extracellular matrix
- metabolic fuelling of the cellular infiltrate.

Amino acids are also used for the synthesis of hepatic acute-phase proteins which mediate systemic inflammatory responses. Recent developments in the field of nutrient pharmacology have focused on the potential for specific amino acids to benefit a range of outcomes, including wound healing, predominantly in patients recovering from surgery, injury and trauma. The roles of two particularly important amino acids, arginine and glutamine, are now described.

Arginine Arginine is a dibasic amino acid which is a precursor of nitric oxide (NO) or endothelial-derived relaxing factor (EDRF). Early clinical studies by Daly & Reynolds (1988) and Barbul et al (1990) found that parenteral feeding with L-arginine improved immune function and wound healing in catabolic patients. More recent studies evaluating the enteral administration of arginine have found net nitrogen retention and protein synthesis in comparisons with isonitrogenous diets (Brittenden et al 1994, Beaumier et al 1995), but no beneficial effects on other outcomes. Heslin et al (1997) compared the administration of a mixed enteral formulation of arginine, RNA and fish oil with standard intravenous crystalloid solutions during postoperative recovery and found no differences in wound-related outcomes/infections, mortality or duration of hospitalization. Further animal investigations suggest that arginine can reduce ischaemia-reperfusion injury in muscle, liver, heart and brain, and also exerts protective haemodynamic effects (Roth 1998).

The effects of arginine on wound healing appear to be mediated via increased growth hormone, prolactin, insulin and glucagon secretion, resulting in enhanced protein synthesis. Production of NO could reduce tissue hypoxia by induction of vascular relaxation. In conclusion, the evidence for routine use of arginine clinically cannot be supported. No specific studies have investigated effects on pressure ulcer formation or treatment, but the work on ischaemia-reperfusion injury is interesting.

Glutamine In humans, glutamine is a non-essential amino acid comprising two-thirds of free intracellular amino acids, of which 75% is located in skeletal muscle (Lin et al 1998). Its high nitrogen content is useful during recovery from injury and trauma, when it is mobilized from skeletal muscle and transported to areas of increased utilization. In healing tissue it forms:

- a substrate for purine and pyrimidine synthesis
- a preferred fuel for fibroblasts, lymphocytes, macrophages
- a precursor of the antioxidant glutathione, which reduces free radical tissue damage
- a precursor of proline and, thereby, collagen in fibroblasts.

Selected clinical studies evaluating glutamine-supplemented parenteral nutrition have found improvements in net nitrogen balance and reduced infectious complications (Kudsk & Minard 1999, Griffiths 1996), but other investigations have failed to demonstrate benefits from enterally administered glutamine (Long & Nelson 1995).

In conclusion, the hypothetical benefits of glutamine on healing outcomes in acute or chronic wounds have not been demonstrated in clinical studies.

Fatty acids

Lipids have major metabolic effects in a variety of tissues and organs, and fulfil key roles in membrane structure and function (Calder & Delkelbaum 1999). In recent years, it has become clear that polyunsaturated essential fatty acids (PUFA) exert wide-ranging effects on inflammatory responses, vascular tone and cellular defence mechanisms through the generation of eicosanoids, notably leukotrienes, prostaglandins and thromboxanes. Dietary fatty acids derived from fish oil (ω-3) and vegetable oil (ω-6), once incorporated into lymphocytes, monocytes and macrophages, generate the eicosanoids of different species. Briefly, metabolism of the n-3 fatty acids gives rise to prostaglandin E_3 and leukotrienes which exert anti-inflammatory and vasodilatory effects; whereas metabolism of n-6 fatty acids to prostaglandins E_2 and I_2 can produce immunosupression and vasoconstriction. Other actions of n-3 fatty acids include closing down cytokine production and thereby pro-inflammatory responses, which can benefit the clinical control of inflammatory diseases (Mayer et al 1998). Although PUFA have the potential to affect wound healing and impair the process in deficiency states, the ratios of n-3 to n-6 fatty acids in the diet which optimize metabolic benefits are unclear. Limited evidence suggests that PUFA improve pressure ulcer healing; Declair (1997) found that PUFA applied topically, in a randomized controlled clinical trial, reduced development of pressure ulcers in comparison with mineral oil. This area warrants further investigation. Further information relevant to the role of PUFA in injury, sepsis and trauma can be found in Edwards & Moldawer (1998) and Redgrave (1999).

MICRONUTRIENTS

The roles of vitamin C, zinc and iron are described below. For a description of the roles of other micronutrients, such as vitamin A, vitamin E, and copper refer to McLaren (1992), Meyer et al (1994), Albina (1994) and Lindemann (1984).

Vitamin C

Evidence from in-vitro and in-vivo animal research has shown that vitamin C is essential for effective wound healing. Key findings are that:

- it acts as a cofactor for hydroxylation of proline and lysine during collagen synthesis
- experimentally induced dietary deficiency of vitamin C leads to decreased wound tensile strength, dehiscence and impaired neoangiogenesis
- together with vitamin E it inhibits oxygen free radical formation, reducing tissue damage
- beneficial effects on complement synthesis and cell-mediated immune function have been reported.

Very few studies have investigated the effects of vitamin C on pressure ulcer risk and healing. However, significantly lower leucocyte vitamin C levels were found in a cohort of elderly patients with fractured neck of femur who developed pressure ulcers, in comparison with those who did not develop ulcers (Goode et al 1992). Small sample size and lack of risk assessment have limited interpretation of this study. A dietetic evaluation by Bergstrom & Braden (1992) found a significantly lower consumption of vitamin C in patients who were at risk of developing grade I pressure ulcers compared with those who did not develop ulcers. In contrast, a community survey by Green et al (1999) found no significant difference in vitamin C intakes between pressure ulcer and control groups in older adult populations. Use of vitamin supplements was reported by 30% of the total sample.

The effects of vitamin C supplements on pressure ulcer healing were investigated by Taylor (1974) in a prospective double-blind controlled trial. Although findings suggested that supplements significantly reduced pressure ulcer area, absence of dietary data and the fact that neither group were clinically vitamin C deficient has limited conclusions of the study.

Zinc

Evidence for the importance of zinc in wound healing can be ascribed to four mechanisms (Solomons 1988):

- trophic effects on all components of the immune system which reduces vulnerability to sepsis
- actions as a cofactor in an extensive number of enzyme systems concerned with protein synthesis
- antibacterial actions directed against some Gram-positive bacteria through inactivation of enzyme systems and bacterial aggregation
- beneficial, stabilizing effects on membrane structure and function

In relation to pressure ulcer risk and healing, very few studies have investigated the influence of zinc status and dietary zinc intakes. In the study by Bergstrom & Braden (1992) no significant differences were detected in serum zinc concentrations and dietary zinc intakes between groups with and without pressure ulcers. Green et al (1999) also found that no significant differences existed in dietary zinc intakes between pressure ulcer and control groups in older adults. However, zinc intakes generally were lower than those recommended in dietary reference values (Department of Health 1991).

The potential for zinc deficiency to influence food intake adversely in older adults by reducing taste acuity should be borne in mind (Sandstead et al 1982).

Iron

Iron depletion resulting from dietary deficiency and chronic blood loss can lead to a hypochronic microcytic anaemia which may compromise wound healing by reducing oxygen transport to tissues, contributing to tissue hypoxia. Iron is also an essential cofactor for the activity of hydroxylases involved in collagen synthesis. Again, studies investigating iron deficiency in patients at risk or with established pressure ulcers are restricted.

Breslow et al (1991) in a prospective investigation of enterally fed nursing home patients found significantly lower haemoglobin levels in patients with pressure ulcers compared with those without. Bergstrom & Braden (1992) found low dietary iron intakes to be associated with pressure ulcer development also in a cohort of elderly nursing home patients.

In summary, the evidence relating dietary micronutrient inadequacy or biochemical status to the development of pressure ulcers is very limited indeed. It is worth noting that:

- plasma levels for some micronutrients are not necessarily a reflection of tissue levels
- metabolic responses to injury sepsis and trauma can lead to depletion of some micronutrients, although plasma levels in the early stages may be normal
- giving supplements to patients with chronic wounds is only likely to benefit established deficiency states.

Advice should be sought from a clinical biochemist if there is reason to suspect micronutrient deficiencies so that appropriate investigations can be initiated. For a fuller discussion of features and diagnosis of deficiency states and micronutrient requirements see Lindemann (1984), Selhub & Rosenberg (1984) and Shenkin (1999).

NUTRITIONAL ASSESSMENT AND SUPPORT

According to Silberman (1989), Taylor & Goodinson-McLaren (1992) and Klein et al (1997), the aims of nutrition support are to achieve the following:

- to provide support which meets individual requirements within an ethical framework of decision making
- to maintain hydration status and haemodynamic stability
- to maintain lean body mass, organ function and immunocompetence
- to replete body composition in malnourished states, prevent the complications of malnutrition, including pressure ulcer development, and promote healing
- to reduce morbidity and mortality associated with medical disorders and their treatment.

The effective management of nutritional support is a cyclic process envisaged in five stages (Fig. 13.3).

Individuals with pressure ulcers represent a heterogeneous group with a range and combination of medical conditions. A detailed discus-

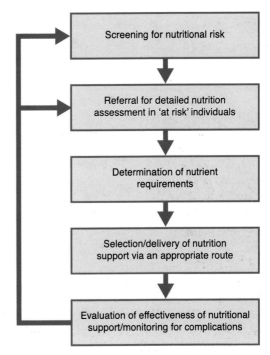

Figure 13.3 Management of nutritional support: key stages.

sion of the management of nutritional support, including artificial nutrition, is beyond the scope of this chapter. Readers will find a detailed discussion on parenteral and enteral nutrition in the classic text of Rombeau & Rolandelli (1997). *Eating Matters* (Bond 1997) addresses nutritional issues in the support of hospitalized older adults, a high risk group for pressure ulcers, from a practical multidisciplinary perspective.

In the UK, the gold standard for management of nutrition support is through a multidisciplinary nutrition support team, who:

- work within terms of reference which are realistic for service needs
- deliver a high-quality, cost-effective, evidence-based service within and across primary and secondary care
- liaise with other professionals and users in the implementation of all stages of nutrition support
- undertake education, research, audit and other activities in accordance with local and national priorities.

Cole & Jones (1995) and McLaren et al (1997) have emphasized the importance of dynamic leadership, flexible approaches concerning work across professional boundaries, the need for clear accountability and referral policies as vital for successful team work. Benefits of nutrition support team work can include more appropriate use of parenteral nutrition and implementation of standards of practice which reduce complications of gastrostomy placement (Mauter et al 1996; Pattison & Young 1997). Core membership usually comprises a dietitian, nurse, doctor and pharmacist, with the co-option of other health professionals as required.

Screening and assessment

Nutritional screening can be defined as a process of identifying individuals at risk of malnutrition who require further comprehensive nutritional assessment and referral (Hunt et al 1985). Nutritional assessment is a more detailed process in which a range of specific methods can be used to identify and quantify impairment of nutritional status, although these terms are often used interchangeably. Protocols or tools can guide the screening and assessment process (McLaren & Green 1998). Protocols outline procedures which should be followed and often include a recommendation for action. Nutritional screening tools (or instruments) are similar to pressure ulcer risk assessment tools, and use risk factors associated with malnutrition to assess the risk of malnutrition. Some nutritional assessment tools are available, for example Subjective Global Assessment (Detsky et al 1987).

The aims of nutritional assessment or screening are as follows (Goodinson & Dickerson 1988):

- to define the nutritional status of an individual at a specific point in time and to evaluate the adequacy of recent nutrient intake
- to identify individuals who require nutritional support
- to evaluate by serial measurements (usually made weekly) the efficacy of nutritional support.

An array of anthropometric, biochemical, physiological, morphological, functional and historical methods can be used to screen for malnutrition and assess nutritional status. Many measurements are affected by non-nutritional factors, and no single, widely available indicator exists. A number of criteria should inform the selection of methods; these include cost, the need for specialist training of personnel in their use, availability and suitability for patients or clients.

In response to recent concern relating to levels of malnutrition, several screening and assessment protocols have been produced by a number of agencies. These encourage nurses and other health care professionals to screen and assess the nutritional status of patients, thus identifying those at risk of malnutrition, so that appropriate nutritional support can be given to improve outcome.

Protocols and standards

The King's Fund report, *A Positive Approach to Nutrition as Treatment*, produced in 1992 described how the nutritional care of patients could be improved (Kings Fund Centre 1992). The report recommends the following nutritional assessment (or screening) for adults:

- height should be recorded once in general practice and hospital
- patients should be regularly weighed to enable weight for height and weight change assessment
- a note of each patient's nutritional status should be mandatory in medical and nursing records
- where malnutrition is detected, an appropriate plan of treatment should be made and its effects monitored.

The RCN document *Nutrition Standards and the Older Adult* was produced in 1993 (RCN 1993). This document outlines standards of nutrition in the older adult (older being defined as over 75 years of age or with a health profile of someone that age). The standards aim to assist all registered nurses to improve the nutritional care of older people. However, the involvement of all members of the multidisciplinary team is seen as essential. Three standards are outlined concerning assessment of past and/or potential difficulties in eating and drinking, enabling the client to eat and drink, and monitoring and evaluating nutritional status and care.

The British Association for Parenteral and Enteral Nutrition (BAPEN) was formed in 1992 as a result of recommendations made by the King's Fund report. The association has set standards for use in clinical practice in nutritional support. BAPEN recommend '... on admission and at regular intervals every patient's nutritional status is assessed in order to identify malnourished patients or those at risk of becoming malnourished' (BAPEN 1996). Several criteria are outlined in order to achieve this. It is recommended that each ward has a guide to the assessment of nutritional status used and that all staff know how to use it. It is advised that nursing records should include sections to record the assessment. A protocol for primary assessment of nutritional status and further components of ongoing nutritional assessment are outlined.

Screening tools

Nutrition screening tools (sometimes termed assessment tools) may also be used to screen for malnutrition. A screening tool aids memory and recording of the information and can be used to give a quantitative assessment of nutritional risk. The purpose of any tool is to identify those at risk of malnutrition and identify the appropriate action. Those designed for use by nurses should be quick and easy to complete because nurses have limited time to assess a patient or client, and nutrition is just one of many aspects of the assessment and planning process. The issues of validity (does the tool measure what it is proposed to measure) and reliability (are the results reproducible) should have been considered in the development of the tool.

A number of screening tools have been developed for use by the nurse (see reviews by McLaren et al 1997, Green & McLaren 1998, Edington 1999). These typically prompt the nurse to ask a number of pertinent questions concerning the patient's or client's nutritional intake and status, for example their normal food intake, appetite and recent weight loss. Further nutritional assessment is made by the nurse, for example BMI and general appearance. Nutritional status is then usually assessed using a simple ordinal scoring system, which when summed indicates risk categories. Screening tools should ideally be used routinely on admission and repeated weekly if there is any change in the patient's condition. Several comprehensive assessment tools have been developed which are very thorough; however, they can take longer to complete, which can be a disadvantage. Examples of screening tools which meet selected criteria for validity and reliability and can be used in older adults are the Mini Nutritional Assessment (Guigoz et al 1994) and the Nutrition Risk Assessment Scale (Nicolaus et al 1995).

Dietary intake and history

A record of food intake over a number of days can provide an insight into dietary quantity and quality. Although this can be carried out and interpreted by nurses, it does not provide an accurate, rapid assessment of nutritional intake. Greater accuracy can be achieved using this method by the dietician.

A dietary history can provide valuable information concerning recent dietary intake. Information concerning a number of factors that may have had an adverse effect on their nutritional status can be obtained from the patient and/or their carer. The content of a history should focus on the normal patterns of eating, diets prescribed, normal weight and patterns of weight change over time, food preferences and drugs or supplements prescribed.

Anthropometric methods

Body mass index can be used to assess malnutrition in adults as described previously. A series of measures of BMI over time gives a far more accurate picture than one single measurement. Although a low BMI will alert the nurse that the person is at risk of malnutrition, a high BMI does not preclude it. Percentage weight loss can be used in conjunction with BMI to give some indication of weight loss.

This can be calculated as:

$$\% \text{ Usual body weight} = \frac{\text{Current weight (kg)}}{\text{Usual weight (kg)}} \times 100$$

This method can rely on self-reports and therefore may be open to error. Practically, measurement of BMI may prove problematic. In the elderly, measurement of height may be difficult due to spine curvature and problems with standing. If standing height cannot be measured accurately, then there is some evidence that it can be estimated from knee height (Chumlea et al 1985, Chumlea & Guo 1992) or arm demispan (Kwok & Whitelaw 1991). A nomogram relating both supine total arm length and seated knee-to-floor height to height is available (Haboubi et al 1990). Measurement of BMI in the elderly may be difficult and sometimes inaccurate: other measurements may be more reliable (Finucane et al 1988). Fluid retention, for example, may limit the accuracy of BMI (Nightingale et al 1996). Ideal body weight (obtained from an ideal weight/height table) may also be useful when assessing individuals with pressure ulcers (Strauss & Margolis 1996).

Biochemical measures

A number of biochemical investigations can give information on nutritional status, although many medical conditions and treatment can affect biochemical measures. The use of any biochemical test should be considered in the light of the patient's medical diagnosis, progress and treatment (Taylor & Goodinson-McLaren 1992, Fogt et al 1995).

The serum proteins albumin, transferrin, retinol-binding protein and thyroxine-binding prealbumin may be used as indicators of nutritional status. In protein-energy malnutrition, the concentrations of these proteins in plasma decrease owing to a reduction in their synthesis by the liver and to a decrease in liver mass. However, plasma levels may not provide a true reflection of nutritional status in acute illness as they can be affected by factors such as acute illness, renal function and administration of whole blood and blood products. Biological half-lives of plasma proteins also vary considerably. Those with a short half-life, e.g. retinol-binding protein, may be more sensitive indicators of malnutrition; in contrast, albumin, with a half-life of 19 days, may not be useful as an indicator of early protein-energy malnutrition in acutely ill patients. In the interpretation of normal and abnormal serum concentrations of plasma proteins in elderly or very young individuals, it is vital to use an appropriate reference range (Eastham 1995).

A range of biochemical investigations can be used to assess macronutrient and micronutrient levels in the body. Nitrogen balance studies may be used to determine whether an individual is gaining or losing tissue protein, i.e. in a state of positive or negative nitrogen balance. If protein is catabolized because of inadequate dietary intake, then a negative balance may result. Assessment of vitamin and mineral status may be useful and encompasses biochemical analysis of urine, plasma and other body tissues. Assessment of levels may be indicated following clinical examination, dietary and medical histories. If a deficiency state is suspected, the clinical biochemist can advise on the use, availability, cost and interpretation of tests.

Once assessment or screening has been carried out, then the decision should be made as to whether the nurse should pay special attention to the patient/client's dietary intake, or whether the patient/client should be referred to the dietitian for more intensive assessment and nutritional support. Referral to the speech therapist and other health care personnel such as the occupational therapist may also be appropriate in swallowing problems and disability affecting eating skills. Nutritional screening and assessment should be considered an ongoing process as nutritional status often changes over time.

Assessment of nutrient requirements

Normally, the dietitian carries out assessment of nutrient requirements. Other health care professionals such as the pharmacist, medical doctor or biochemist may also have input:

- Energy requirements can be estimated using indirect calorimetry, predictive equations, nomograms and reference tables.
- Nitrogen (protein) requirements can be assessed using nitrogen balance studies, reference tables.
- Micronutrient requirements can be estimated using a range of reference tables and biochemical methods.

Further information on appropriate application of the above can be found in Silberman (1989), Department of Health (1991), Taylor & Goodinson-McLaren (1992), Bender & Bender (1997), Rombeau & Rolandelli (1997) and Shenkin (1999). Nutrient requirements are increased in injury, trauma, sepsis following surgery and in a number of medical conditions. Bonnefoy et al (1995) found that some patients with pressure ulcers sustained a metabolic response to injury marked by elevated plasma cytokine levels; hence macronutrient and micronutrient requirements may be increased in these individuals.

Breslow et al (1991) showed that patients with pressure ulcers had a low body weight, serum albumin and haemoglobin, despite being naso-gastrically fed to meet estimated requirements. A recent study demonstrated that individuals with quadriplegia and pressure ulcers had an elevated metabolic rate compared with individuals with quadriplegia alone (Liu et al 1996). Assessment of nutrient requirements should therefore continue throughout the treatment course and be informed by progressive healing and ulcer severity, medical diagnosis and other factors known to affect needs (Osterweil et al 1995).

Approaches to nutritional support

Delivery of nutritional support requires a consideration of appropriate routes, preparation, timing and prevention of complications that can result from the use of artificial techniques. If the gut is functional, then oral feeding or use of enteral catheters may be indicated. If the gut is non-functional then intravenous (parenteral) feeding via the central or peripheral route can be used; occasionally, in selected individuals, combined enteral and parenteral approaches may be appropriate and necessary. Clearly, patients with pressure ulcers present a spectrum of medical diagnoses, treatment groups and have individual needs which are beyond the scope of this text; readers will find further information in the references cited previously. Contemporary views on nutrition support are that it should be given promptly and that the enteral route is preferable and associated with fewer complications (Klein et al 1997, Green 1999). In chronically malnourished individuals, preliminary correction of fluid and electrolyte imbalances with initial slow rates of nutrient repletion are necessary to avoid hypophosphataemia and 'refeeding syndrome'.

Oral delivery of nutritional support

Food supplements can be used to complement dietary intake in order to meet nutritional requirements; rarely, they may be used for a longer period of time to replace a normal diet. The use of food supplements can markedly improve the nutritional status of malnourished patients or clients (McWhirter & Pennington 1996). Food supplements usually comprise milk or fruit-flavoured energy and nutrient-dense beverages, often termed sip feeds. Nutrient-rich puddings and soups may also be used to enrich the quality of the hospital meal. Food supplements are normally prescribed by the dietician who assesses the nutritional needs of the individual patient and prescribes a food supplement if appropriate. In some areas certain food supplements can be given without the dietitian's specific prescription to supplement the diet taken in hospital. Specific guidelines should be available to indicate when it is appropriate to use these supplements.

The nurse should ensure that each patient or client receives and consumes the correct supplement at the appropriate time. It is important that food supplements are given when the dietitian advises. For example, beverage supplements are often prescribed mid-morning, mid-afternoon and at bedtime. If these supplements are taken at meal times they may be used as a substitute for food instead of as a supplement, thereby decreasing the amount of food eaten. Food supplements should not be given in excess of that prescribed as they contain relatively high concentrations of nutrients, which might be deleterious in excess (Taylor & Goodinson-McLaren 1992). The amount of the supplement consumed should be recorded so the effectiveness of the prescription of dietary supplements can be assessed. Positive encouragement to eat or drink the entire food supplement can increase intake. Supplement not consumed at the recommended time should be discarded or stored appropriately. Some individuals may not tolerate the supplements (Stableforth 1986), which should be noted and reported to the dietitian. Vitamin or mineral supplements may be prescribed if there is evidence of a specific deficiency. A multivitamin supplement may be considered necessary by the health care team if dietary intake of energy, protein, fat and carbohydrate is adequate but the diet is considered to be limited and therefore lacking in micronutrients.

Enteral and parenteral nutrition

Artificial nutrition support can be life sustaining and has revolutionized treatment of the critically ill, but it is not without potential complications. Approaches, routes and indications are summarized below (Guenter et al 1997, Lord 1997).

Enteral nutrition   Enteral nutrition (EN) is administered via a catheter (i.e. nasogastric, gastrostomy, jejeunostomy). EN route selection is determined by the level of alimentary tract function, accessibility to the tract, practicality of using it and patient preference; nutrients must be delivered distal to any abnormality and sufficiently proximal for complete absorption. Indicators for using EN can include neurological and obstructive dysphagia, oropharyngeal obstruction, inflammation and trauma, mild inflammatory bowel disease and malabsorption, burns, chemotherapy, radiation therapy and organ transplantation. EN is contraindicated in paralytic ileus; intestinal obstruction beyond the duodenum; intractable vomiting, diarrhoea and gut bleeding; ischaemia; or severe inflammatory bowel disease.

Parenteral nutrition   In contrast to enteral nutrition, parenteral nutrition can be used where acute, temporary or long-term intestinal failure is present due to the following (Galica 1997):

- gut infarction
- pancreatitis, fistulas
- following gut resection
- cancer, trauma, radiation enteritis precluding use of the gut
- hypercatabolic states.

It is contraindicated where the gut is functional/accessible, where less than 5 days use is anticipated, where risks are judged to exceed benefits and if no therapeutic or palliative purpose is served.

CONCLUSION

Nutritional status and dietary intake have been shown to be associated with the presence and healing of pressure ulcers. Therefore, it is reasonable to suggest that assessment or screening for malnutrition or risk of malnutrition should be considered a part of the nursing assessment of the patient/client with a pressure ulcer. Simple nutritional assessment and screening can be carried out by the nurse to identify patients/clients who are malnourished or at risk of malnourishment. They can then be referred to another health care professional (usually the dietitian), where appropriate, for a thorough assessment and subsequent plan of care. People become malnourished or are at risk of malnourishment for a variety of reasons. It is important to determine the reasons why dietary intake may be poor or inadequate, so an appropriate plan of care can then be formulated.

The 'responsibility for nutritional assessment and support in wound management … is not the domain of one individual, and a multidisciplinary team approach must be adopted' (Wells 1994).

CASE STUDY 13.1

Mr David Clement (pseudonym) aged 88 years was admitted to the acute geriatric assessment unit of his local hospital after a home visit by the GP, made at the request of a next door neighbour. He had cardiac failure of 5 years' duration, which was controlled with diuretics, cardiac glycosides and hypotensive drugs and had been discharged home after partial recovery from a stroke 18 months previously. The stroke had resulted in a residual left-sided paresis affecting his arm and leg, restricting mobility.

Since the sudden death of his wife 8 months previously, the next door neighbour had noticed that he had become very withdrawn, apathetic, progressively unkempt and dishevelled. He appeared to have lost weight and had become extremely breathless. A neighbour did his shopping for food and other household items since he had no immediate family in the locality. They called in the GP when they found Mr Clements in a confused, disoriented state one morning and feared he had suffered another stroke.

On admission to the geriatric assessment unit he was hypertensive (180/120 mmHg), dyspnoeic (respirations 28/min), cyanosed with marked sacral and peripheral oedema present. Biochemical and haematological investigations confirmed a serum albumin concentration of 29 g/L and haemoglobin of 9 g/dl. Body mass index was 18, Waterlow score 18 and Mini Nutritional Assessment score 7. He appeared depressed, withdrawn and disoriented. His skin was dry, flaky and the sacral area was red but unbroken. Mr Clement was chairbound with a marked left-sided paresis but the neurological assessment did not suggest that a further stroke had occurred.

1 Identify the features which could be indicative of malnutrition and pressure ulcer risk.

2 Why has this individual become malnourished with loss of control of his cardiac failure?

3 Identify the immediate priorities in management from the perspectives of tissue viability and nutrition support.

4 List the methods which could be used to assess nutritional status. Is the measurement of serum albumin a reliable nutritional risk indicator here?

5 Identify the health professionals with whom liaison/referral are necessary to resolve the patient's nutritional problems.

6 What form of nutritional support is indicated in this case?

SELF-ASSESSMENT QUESTIONS

1 Define the terms undernutrition, protein-energy malnutrition and obesity.

2 List the effects of malnutrition on body systems which can impair wound healing. Which specific risk factors can contribute to pressure ulcer development?

3 How is body mass index calculated? What points should be taken into account when interpreting measurements made in older adults?

4 List the reasons why older adults may become malnourished. Which risk factors are also common to the development of pressure ulcers?

5 Differentiate between nutritional screening and assessment.

6 Briefly describe anthropometric and biochemical methods of nutritional assessment. What other factors can affect the measurements obtained?

7 Compare and contrast the roles of glucose, amino acids and fatty acids in tissue repair.

8 Summarize the key roles of vitamin C and zinc in wound healing.

9 List the aims of nutrition support and stages in its provision.

10 Compare and contrast the indications for using parenteral and enteral nutrition.

11 Briefly describe the aims, membership and operation of a nutrition support team.

FURTHER READING

1. Bond S 1997 Eating matters. Centre for Health Services Research, University of Newcastle-upon-Tyne
   An excellent review of practical nutritional issues related to the multidisciplinary care of older adults in hospital. It covers each aspect of dietary management, including screening, assessment, determination of nutrient requirements, resolution of distressing symptoms affecting eating, and provision of appropriate meals. Aspects of quality are addressed in relation to audit, development of evidence-based standards and guidelines for nutrition support. It contains case studies and a wealth of information on support agencies.
2. Morley J E, Glick Z, Rubenstein L Z 1995 Geriatric nutrition: a comprehensive review, 2nd edn. Raven Press, New York
   An authoritative review of nutritional issues in old age, covering effects of ageing, nutritional deficiencies, systems malfunction and nutrition, and a range of special topics including pressure ulcers and nutrition.
3. Allison S 1999 Hospital food as treatment. A report by a working party of the British Association for Parenteral and Enteral Nutrition. BAPEN Publications, Maidenhead
4. Sizer T 1996 Standards and Guidelines for Nutritional Support of Patients in Hospitals. A report by a working party of the British Association for Parenteral and Enteral Nutrition. BAPEN Publications, Maidenhead
5. Silk 1994 Organisation of Nutrition Support in Hospitals. Report by a working party of the British Association for Parenteral and Enteral Nutrition. BAPEN Publications, Maidenhead
6. Lennard-Jones J E 1998 Ethical and legal aspects of clinical hydration and nutritional support. Report by a working party of the British Association for Parenteral and Enteral Nutrition. BAPEN Publications, Maidenhead
   Reading sources 3–6 above are from an excellent series of monographs produced by BAPEN for clinical practitioners. They are accessibly written, with substantive research references and an emphasis on practical applications.
7. Rombeau J L, Rolandelli R H (eds) 1997 Clinical nutrition: enteral and tube feeding, 3rd edn. W B Saunders, London
   A comprehensive text on the use of artificial nutrition.

REFERENCES

Albina J E 1994 Nutrition and wound healing. Journal of Parenteral and Enteral Nutrition 18(4):367–376

Allman R M, Laprade C A, Noel L B et al 1986 Pressure sores among hospitalised patients. Annals of Internal Medicine 105:337–342

BAPEN 1996 Standards and guidelines for nutritional support of patients in hospitals. A report by a working party of the British Association for Parenteral and Enteral Nutrition. BAPEN Publications, Maidenhead

Barbenel J C, Jordan H M, Nicol S M, Clark M O 1977 Incidence of pressure sores in the greater Glasgow Health Board Area. Lancet ii: 548–550

Barbul A, Lazaron S A, Efron D T 1990 Arginine enhances wound healing and lymphocyte response in humans. Surgery 19(8):331–337

Beaumier L, Custillo L, Ajami A M, Young V R 1995 Urea cycle intermediates kinetics and nitrate excretion at 'normal' and 'therapeutic' intakes of arginine in humans. Endocrinology and Metabolism 269(1): E884–896

Bender D A, Bender A E 1997 Nutrition: a reference handbook. Oxford University Press, Oxford

Bergstrom N, Braden B 1992 A prospective study of pressure sore risk among institutionalised elderly. Journal of the American Geriatric Society 40:747–758

Bergstrom N, Demuth P J, Braden B J 1987 A clinical trial of the Braden Scale for predicting pressure sore risk. Nursing Clinics of North America 22:417–428

Berlowitz D R, Wilking S V B 1989 Risk factors for pressure sores: a comparison of cross-sectional and cohort-derived data. Journal of the American Geriatrics Society 37:1043–1050

Bond S 1997 Eating matters. Centre for Health Services Research Publications, University of Newcastle-upon-Tyne, Newcastle-upon-Tyne

Bonnefoy M, Coulon L, Bievenu J 1995 Implications of cytokines in aggravating malnutrition and hypercatabolism in elderly patients with severe pressure sores. Age and Ageing 24:37–42

Breslow R 1991 Nutritional status and dietary intake of patients with pressure ulcers: review of research literature 1943–1989. Decubitus 4(1):16–21

Breslow R A & Bergstrom N 1994 Nutritional prediction of pressure sores. Journal of the Dietetic Association 94(11):1301–1304

Breslow R A, Hallfrisch J, Goldberg A P 1991 Malnutrition in tube fed nursing home patients with pressure sores. Journal of Parenteral and Enteral Nutrition, 15(6):663–668

Breslow R A, Hallfrisch J, Guy D G et al 1993 The importance of dietary protein in healing pressure sores. Journal of the American Geriatrics Society 41:357–362

Brittenden J, Heys S D, Ross J, Park K G M, Cremin O 1994 Nutritional pharmacology: effects of L arginine on host defenses. Clinical Science 86:123–132

Calder P C, Delkelbaum R J 1999 Dietary lipids: more than just a source of calories. Current Opinion in Clinical Nutrition and Metabolic Care 2:105–107

Chumlea W C, Guo S 1992 Equations for predicting stature in white and black elderly individuals. Journal of Gerontology 47(6):M197–M203

Chumlea W C, Roche A F, Steinbaugh M L 1985 Estimating stature from knee height for persons 60 to 90 years of age. Journal of the American Geriatrics Society 33(2):116–120

Cole K D, Jones F A 1995 Interdisciplinary teams for the solution of nutritional problems. In: Morley J E, Glide Z, Rubenstein L Z (eds) Geriatric nutrition, 2nd edn. Raven Press, New York, pp. 367–376

Daly J M, Reynolds J 1988 Immune and metabolic effects of arginine in the surgical patient. Annals of Surgery 208:512–552

De Groot C P G M, Enzi G, Perdigao A L, Deurenberg P 1996 Longitudinal changes in anthropometric characteristics of elderly Europeans. European Journal of Clinical Nutrition 50(S2):S9–S15

Declair V 1997 The usefulness of topical application of essential fatty acids (EFA) to prevent pressure ulcers. Ostomy/Wound Management 43(5):48–52, 54

Department of Health (DoH) 1991 Dietary reference values for food, energy and nutrients for the United Kingdom. HMSO, London

Detsky A S, McLaughlin J R, Baker J P et al 1987 What is subjective global assessment of nutritional status? Journal of Enteral and Parenteral Nutrition 11(1):8–13

Eastham R D 1995 Biochemical values in clinical medicine, 7th edn. Churchill Livingstone, Edinburgh

Edington J 1999 Problems of Nutritional assessment in the community. Proceedings of nutritional Assessment 58:47–51

Edwards P D, Moldawer L L 1998 Role of cytokines in the metabolic response to stress. Current Opinion in Clinical Nutrition and Metabolic Care 1(2):187–190

Ek A-C 1987 Prediction of pressure sore development. Scandinavian Journal of Caring Sciences 1(2):77–84

Ek A-C, Unosson M, Larsson J, von Schenck H, Bjurulf P 1991 The development and healing of pressure sores related to the nutritional state. Clinical Nutrition 10:245–250

Falcone P A, Caldwell M D 1990 Wound metabolism. Clinics in Plastic Surgery 17:443–456

Finucane P, Rudra T, Hsu R, Tomlinson K, Hutton R D, Pathy M S 1988 Markers of the nutritional status in acutely ill elderly patients. Gerontology 34(5–6):304–310

Finucane T E 1995 Malnutrition, tube feeding and pressure sores: data are incomplete. Journal of the American Geriatrics Society 43(4):447–451

Fogt E J, Bell S J, Blackburn G L 1995 Nutrition assessment of the elderly. In: Morley J E, Glick Z, Rubenstein L Z (eds) Geriatric nutrition, 2nd edn. Raven Press, New York, pp. 51–62

Galica L A 1997 Parenteral nutrition. Nursing Clinics of North America 33:705–717

Gilchrist B, Morison M 1997 Wound infection. In: Morison M, Moffatt C, Bridel-Nixon J, Bale S (eds) Nursing management of chronic wounds, 2nd edn. Mosby, London, pp. 53–67

Gilmore S A, Robinson G, Posthauer M E, Raymond J 1995 Clinical indicators associated with unintentional weight loss and pressure ulcers in elderly residents of nursing home facilities. Journal of the American Dietetic Association 95:984–992

Goode H F, Burns E, Walker B I 1992 Vitamin C depletion and pressure sores in elderly patients with femoral neck fracture. British Medical Journal 305:925–927

Goodinson S M, Dickerson J W T D 1988 Assessment of nutritional status. In: Dickerson J W T D, Lee H A (eds) Nutrition in the clinical management of disease, 2nd edn. Edward Arnold, London, pp. 456–485

Green C J 1999 Existence, causes and consequences of disease-related malnutrition in the hospital and the community, and clinical and financial benefits of nutritional intervention. Clinical Nutrition 18(2):3–28

Green S M, McLaren S 1998 Nutritional assessment and screening: instrument selection. British Journal of Community Nursing 3:233–242

Green S M, Winterberg H, Franks P J, Moffatt C J, Eberhardie C, McLaren S 1999 Dietary intake of adults, with and without pressure sores, receiving community nursing services. Journal of Wound Care 8(7):325–330

Griffiths 1999 Glutamine: establishing clinical indications. Current Opinion in Clinical Nutrition and Metabolic Care 2:177–182

Guenter P, Jones S, Ericson M 1997 Enteral nutrition therapy. Nursing Clinics of North America 32(4):651–667

Guigoz Y, Velas B, Gary P J 1994 Mini-nutritional assessment: a practical assessment tool for grading the nutritional state of elderly patients. Facts and Research in Gerontology 4(Suppl 2):15–59

Guralnik J M, Harris T B, White L R, Cornoni-Huntley J C 1988 Occurrence and predictors of pressure sores in the National Health and Nutrition Examination Survey follow-up. Journal of the American Geriatrics Society 36:807–812

Haboubi N Y, Hudson P R, Pathy M S 1990 Measurement of height in the elderly. Journal of the American Geriatrics Society 38:1008–1010

Heslin M J, Latkany L, Leung D, Brooks A D, Hockwald S N, Pisters P W 1997 A prospective randomised trial of early enteral feeding after resection of upper GI malignancy. Annals of Surgery 226:567–580

Hunt D R, Maslovitz A, Rowlands B J, Brooks B 1985 A simple-nutrition screening procedure for hospital patients. Journal of the American Dietetic Association 85(3):332–335

Hunt T K, Zelderfeldt B 1969 Nutrition and environmental aspects of wound healing. In: Dunphy J E, van Winkle W (eds) Repair and regeneration. McGraw-Hill, New York

Keller 1993 Malnutrition in institutionalised elderly: how and why. Journal of the American Geriatrics Society 41(11):1212–1218

Kemp M G, Keithley J K, Smith D W, Morreale B 1990 Factors that contribute to pressure sores in surgical patients. Research in Nursing and Health 13:293–301

King's Fund Centre 1992 A positive approach to nutrition as treatment. Report of a working party chaired by Professor Lennard-Jones on the role of enteral and parenteral feeding in hospital and at home. Multiplex Medway Ltd, London

Klein S, Kinney J, Jeejeebhoy K, Alpers D, Hellerstein M, Murray M 1997 Nutritional support in clinical practice: review of published data and recommendations for future research directions. Journal of Parenteral and Enteral Nutrition 21(3):133–156

Kudsk K A, Minard G 1996 A randomised trial of isonitrogenous enteral diets after severe trauma: an immune enhancing diet reduces septic complications. Annals of Surgery 224:531–543

Kushner R F 1993 Body weight and mortality. Nutrition Reviews 51(5):127–136

Kwok T, Whitelaw M N 1991 The use of armspan in nutritional assessment of the elderly. Journal of the American Geriatrics Society 39(5):492–496

Lewis B 1998 Nutrient intake and the risk of pressure sore development in older patients. Journal of Wound Care 7(1):31–35

Lin E, Goncalves J A, Lowry S F 1998 Effect of nutritional pharmacology in surgical patients. Current Opinion in Clinical Nutrition and Metabolic Care 1:41–50

Lindemann R D 1984 Assessment of trace element depletion. In: Wright R, Heymsfield S (eds) Nutritional assessment. Blackwell Scientific, Oxford, pp. 239–261

Liu M H, Spungen A M, Fink L, Losada M, Bauman W A 1996 Increased energy needs in patients with quadriplegia and pressure ulcers. Advanced Wound Care 9(3):41–45

Long C L, Nelson K M 1995 Glutamine supplementation of enteral nutrition: impact on whole body protein kinetics and glucose metabolism in critically ill patients. Journal of Parenteral and Enteral Nutrition 19:470–476

Lord L M 1997 Enteral access devices. Nursing Clinics of North America 32(4):685–703

McLaren S 1992 Nutrition and wound healing. In: Proceedings of the 2nd European Conference on Advances in Wound Management. Emap Healthcare, Cardiff, pp. 67–78

McLaren S 1997 Nutritional factors in wound healing. In: Morison M, Moffatt C, Bridel-Nixon J, Bale S (eds) Nursing management of chronic wounds, 2nd edn. Mosby, London, pp. 27–51

McLaren S, Green S 1998 Nutritional screening and assessment. Nursing Standard 12(48):26–29

McLaren S, Holmes S, Green S, Bond S 1997 An overview of nutritional issues relating to the care of older people in hospital. In: Bond S (ed) Eating matters. The Centre for Health Services Research, University of Newcastle-upon-Tyne, Newcastle-upon-Tyne

McWhirter J P, Pennington C K 1994 Incidence and recognition of malnutrition in hospital. British Medical Journal 308:945–948

McWhirter J P, Pennington C R 1996 A comparison between oral and nasogastric nutritional supplements in malnourished patients. Nutrition 12(7–8):502–506

Mauter J, Weibanm F, Turner J 1996 Reducing the inappropriate use of parenteral nutrition in an acute care teaching hospital. Journal of Parenteral and Enteral Nutrition 20(4):272–274

Mayer K, Seeger W, Grimminger F 1998 Clinical use of lipids to control inflammatory disease. Current Opinion in Clinical Nutrition and Metabolic Care 1(2):179–184

Meaume S, Merlin L, Ramamonjisoa M 1994 Major risk factors associated with pressure sores in geriatric patients. A study of 87 hospitalised elderly people with decubitus ulcers. In: Cherry G N, Leaper D J, Lawrence J C, Milward P (eds) Proceedings of the Fourth European Conference on Wound Management. Macmillan, London, pp. 39–42

Melcher R E, Longe R I, Gelbart A O 1988 Pressure sores in the elderly. Postgraduate Medicine 3:299–308

Meyer N A, Muller M J, Herndon D N 1994 Nutrient support of the healing wound. New Horizons 2(2):202–214

Moolten S E 1972 Bedsores in the chronically ill patient. Archive of Phys Medical Rehabi 53:430–438

Morley J E 1995 Anorexia of ageing and protein-energy under-nutrition. In: Morley J E, Glick Z, Rubenstein L Z (eds) Geriatric nutrition: a comprehensive review. Raven Press, New York, pp. 75–78

Muhlethaler R, Stuck A E, Minder C E, Frey B 1995 The prognostic significance of protein energy malnutrition in geriatric patients. Age and Ageing 24:193–197

Mulholland J H, Tui C, Wright A M, Vinci V, Shafiroff B 1943 Protein metabolism and bed sores. Annals of Surgery 118(6):1015–1023

Myers S A, Takiguchi S, Slavish S, Rose C L 1990 Consistent wound care and nutritional support in treatment. Decubitus 3(3):16–28

Nicolaus T, Bach M, Siezen S, Volkert D, Oster P, Schlierf G 1995 Assessment of nutritional risk in the elderly. Annals of Nutrition and Metabolism 39:340–345

Nightingale J M D, Walsh N, Bullock M E, Wicks A C 1996 Three simple methods of detecting malnutrition on medical wards. Journal of the Royal Society of Medicine 89:144–148

Osterweil D, Wendt P F, Ferrell 1995 Pressure ulcers and nutrition. In: Morley J E, Glick Z, Rubenstein L Z (eds) Geriatric nutrition. Raven Press, New York, pp. 335–342

Pattison D, Young A 1997 Effects of a multidisciplinary care team on the management of gastrostomy feeding. Journal of Human Nutrition and Dietetics 10:103–109

Perneger T V, Heliot C, Rae A C, Borst F, Gaspoz J M 1998 Hospital-acquired pressure ulcers: risk factors and use of preventive devices. Archives of Internal Medicine 158(17):1940–1945

Pinchcofsky-Devin G D, Kaminski M V 1986 Correlation of pressure sores and nutritional status. Journal of the American Geriatric Society 34:435–440

Potter J, Klipstein K, Reilly J J, Roberts M 1995 The nutritional status and clinical course of acute admissions to a geriatric unit. Age and Ageing 24:131–136

RCN 1993 Dynamic quality improvement programme. Nutrition standards and the older adult. Royal College of Nursing, London

Redgrave T G 1999 Lipids in enteral nutrition. Current Opinion in Clinical Nutrition and Metabolic Care 2(2):147–152

Rissanen A, Heliovaara M, Knekt P, Aromaa A, Reunanen A, Maatela J 1989 Weight and mortality in Finnish men. Journal of Clinical Epidemiology 42:781–789

Rissanen A, Heliovaara M, Knekt P, Aromaa A, Reunanen A, Maatela J 1991 Weight and mortality in Finnish women. Journal of Clinical Epidemiology 44:787–795

Rombeau J L, Rolandelli R H (eds) 1997 Clinical nutrition: enteral and tube feeding, 3rd edn. W B Saunders, London

Roth E 1998 The impact of L-arginine-nitric oxide metabolism on ischaemia-reperfusion injury. Current Opinion in Clinical Nutrition and Metabolic Care 1:97–99

Ruberg R 1984 Role of nutrition in wound healing. Surgical Clinics of North America 64:705–714

Sandstead H H, Henriksen L K, Greger J, Prasad A S, Good R A 1982 Zinc nutriture in the elderly in relation to taste acuity, immune response and wound healing. American Journal of Clinical Nutrition, 1046–1059

Schue R M, Langemo D K 1998 Pressure ulcer prevalence and incidence and a modification of the Braden Scale for a rehabilitation unit. Journal of Wound, Ostomy and Continence Nursing 25(1):36–43

Selhub J, Rosenberg I 1984 Evaluation of vitamin deficiency states. In: Wright R, Heymsfield S (eds) Nutritional assessment. Blackwell Scientific, Oxford, pp. 209–238

Shenkin A 1999 Why are vitamins and trace elements needed? In Proceedings of 21st ESPEN Congress Educational Supplement. Stockholm, pp. 75–88

Silberman J 1989 Parenteral and enteral nutrition. Appleton & Lange, New York

Sitton-Kent L, Gilchrist B 1993 The intake of nutrients by hospitalised pensioners with chronic wounds. Journal of Advanced Nursing 18:1962–1967

Solomons N W 1988 Zinc and copper. In: Shils M E (ed.) Modern nutrition in health and disease. Lea and Febiger, Philadelphia, pp. 239–244

Stableforth P G 1986 Supplement feeds and nitrogen and calorie balance following femoral neck fracture. British Journal of Surgery 73(8):651–655

Stordy J 1988 Obesity: management in the treatment of disease. In: Dickerson J W T, Lee T A (eds) Nutrition in the clinical management of disease. Edward Arnold, London, pp. 145–166

Stratton R J, Elia M 1999 A critical systematic analysis of the use of oral nutritional supplements in the community. Clinical Nutrition 18:29–84

Strauss E A, Margolis D J 1996 Malnutrition in patients with pressure ulcers: morbidity, mortality and clinically practical assessments. Advances in Wound Care 9(5):37–40

Tayback M, Kumanyika S, Chee E 1990 Body weight as a risk factor in the elderly. Archives of Internal Medicine 150(5):1065–1072

Taylor S, Goodinson-McLaren 1992 Nutritional support: a team approach. Wolfe Publishing, London

Taylor T V 1974 Ascorbic acid supplementation in the treatment of pressure sores. Lancet ii:544–546

Telfer N R, Moy R L 1993 Drug and nutrient aspects of wound healing. Dermatologic Clinics 11(4):729–737

Thomas D R 1997 The role of nutrition in prevention and healing of pressure ulcers. Clinics in Geriatric Medicine 13(3):497–511

Ward M W N 1982 Effects of subclinical malnutrition and refeeding on the healing of experimental colonic anastomoses. British Journal of Surgery 69:308

Wells L 1994 At the front line of care. The importance of nutrition in wound management. Professional Nurse 9(8):525–526, 528–530

Zulkowski K 1998 MDS+ RAP items associated with pressure ulcer prevalence in newly institutionalised elderly: study 1. Ostomy/Wound Management 44(11):40–44, 46–48, 50

14 *Barbara Pieper*
Patient education

INTRODUCTION

Patient and caregiver education is a cornerstone for the prevention and treatment of pressure ulcers. It is a process of assisting patients and caregivers to learn and incorporate health-related behaviour into daily life. Patients have a right to participate and make decisions about their care but they need knowledge if they are to do so in an informed way. However, debilitation, which is a primary factor for placing a patient at risk for pressure ulcers, may severely hamper the achievement of learning.

Goals of patient education include enabling patients to gain an understanding of the disease process, to regain health, to minimize dysfunction or further loss, and to shorten the length of hospital stay (Barnes 1987). For pressure ulcer prevention, education needs to be immediate, relevant, intense and motivational. The learner needs to both cognitively understand and effectively perceive their susceptibility to pressure ulcers, the likely cost to themselves of pressure ulcers if acquired, the efficacy of skin care and barriers to skin care (Dai & Catanzaro 1987). Ideally, the person should feel empowered, and change should be viewed as worthwhile and of benefit.

Pressure ulcer education by health care professionals can be patchy and inadequate. Numerous health care providers are involved in pressure ulcer education, including the nurse, physician, physical therapist and occupational therapist. Teaching involves interpersonal interactions in a trusting relationship between the patient and

caregiver and the health care clinician, and patients and caregivers need to be encouraged, listened to and respected.

In this chapter the concept of empowerment is briefly reviewed, together with the advantages and disadvantages of a number of approaches to teaching and learning. There is a growing body of evidence to suggest that the distribution of educational materials to patients is not enough.

EMPOWERMENT

In the last three decades there has been a fundamental shift in health promotion away from a 'top-down' biomedical approach, which assumes that health care professionals always know best, towards a 'bottom-up' approach which emphasizes partnership, empowerment of the individual, and respect for the individual's rights to self-determination and autonomy. Empowerment is fundamental to a client-centred approach, with its emphasis on mutuality, egalitarianism and shared responsibility. Clients are viewed as their own experts rather than as passive recipients of advice, and health care professionals are regarded as facilitators rather than as experts whose views should not be challenged.

Empowerment is concerned with assisting the individual to develop proactive healthy behaviours for themselves (Brown 1997, Florian & Elad 1998). It involves enhancing perceived control and self-efficacy over the course of life events and influencing life conditions through problem solving, coping and effective use of resources. Empowerment is not 'given' to a person (Pellino et al 1998, Walker, 1998), it is a participative process through which a nurse and client work together to change unhealthy behaviours (Ellis-Stoll & Popkess-Vawter 1998). The patient is an active learner and teaching goes beyond the treatment plan and technical procedural skills (Wellard et al 1998). The patient is a problem solver and the nurse is a resource; both share responsibility for treatment and outcomes. The nurse's teaching goes beyond giving information and the patient helps to identify problems and learning needs.

Effective communication may improve outcomes of care, patient satisfaction and adherence to care recommendations. Teaching fosters increased patient confidence in the management of a health condition (Wellard et al 1998) and knowledge enables the patient to make informed choices about actions and activities (Walker 1998).

Nurses may vary in their beliefs about their role in patient education. Kruger (1991) examined nurses' perceptions of responsibility for patient education and the level of its achievement. Nurses believed that they should hold a high level of responsibility for patient education. However, the overall achievement of patient education activities was rated low. To improve teaching, nurses need increased knowledge about patient teaching, time for teaching and accessible patient teaching kits (Kruger 1991, Wellard et al 1998).

WHAT THE LEARNER BRINGS TO THE SITUATION

To prevent pressure ulcers, a learner needs to aspire to acquire new knowledge and to recognize a gap between the status quo and the desired state. In addition to the cognitive information about pressure ulcer prevention and treatment, affective considerations, such as perceptions, expectations and values, as well as psychomotor abilities and financial and social considerations must be considered. For example, many paraplegic individuals are physically able to prevent pressure ulcers but still develop them. Patients change over their disability course; education,

assessment and evaluation must be lifelong. Health professionals should not assume that patients/caregivers associate the same meaning with a medical word or phrase. A 'sore' may be perceived as a scraped knee that heals in an expedient manner. Patients may assume that skills that are most difficult to perform are the most important ones to do; since it may appear to be basic, skin care may be ignored. When patients receive reinforcement for performing a skill, they sense its importance; health care providers need to praise pressure ulcer preventive skills and demonstrate their importance in care.

Olshansky (1994) identified two groups of persons with pressure ulcers: passive and active. The passive pressure ulcer group is dependent upon others for care and has no control over the development or treatment of pressure ulcers (i.e. the bedridden patient or the person with quadriplegia). Caregivers are essential for the passive group. The active group has some control over the development of pressure ulcers. Those in the active group need to be asked if they want to prevent pressure ulcers; this involves a psychosocial assessment. The teacher must be ready to deal with hostility, rage, loss, pain and self-esteem.

Readiness to learn is critical

Readiness can be impaired by the person's physical health, pain, disturbed sleep and psychosocial factors. Goals for learning must be realistic and include short-, intermediate- and long-term objectives; they should be mutually determined by the patient, caregiver and health care clinician. There may at times be discrepancies between the patient's and clinician's goals, but it still may be possible to achieve the same outcome of care (Maklebust & Magnan 1992). Revisions of goals are a valuable part of education.

The information necessary for pressure ulcer prevention and treatment is complex. The person must learn core information, be able to discriminate relevant cues and decide upon a course of action (Andberg et al 1983). Decision making may be constrained by the person's situation, attitude and/or social pressure. Poor reading skills make it difficult to analyse instructions and to ask questions (Ayello 1993). It is possible that those with poor reading skills may not have the ability to synthesize information (Ayello 1993). Most patient educational materials are written two grade levels above the average grade achieved by the patient (Yasenchak & Bridle 1993). The patient's grade level may be inaccurate owing to social promotion in school, inaccurate history or reporting, and loss of reading skill over time through disuse. A low literacy level does not mean that a person cannot learn, but creative approaches must be used to help with learning. Written materials, such as manuals and booklets, should be secondary sources of information. When teaching patients with low literacy levels it helps to:

- teach the smallest amount of information possible
- use simple language
- avoid complex and ambiguous information and medical jargon
- use pictures and graphics
- share and learn from the experiences of other patients.

The special needs of children

Because of the growing number of children with chronic illness, infants and children may develop pressure ulcers yet they may be overlooked because of the number of other childhood skin problems (Quigley & Curley 1996). The primary pressure ulcer site for infants and toddlers is the occipital region and for children, the sacrum (Quigley & Curley 1996). Education of the child in terms of pressure ulcer prevention is dependent upon the child's physical, cognitive and psychosocial developmental level. For infants and toddlers, generally the parents are the primary learners. School-age children may be more independent and able to learn pressure ulcer prevention techniques such as weight shifting while sitting or repositioning while lying in bed. Adolescents are able to understand health as a concept, desire to assert independence and are concerned about privacy, personal

space and confidentiality (Whitman 1992). The child's developmental level will affect how teaching is done. Pictures are critical components of teaching programmes; words and symbols are used as a child is able to comprehend them. Because of a child's exposure to television and computers, the use of videotapes and computer programs may enhance interest in maintenance of skin integrity. The gross and fine motor abilities will impact if the child is able to assist with technical aspects of care such as weight shifting or wound care.

The adult learner

Learning by the adult is determined by life tasks, roles and immediate problems (Whitman 1992). In adulthood, the person generally reaches peak physical ability and cognitive capacity and is able to learn formally and informally. Adulthood should also be examined in terms of the developmental tasks of the person depending upon age, physical maturity, and cognitive and psychosocial development. An illness that affects mobility and thus increases risk for pressure ulcer development may negatively affect the adult's lifestyle and the stress of the life change may affect readiness to learn. The teaching method for adults should match their learning style. Adults resist learning non-relevant material, may need time to complete learning tasks and may resist changing established practices (Whitman 1992). Adults are concerned about time needed for education since it competes with time for work, family and other activities.

The special needs of older patients and caregivers

Older patients at risk of pressure ulcers may be quite debilitated. It is a myth that pressure ulcers are to be expected and unavoidable with ageing. Physiologically, older patients have weakened epidermal junctions in the skin and decreased subcutaneous fat so that skin may more easily break down. Older patients/caregivers need to be educated about pressure ulcer prevention. Baharestani (1994) identified reasons why older patients/caregivers receive suboptimal care and teaching:

1 clinician views patient education for older adults as futile since cognitive ability may decline with ageing
2 health care focus on disease
3 lack of understanding of older patients
4 myths about ageing
5 fear about ageing and death, and
6 stereotyping older adults instead of working with them as individuals.

The elderly are less likely to challenge authority figures, less likely to ask questions, less inclined to take a participatory or controlling role in the health care process and less effective in getting the physician to attend to their health concerns than younger patients (Maly et al 1998). Older adults weigh the costs and benefits of care in terms of improving quality of life, comfort and/or mobility. As with any learner, the teacher should maximize the older person's strengths during teaching sessions. The older adult should be treated with respect; first names should not be used unless requested by the person.

Physiological changes with ageing may affect teaching the older adult. Because memory and memory storage changes with age, older adults need more time to process information during a teaching session. Older adults take longer to arrive at an awareness level of the content and longer for the stimulus of what is being taught to clear before moving to another topic. Teaching content is best presented slowly, using pneumonic devices. Short specific instructions, repetition and hands-on participation are important teaching strategies. Frequent breaks are helpful.

It should be noted that visual acuity, glare tolerance, ability to adapt to light and dark and peripheral vision all decrease with ageing. Written materials should therefore have a large type size, solid print, short sentences and be in colours that provide distinct contrasts. Paper should be glare free. The educator should consider the glare in the room from the windows and floor. The older adult should be able to see the teacher's face. Older adults may learn better with one-on-one instruction since peripheral vision is impaired for group participation.

With changes to hearing, words begin to sound distorted and conversation is difficult to understand; background noise makes hearing worse. The teacher should slow the rate of speech, use a lower voice pitch and speak slightly louder. It is best to face the person directly. Background noises need to be decreased, e.g. by turning off the television and radio and closing doors to block out noisy areas.

The special needs of the spinal cord injured patient

Spinal cord injury is associated with a high incidence of pressure ulcers. Education should include a concise and coherent core of information about skin care problems among the spinal cord injured and the need for self-responsibility. The patient needs to find personal relevance in skin care activities; the staff then becomes a resource (Andberg et al 1983). Dover and colleagues (1992) suggest a comprehensive educational programme reinforced by all staff across inpatient, outpatient and community settings. Attention to detail and regular follow-up may decrease the incidence of pressure ulcers.

Rehabilitation nurses and others have examined skin care education for the spinal cord injured. Dai & Catanzaro (1987) noted that perceived severity of pressure ulcers and perceived efficacy of skin care were positively related to compliance with skin care. Perceived susceptibility did not correlate significantly with compliance. Factors modifying skin care included the patient's actual skin condition, advice from others, patient–practitioner relationship, demographic, sociopsychologic variables, and prior experiences with skin care. LaMantia and coworkers (1987) noted that spinal cord injured patients could maintain healed skin for the first 3 months, but an additional percentage reopened between 3 months and 1 year. Rodriguez & Garber (1994) studied men with spinal cord injuries who had developed pressure ulcers in the past but whose skin was intact when the study began. Most (82%) believed that they were not likely to develop another ulcer in the coming years, 61% believed that pressure ulcers were very serious and 72.5% used weight shifts and turning as the most performed activity to prevent pressure ulcers. Only 29% avoided sitting for too long, 24% inspected the skin, 21% used a wheelchair cushion and 18% used a careful transfer technique. Rodriguez & Garber (1994) reported a discrepancy between what patients with spinal cord injury knew about pressure ulcer prevention and what they practised. Knowledge retained was incomplete and had not been translated into effective strategies for preventing recurrence. Unfortunately, no patient asked for either additional information about skin care or to be re-evaluated for pressure-related problems. Continued education is necessary since patients are discharged when they have achieved medical stability and have only a modest degree of functional independence.

Involving the family

Family members are often care providers for an ill or disabled member. Roles within a family may change with care of an ill member; communication among and between family members is therefore critical. The family's reaction and perception of an illness, and its priority learning needs are critical components of the nurse's assessment (Viggiani 1997). For the person with impaired mobility, pressure ulcer prevention is probably only one component of care the family is learning. The nurse and family must decide upon mutual goals for the care, and the availability of the family to be part of teaching sessions must always be considered.

PSYCHOSOCIAL FACTORS AFFECTING TEACHING AND LEARNING

Culture

Culture is an integral part of a person's life and includes knowledge, beliefs, values, morals, customs, traditions and habits (Bastable 1997). Cultural assessment of a patient and family may provide information which will affect teaching. Culture may affect the way someone perceives a health problem, treatment options, attitudes and reactions to the illness, and readiness to learn

KEY POINTS

SOME GENERAL PRINCIPLES

- ◆ Empowering the patient/caregiver enhances learning
- ◆ The patient and caregiver need to be assessed in terms of learning needs and preferred learning style
- ◆ The patient's/caregiver's culture, educational level, family structure and income may affect teaching and learning
- ◆ Teaching usually needs repetition and reinforcement over time
- ◆ Patients/caregivers who are elderly or have a physical or mental disability or low literacy may still be capable of learning
- ◆ Patients/caregivers may participate in educational programmes in a variety of settings
- ◆ Numerous teaching methods and materials are available – no single method is effective for every learner and each has advantages and disadvantages
- ◆ Teaching methods and materials need to be critically selected to match the teacher's, learner's and institution's needs
- ◆ Use of multiple teaching methods and materials enhances learning
- ◆ Evaluation of the teaching in terms of the learner, teacher, and outcomes is critical and may stimulate research.

(Bastable 1997). Nurses need to be culturally sensitive. This may include teaching with an interpreter; providing written and audiovisual materials in an appropriate language; incorporating folk and religious practices in care if not harmful; respecting the family leadership; and demonstrating sensitivity for privacy and exposure of the body. Working within a patient's culture in terms of pressure ulcer prevention may empower the patient and family.

Socioeconomic status

Socioeconomic status includes income, educational level and family structure (Bastable 1997). Poverty may affect educational level, lifestyle and health care options for patients and their families. Stereotyping a patient and family, however, because they are low income, is unacceptable. The nurse must assess literacy level and availability of resources prior to teaching pressure ulcer prevention; strengths and weakness for learning should be noted.

KEY POINTS

THE EDUCATION PROCESS

- ◆ Pressure ulcer prevention teaching needs to begin at admission and be relevant, intense and motivational so as to empower the patient/caregiver in maintaining healthy skin. Goals of teaching should match the person's readiness to learn

- ◆ Pressure ulcer prevention teaching must be reinforced over time, such as during subsequent home visits or outpatient clinic visits

- ◆ The nurse should carefully listen to the patient/caregiver since they may have a different understanding as to what a pressure ulcer is

- ◆ The nurse should demonstrate pressure ulcer preventive care to patients because it reinforces its importance and allows the patient to see an expert performing care

- ◆ The nurse should consider growth and developmental issues of childhood, adulthood and old age when considering teaching strategies and methods

- ◆ Culture and socioeconomic status may affect who is allowed to be a caregiver, treatment options and attitude and reactions to illness. The nurse needs to assess the patient/caregiver and provide culturally competent care. Stereotyping of a patient or family should be avoided

- ◆ The nurse should try to use more than one teaching method, i.e. lecture, one to one, group discussion, demonstration and return demonstration, and role play

- ◆ The nurse should critically review and use a variety of teaching materials, i.e. written materials, slides, overhead transparencies, computer-generated images, videotapes, television, flip charts, flannel boards, chalkboards, markerboards, computers and contracts. A teacher will be proficient in the use of some, but probably not all of the materials

- ◆ The nurse needs to evaluate each patient teaching episode for its potential outcomes, modify the teaching as necessary and continue to teach.

PATIENT EDUCATIONAL SETTINGS

Generally, clinicians think of acute care and rehabilitative settings as primary areas for patient education. Yet patients in these settings may be in pain and coping with a new diagnosis and therapies. Since the length of stay is short, there is urgency to teach pressure ulcer prevention as well as other aspects of care. Teaching materials need to be readily available so that teaching can be done whenever the nurse is in the patient's room. (Panel for the Prediction and Prevention of Pressure Ulcers in Adults 1992, Bergstrom et al 1994). Inpatient settings provide opportunities for the initial assessment of patient/caregiver learning needs and resources and supervised skill practice.

APPROACHES TO TEACHING AND LEARNING

Methods of teaching and learning

The teacher usually selects the method of instruction after careful assessment of the learner's needs, through a process of consultation and negotiation. Methods are the techniques the teacher uses to present the content to the learner. No one method of teaching is best; generally, multiple teaching methods enhance learning. The method selected is often dependent upon the teacher's preference, how active the learner is to be, class size, characteristics of the learner such as age, ethnicity, culture, educational background, and the setting (Fitzgerald 1997). Table 14.1 summarizes a number of approaches.

The method of instruction selected should help the patient and/or caregiver meet the objectives of the learning experience. Learning objectives should be mutually determined to empower the person in terms of health promotion for skin integrity. The learner must be an active participant in the teaching and stimulated to learn by the method; thus, the person's literacy level, physical and emotional developmental level, and sociocultural factors must be assessed. The teaching method must be accessible to the learner

Table 14.1 Advantages and disadvantages of a number of methods of teaching and learning	
Advantages	Disadvantages
One-to-one instruction	
• Individualized	• Learners may feel they are being quizzed
• Learner and teacher actively involved	• Labour-intensive and time-consuming for the teacher
• Mutual goal setting	• Learner not exposed to others with same problem for sharing ideas
• Proceeds at pace of learner; suited to persons with low literacy	
Lecture	
• Presented to a group; cost and time effective	• Learner is often passive
• Good for presenting basic and foundational content	• Psychomotor skills are not learned
• Teacher available to answer questions	• Does not account for variations in learners
• Method generally associated with learning	• Follows a structured schedule
• Effective for a motivating, high-energy teacher	• Needs to be planned; learner must plan to attend
	• Associated with being in school
	• Difficult for some persons to hear
	• Teacher may not be comfortable with it
	• Ineffective for affective and psychomotor learning
Demonstration return demonstration	
• Active participation of the learner	• Time-consuming
• Able to watch person with expertise and ask questions	• Teacher and learner must be available at the same time
• Able to learn safety measures	• Setting must have equipment available for practice
• Individualized learning	• Equipment must match what learner will use
• Gain confidence before performing a skill on a person	• Practice should be supervised
• Teacher is a coach	
• Praise is important	
Role play	
• Stimulates affective learning	• Discomfort in performing in front of others
• Active involvement of the learner	• Some may exaggerate a role
• Dramatization of a situation	• Takes time
	• Group size may limit effectiveness
Group discussion	
• Active involvement of the learner	• Teacher may not feel comfortable with the method
• May learn from others sharing information	• Group may wander aimlessly
• Teacher helps to keep group focused	• Learner may feel uncomfortable or shy in a group
• May learn how to respond to situations	• Participants may monopolize a group or make others feel uncomfortable
• Groups generally limited to no more than 20	• Must attend at a structured time
• Effective use of time	• Takes more time to present information than a lecture
• May improve coping mechanisms	
• May increase self-confidence	

and presented within a reasonable time-frame. Enthusiasm, humour, examples, problem-solving activities, positive reinforcement and feedback, repetition and questioning often enhance the teaching method being used. In addition, the cost effectiveness of the teaching for the patient and the health care agency must be considered.

Issues of transfer of newly learned skills to the home environment have been identified as a research priority (Gordon et al 1996). Most elderly people live at home; without carers many elderly would require institutionalization (Baharestani 1994). In the patient's home, a priority is placed on quality of life (Benbow 1996). Sharing the work relieves the burden on the primary caregiver and decreases caregiver strain; it is important that all caregivers should be involved in pressure ulcer education. Ayello et al (1997) noted factors that inhibit or enhance learning by home caregivers:

- the person's physical ability to perform a task
- the culture's effect on performing care
- financial resources
- cognitive impairment
- ability to retain information, and
- gender-affected teaching situations.

Baharestani (1994) identified themes in elderly wives' caregiving in the home when a husband had a Stage III or IV pressure ulcer. Difficulty with caregiving included fatigue from the physical care, the emotional strain of seeing the husband debilitated, safety issues with care and financial concerns. Caregivers were frail and disregarded their own health. They had limited socialization and social support from others. Caregivers had limited knowledge about caregiving and often learned skills by experience. To reach and educate caregivers, educational television, social security checks with freephone numbers for obtaining educational literature, counselling and assistance, and free phone numbers to answer caregiver questions may be helpful (Baharestani 1994).

Materials as an aid to teaching and learning

Teaching materials are resources and tools that help to communicate the content being taught.

Teaching materials should complement the method of teaching. Teaching materials should progress from the known to unknown, maximize the patient's/caregiver's involvement and be logically organized. Teaching materials may be used in individual or group sessions. Constraints of teaching materials should be considered, such as time for use, preparation time, time commitment of the caregiver, the illness acuity of the patient, the environment in which the materials are to be used and the size of the group. Evaluation of teaching materials is done in terms of outcomes, such as the patient's/caregiver's knowledge, attitudes and skills. Table 14.2 summarizes a number of forms for instructional materials. Some of the most commonly used media are described below.

Written materials (booklets, pamphlets, handouts)

Written materials are a potentially important resource for the patient and caregiver because they are there when the clinician is not. Written materials supplement and reinforce verbal explanations. They are the medium generally preferred for understanding complex concepts and relationships. Patients/caregivers have control over how fast they read and understand the material. Written materials are the most widely used teaching material and are familiar and acceptable to the public.

Poorly written materials can impede the learning process. They may tell a person what to do yet not involve the person. The longer and more complicated they are, the less likely they are to be read. The person must be able to read well enough to understand and interpret what is read and use the information as it was intended (Ayello 1993). Written materials may not match the person in terms of gender, ethnicity or age, thus making it difficult for the person to identify with what is being taught. Written materials should not merely be left with the patient but used to augment interaction with a teacher.

Written materials should be evaluated before they are used. It is important to consider the

Table 14.2 Advantages and disadvantages of a number of forms of presenting instructional materials

Advantages	Disadvantages
Written materials	
• Augment interaction with the teacher	• May overwhelm the learner
• Readily available at any time for the learner	• May be poorly developed and not match criteria for written materials
• Reinforce content	• Time-consuming to create well
• Widely accepted and familiar to the general public	
• Readily updated	
• Can be personalized to a setting, person, situation	
Slides/overheads/computer images	
• Good augmentation for a lecture	• Room needs to be darkened to some degree, so some persons may fall asleep or lose interest
• Focus the learning	• Teacher may not know how to handle basic mechanical problems with the equipment
• May be organized in the order to match the teaching	• Teacher must be careful where standing, so as to not block the image
• Readily updated and created	• May be poorly made – type too small, too much information, colour difficult to see
• May go backwards and forwards	• Equipment may generate noise and make hearing difficult
• Generally inexpensive	• Generally do not project action
Videotapes/television	
• Comfortable media for many learners	• Television does not allow a programme to be stopped or replayed
• May visualize a skill/technique of care	• Programmes may be too long
• Provides action	• May not have a programme tape to match the learning need
• Videotapes allow viewing of all or part of a programme at the learner's pace and repetition is possible	• Need access to a television and video player
• Videotapes may be viewed at any time and at varied locations	• Learner may be uncomfortable with video player equipment
• Less time for the teacher since a person may view it alone	• May need cable, satellite television access for some information
	• Learner may be easily distracted and miss parts of programmes
	• Teacher may not be present to answer questions or summarize content
	• Programme may not accurately show the content
Flip charts/flannel boards	
• Creative	• Learner may not relate to poorly written stories
• Interactively involves the learner	• Words or pictures may be too difficult to see
• Visualizing a story is effective with children	• May contain too much information and clutter
• Stories written to specifically match a situation	• May not match the person's learning level
Chalkboards/markerboards	
• Inexpensive	• Writing may be illegible
• Help to focus a presentation/discussion	• Writing/diagrams may be too small for all to see
• Display a simple message	• Teacher's back is to the audience
• Display steps to a procedure	• Information is lost with erasing
• Quickly created	• May add time to teaching
• Errors quickly erased	
• Encourage learner participation	
Computer/computer-assisted instruction (CAI)	
• Wide availability of teaching materials and methods – games, simulations	• Equipment may not be accessible
• May chat with experts or other persons with the same condition	• Fear of technology and using a computer
	• Cost of computer and Internet access may be too high

Table 14.2 *Continued*	
Advantages	Disadvantages
• May see pictures and read articles • Provides information about professional and lay groups • May progress at own pace and at any time • With CAI, the teacher can see where the learner is having problems • Access to persons of various cultures and languages • Reduces feelings of isolation • Access to information that a learner may want to keep confidential	• Lack of educational programs to match learning goals • CAI programs too complex to use • CAI programs time-consuming and expensive to develop • May not be appropriate for someone with low literacy
Self-study modules • Promote individual learning • May be individualized to the learner • Able to complete at any time • Promotes distant learning	• Independent learning is not effective for some learners • Literacy level may be too high • May lack interaction with a teacher for questions • Modules difficult and time-consuming to create • Modules use technology that may not be available for some learners
Learning contracts • Mutually negotiated between the learner and teacher • Provide direction, goals and evaluation criteria • Learner may feel committed and accountable • Usually include a reward	• Teacher/learner may not feel comfortable with the method • Objectives and dates may need to be renegotiated as learning progresses • May be incorrectly written – lack content, time frame, performance expectations, terms of contract, criteria for evaluation

audience. Who, in terms of age, sex, literacy level and racial/ethnic background will use the materials? What is the length of the material? Will the materials overwhelm the learner or do they stimulate the learner? One should consider the reading level of the materials, illustrations, paper and print colour, type size and style, layout and appearance, and clarity. Considerations for the development of written materials are presented in Table 14.3. In summary, written materials should enhance the educator's teaching and be appropriate for the situation and the learner.

Videotapes and television

Videotapes and television allow people to learn using a medium that they are familiar and generally comfortable with (Redman 1997). Videotape programmes allow the learner to visualize a skill. Information moves in an active way to encourage attention to what is being taught. It is a flexible medium since the learner may view all or part of the tape as often as desired. Videotapes need to be kept short, preferably 5–20 min (Hainsworth 1997). The patient or caregiver may be taped so that the person views the self-performing of a skill for reinforcement of content. Disadvantages of videotapes include the lack of compatibility of content with the learning goals, and the cost and time to develop tapes. Some individuals may not have equipment to view tapes. The person also needs to be able to hear the tape or captions need to be provided for the hearing-impaired person. Videotaping should be used as an adjunct to traditional teaching methods so that the learner has an opportunity to talk with the teacher.

Computer-assisted learning

Computer education may include the Internet and computer-assisted instruction (CAI). Use of the World Wide Web is helpful for some patients/ caregivers in learning. Computer

Table 14.3 Considerations when developing written materials

Words
- Use words consistently, e.g. pressure ulcer
- Use short words – one or two syllables
- Use common words
- Avoid compound words
- Avoid words with prefixes and suffixes
- Avoid abbreviations and symbols
- Avoid jargon, slang and cliches
- Define medical terms

Sentences
- Keep length short
- Use active instead of passive voice
- Use conversational style – you and yours

Paragraphs
- Start with a strong topic sentence
- Have one idea/message
- Give examples
- Do not 'talk down' to the reader

Graphics
- Use simple diagrams/illustrations with titles and captions
- Avoid cartoons if they trivialize the message or insult the reader
- Provide sufficient picture of a body part so that it is identifiable
- Show only the correct way to do things

Layout
- Aim to make the material 'eye catching'
- Allow white space; do not crowd pages
- Highlight with bold or underlining
- Use colour consistently
- Use dull finish instead of high-gloss paper
- Use white/off-white paper
- Use black type; red, yellow, blue, orange and pastel colours are not easily seen
- Use headings to divide sections
- Avoid all capital letters
- Avoid italics, script and fancy lettering
- Use simple type style – serif
- Use large font size; 14–18 print size
- Use bullets for key points
- Organize content in chunks
- Consider flow for pamphlets that are folded/unfolded

General
- Provide information; do not assume that the person is an expert
- Consider ethnic/cultural/gender sensitivity
- Avoid a high reading level; best to keep at 8th grade or lower
- Use a reading level formula: Fog Index, SMOG formula, Fry Readability Graph-Extended
- Use numbers and statistics sparingly
- Have supplemental information to augment written work – videotapes, audio tapes, models, etc.
- Allow space to personalize information
- Write in a positive manner

resources may allow the patient/caregiver to learn about specific treatments, chat with wound care experts, feel less isolated, read articles about pressure ulcer prevention and treatment, find information about confidential topics, and also provide information about various organizations and groups that have an interest in pressure ulcer prevention and treatment (Ayello et al 1997, Redman 1997). Professional organizations with computer access include, but are not limited to, the Wound, Ostomy and Continence Nurses Society, Association for the Advancement of Wound Care, Dermatology Nurses Association, American Academy of Dermatologists and the National Pressure Ulcer Advisory Panel. It is implicit that the person must have access to a computer and the Internet and be comfortable in using both.

CAI may help to teach and reinforce cognitive information. Games or instructional materials can be developed about pressure ulcer preven-tion and the patient/caregiver can work through the programs at an individualized pace. Inter-active programs can immediately provide feed-back to the learner. Some CAI allows the educator to obtain information about where the person is having difficulty and enhance teaching in that area. Disadvantages of CAI include the method not being of interest to the learner, lack of programs to match the learning goals, the complexity and time-consuming nature of devel-oping programs, the quality of the programs and the expense. Individuals with low literacy levels and some disabilities may not be able to com-plete computer programs.

DEVELOPING LEARNING CONTRACTS

Learning contracts encourage active participa-tion by the learner, improve teacher–learner com-munication and enhance learner expressiveness and creativity (Bastable & Sculco 1997). Learning contracts are a mutually negotiated agreement and are generally written. They empower the learner because they emphasize direction, mutual goal setting and mutual evaluation. Because of active involvement, the learner may feel committed and accountable for learning. There is usually some type of reward for following the contract. A tangible reward for pressure ulcer prevention is the person's skin remaining intact, thus avoiding the pain and disfigurement of a pressure ulcer; they are also praised for their management.

Contracts need to include the content to be learned, the time-frame to learn the content, the performance expectations, terms of the contract and the criteria for evaluation (Bastable & Sculco 1997). Because both the educator and learner play active roles in contract learning, they must feel comfortable with this method. The learner's current abilities and learning needs must be considered and objectives and dates may need to be renegotiated from time to time.

EVALUATION OF LEARNING

Evaluation of the educational experience is a critical component of patient and caregiver education. The learner needs to be evaluated with regard to the objectives and goals of the educational programme. Criteria need to be developed to evaluate learning successfully: for example, the learner may verbalize knowledge or perform a skill. The teaching methods and materials also need to be evaluated by the teacher and learner in terms of their qualities and their impact on the learner. The entire patient and staff educational programme in a care setting needs to be evaluated. Since research about patient education is limited, evaluation may lead to research and further refinement of teaching (Redman 1997).

LEGAL CONCERNS

Health care settings need to have programmes for the prevention and treatment of pressure ulcers. The management within a facility must decide who is responsible for seeing that the prevention programmes are carried out and who is accountable when a patient develops a pressure ulcer (Olshansky 1994). An issue in medical malpractice is whether the clinician met the standard of care: namely, that exercised by others in the same line of practice under the same or similar circumstances (Murphy 1997). This includes failure to do something that should have been done, such as patient teaching. Documentation is critical and should be detailed. Documentation shows communication and continuity among those involved in the care. Teaching that was done and the person's response to teaching are important.

In order to implement teaching, the practitioner must be knowledgeable about pressure ulcer prevention and treatment. Quality assurance programmes have validated the belief that staff education is beneficial in preventing pressure ulcers, yet nurses' knowledge of pressure ulcers may be lacking (Hunter et al 1995, Pieper & Mott 1995, Pieper & Mattern 1997). Guidelines document the educational content for pressure ulcer prevention and care (Panel for the Prediction and Prevention of Pressure Ulcers in Adults 1992, Bergstrom et al 1994). Care practices also change; thus, practitioners, like patients/caregivers, need updating and reinforcement of pressure ulcer prevention and treatment knowledge.

CONCLUSIONS

Patient education is a critical component of pressure ulcer prevention and treatment. The form that patient education takes should be mutually determined by the patient and the nurse so that the patient is empowered to strive toward well-being. Patient education about pressure ulcer prevention can occur throughout their life. At times a family member is the primary care provider and must be included in all teaching. The nurse needs to consider the patient's culture, developmental level, physical ability and economic status during the educational process. Instructional methods are numerous and varied and the methods and materials should be selected to meet the patient's learning needs, bearing in mind constraints of availability and expense. Teaching methods and materials must be continuously evaluated and updated. In addition to the patient and caregiver, nurses must also continuously update their knowledge level so that accurate information is given. Patient education is a never-ending process and must be continually reinforced.

CASE STUDY 14.1

Mr Allan is 70 years old and had a stroke 1 week ago. He has a history of diabetes mellitus, arthritis and hypertension. He currently has left hemiplegia.

Before the stroke, he was very independent and enjoyed gardening. He has been married for 45 years and resides in a single-story home. He is well nourished and is able to feed himself. He has a great deal of difficulty in transferring from the bed to the chair and in repositioning himself in bed. Mr Allan has decided to return home for rehabilitation and his wife has agreed to assist him with his care. Their insurance will pay for a home care nurse for a limited amount of time.

The nurse met with Mr and Mrs Allan to assess their learning needs. They stated that they did not have difficulty learning about the care and treatment of Mr Allan's other health conditions and do follow his medication regimens. They like to be part of the care decisions that are made. Mr Allan likes to read gardening books. They rarely attend concerts or plays because they have too much difficulty hearing. They watch some television and some films on VCR. Mr Allan

describes himself as a quiet person and feels uncomfortable participating in a group. They have a friend who became disabled but who never discussed with him how he handles his care. Mr Allan is frightened about not being able to perform his own care, but wants to learn what is best for him.

1 What has the nurse learned about Mr and Mrs Allan regarding empowerment for pressure ulcer prevention teaching?

2 What assessment information is important for selecting a teaching method?

3 Which instructional methods are likely to work best for them to learn about pressure ulcer prevention?

4 Which instructional materials may work best for them to learn about pressure ulcer prevention?

5 What are considerations for instructional materials?

6 What are general issues regarding pressure ulcer prevention teaching for this family?

SELF-ASSESSMENT QUESTIONS

1 What factors should the nurse take into account when teaching older patients?

2 Describe the special challenges associated with developing an education programme for patients with spinal cord injuries.

3 What methods might you use to teach the principles of pressure ulcer prevention to patients with low literacy levels?

4 What are the key qualities to consider when evaluating or developing written materials?

REFERENCES

Andberg M M, Rudolph A, Anderson T 1983 Improving skin care through patient and family training. Topics in Clinical Nursing 5(2):45–54

Ayello E A 1993 A critique of the AHCPRs 'Preventing Pressure Ulcers – A Patient's Guide' as a written instructional tool. Decubitus 6(3):44–50

Ayello E A, Mezey M, Amella E J 1997 Educational assessment and teaching of older clients with pressure ulcers. Clinical Geriatric Medicine 13(3):483–496

Baharestani M M 1994 The lived experience of wives caring for their frail homebound, elderly husbands with pressure ulcers. Advances in Wound Care 7(3):40–52

Barnes S H 1987 Patient/family education for the patient with a pressure necrosis. Nursing Clinics of North America 22(2):463–474

Bastable S B 1997 Gender, socioeconomic, and cultural attributes of the learner. In: Bastable S B (ed.) Nurse as educator principles of teaching and learning. Jones and Bartlett, Sudbury, pp. 176–203

Bastable S B, Sculco C D 1997 Educational objectives. In: Bastable S B (ed.) Nurse as educator principles of teaching and learning. Jones and Bartlett, Sudbury, pp. 237–260

Benbow M 1996 Pressure sore guidelines: patient/carer involvement and education. British Journal of Nursing 5(3):182–186

Bergstrom N, Bennett M A, Carlson C E et al 1994 Treatment of pressure ulcers. Clinical practice guideline, no. 15. AHCPR publications no. 95–0652, US Department of Health and Human Services. Public Health Services, Agency for Health Care Policy and Research, Rockville

Brown F 1997 Patient empowerment through education. Professional Nurse 3(Suppl):S4–S6

Dai Y T, Catanzaro M 1987 Health beliefs and compliance with a skin care regimen. Rehabilitation Nursing 12(1):13–16

Dover H, Pickard W, Swain I et al 1992 The effectiveness of a pressure clinic in preventing pressure sores. Paraplegia 30(4):267–272

Ellis-Stoll C C, Popkess-Vawter S 1998 A concept analysis on the process of empowerment. Advances in Nursing Science 21(12):62–68

Fitzgerald K 1997 Instructional methods selection, use, and evaluation. In: Bastable S B (ed.) Nurse as educator principles of teaching and learning. Jones and Bartlett, Sudbury, pp. 261–286

Florian V, Elad D 1998 The impact of mothers' sense of empowerment on the metabolic control of their children with juvenile diabetes. Journal of Pediatric Psychology 23(4):239–247

Gordon D L, Sawin K J, Basta S M 1996 Developing research priorities for rehabilitation nursing. Rehabilitation Nursing 5(2):60–66

Hainsworth D S 1997 Instructional materials. In: Bastable S B (ed.) Nurse as educator principles of teaching and learning. Jones and Bartlett, Sudbury, pp. 287–317

Hunter S M, Langemo D K, Olson B et al 1995 The effectiveness of skin care protocols for pressure ulcers. Rehabilitation Nursing 20(5):250–255

Kruger S 1991 The patient educator role in nursing. Applied Nursing Research 4(1):19–24

LaMantia J G, Hirschwald J F, Goodman C L et al 1987 A program design to reduce chronic readmissions for pressure sores. Rehabilitation Nursing 12(1):22–25

Maklebust J, Magnan M A 1992 Approaches to patient and family education for pressure ulcer management. Decubitus 5(7):18–28

Maly R C, Frank J C, Marshall G N et al 1998 Perceived efficacy in patient–physician interactions (PEPPI): validation of an instrument in older persons. Journal of the American Geriatric Society 46(7):889–894

Murphy R N 1997 Legal and practical impact of clinical practice guidelines on nursing and medical practice. Nurse Practitioner 22(3):138,147–148

Olshansky K 1994 Essay on knowledge, caring, and psychological factors in prevention and treatment of pressure ulcers. Advances in Wound Care 7(3):64–68

Panel for the Prediction and Prevention of Pressure Ulcers in Adults 1992 Pressure ulcers in adults: prediction and prevention. Clinical practice guideline, no. 3. AHCPR publication no. 92–0047. Agency for Health Care Policy and Research, Public Health Service, US Department of Health and Human Services, Rockville

Pellino T, Tluczek A, Collins M et al 1998 Increasing self-efficacy through empowerment: preoperative education for orthopaedic patients. Orthopaedic Nursing 17(4):48–59

Pieper B, Mattern J C 1997 Critical care nurses' knowledge of pressure ulcer prevention, staging and description. Ostomy/Wound Management 43(2):22–31

Pieper B, Mott M 1995 Nurses' knowledge of pressure ulcer prevention, staging, and description. Advances in Wound Care 8(3):34–48

Quigley S M, Curley M A Q 1996 Skin integrity in the pediatric population: preventing and managing pressure ulcers. Journal of Social and Pediatric Nursing 1(1):7–18

Redman B K 1997 Evaluation and research in patient education. In Redman B K (ed.) The practice of patient education. Mosby, St Louis, pp. 69–90

Rodriguez G P, Garber M A 1994 Prospective study of pressure ulcer risk in spinal cord injury patients. Paraplegia 32(3):150–158

Viggiani K 1997 Special populations. In: Bastable S B (ed.) Nurse as educator principles of teaching and learning. Jones and Bartlett, Sudbury, pp. 204–233

Walker R 1998 Diabetes: reflecting on empowerment. Nursing Standard 12(23):49–56

Wellard S J, Turner D S, Bethune E 1998 Nurses as patient-teachers: exploring current expressions of the role. Contemporary Nurse 7(1):12–17

Whitman N I 1992 Developmental characteristics. In: Whitman N I, Graham B A, Gleit C J, Boyd M D (eds) Teaching in nursing practice. Appleton & Lange, Norwalk, pp. 115–131

Yasenchak P, Bridle M J 1993 A low-literacy skin care manual for spinal cord injury patients. Patient Education and Counselling 22(1):1–5

15 *Patricia R Boynton*
Quality assurance and audit

INTRODUCTION

Health care as an industry has moved from its historical mission of service to operating as a business. Rapid changes in health care and technology combined with progressive rises in average patient age, patient acuity and prevalence of chronic illness have escalated health care costs. In the USA, UK and Europe, various strategic initiatives have emerged at governmental level to control expenditures and service utilization, while preserving and/or enhancing quality. This has, in part, been due to a recognition that there is an unacceptable variation in both quality and cost among health care institutions and in different geographical areas. Any effective system of quality management mediates both variances and conflicting goals, and fosters high-quality, efficient and cost-effective care delivery.

This chapter traces the development of quality management in business, the application of quality principles to health care, explores concepts of quality assurance and audit, and makes special reference to quality issues associated with the prevention and treatment of pressure ulcers.

OVERVIEW OF QUALITY MANAGEMENT

Quality is elusive to define and a challenge to achieve. *Webster's Collegiate Dictionary* (1976) describes quality as, 'a peculiar and essential character; a degree of excellence; superiority in kind'. W. Edwards Deming, an American statistician who revolutionized Japanese industry after World War II stated, 'The difficulty in defining quality is to translate future needs of the user into measurable characteristics, so that a product can be designed and turned out to give satisfaction at a price that the user will pay' (Deming 1986).

In the early twentieth century, growing demand for quality products led to inspection of work. Workers learned skills, put them into practice, then products were inspected by supervisors trained in quality control. Output that failed to meet expectations was reworked, leading to delays, repetition, and the blaming of workers for the problems. While quality control added costs to finished products, inspection was the major means for protecting consumers from defective products.

In the mid 1920s, the young Deming learned that management of work processes is more effective than inspection of products. He subsequently promoted and taught management of systems versus people, noting, 'Quality is not about control – it is about enabling people to succeed' (Deming 1986). Deming's philosophy focused on reducing variations in products/outcomes by doing the right thing the first time. His philosophy was that quality should be built in to the production process rather than depending on inspection to find flaws in the product arising from that process. Insisting that people work harder was an outdated concept for Deming, rather they should be encouraged to work 'smarter'. He taught students that quality emerges from effective leadership/management, active participation of employees at all levels and extensive communication. While Deming was a

BOX 15.1 DEFINITIONS OF TERMS

Algorithm: A rule of procedure for solving a problem (Webster 1976). A decision-tree is an example of an algorithm.

Benchmarking: Tool that promotes best practice or the gold standard of care. Collaborative benchmarking is the process of learning and changing through comparisons with other similar organizations/situations (Bankett et al 1996).

Consensus statements: Formal summaries of the existing knowledge/literature. They tend to be general and usually include information that is not controversial (McGuckin et al 1996).

Critical/clinical path: A written sequence of clinical responses or events that guides a patient with a defined problem towards an expected outcome (Barr & Cuzzell 1996). The paths identify goals of patient care and list the sequence and timing of events and activities to meet goals. The focus is on how care decisions are implemented. Paths allow for benchmarking.

Guidelines: Begin with a consensus statement and include peer review. They are usually developed by professional organizations that address specific conditions, or by governmental bodies. Guidelines tend not to be validated and may have limited impact on care delivery (McGuckin et al 1996).

Indicators: Quantitative measures used to monitor and evaluate important governance, management, clinical and support functions affecting patient outcomes. Indicators may relate to structure, process or outcomes (JCAHO 1992).

Policy: A statement of rule that recurrently affects work delivery. A policy is a structure standard.

Procedure: A procedure describes a technique for achieving an objective. Procedures are process standards. They allow for discretion in application (McGuckin et al 1996).

Protocol: A collection of activities involving collaboration of methods and techniques among care providers so that a specific goal can be attained (McGuckin et al 1996).

Standards of care: Standards of patient care provide a model of practice formulated from usual and customary care resulting in positive outcomes and maintaining consistent quality. Standards of care serve as a broad structure for individualized care plans. Nursing standards focus on documented assessment, intervention, patient and caregiver education, staff education and competence, discharge planning, resource utilization and a multidisciplinary approach.

Variance: Deviation or detour from the expected course of events outlined by a standard or pathway (Barr & Cuzzell 1996).

legend in Japan, he was generally ignored by American businesses until late in the twentieth century.

With time, quality management has evolved. Many terms or labels overlap and are used interchangeably. Most share common concepts, but there are important distinctions. A summary of some useful definitions is given in Box 15.1.

Quality assurance (QA) involves a process of systematic monitoring that has traditionally stressed survey, review, citation and outcomes. QA strategies in both the USA and the UK have evolved to standard setting, data collection and analysis of work processes, followed by action plans to improve compliance with standards and to positively affect outcomes. Evaluation of change determines effectiveness in achieving desired outcomes (Gawron 1993) (Box 15.2).

The model currently used by the Joint Commission on Accreditation of Healthcare

BOX 15.2 EVOLVING CONCEPTS OF QUALITY MANAGEMENT (ADAPTED FROM BERWICK ET AL 1990)

Outdated quality control	Effective quality management
Work standards	Teams/change agents to brainstorm/lead
Inspection	Scientific investigation of processes
Surveillance	Planned, evidence-based change
Blame	Implementation
Incentives to improve	Customer–provider communication
	Evaluate and monitor outcomes
	Recognize and celebrate success

Organizations (JCAHO) which surveys selected American health care facilities is continuous quality improvement (CQI) and involves a multidisciplinary approach (Dealey 1996). CQI uncovers current concerns with overall delivery systems of a business, industry or institution, then devises corrective actions. The focus is ongoing monitoring, evaluation and improvement of processes.

Total quality management/total quality improvement (TQM/TQI) is the application of quantitative methods (tools) and human resources to improve materials, work processes, products and services, and customer satisfaction (JCAHO 1992). It is an even larger concept than CQI. With TQM/TQI, quality improvement activities are integrated with management systems throughout an organization, with all functions focused on satisfying customer needs. Historical quality control is but one tool of TQM (Berwick et al 1990).

Regardless of which model is used, the principles of quality improvement reflect responsible, dedicated leadership and management as key to empowering employees and achieving quality throughout an organization. Quality outcomes depend upon long-term vision rather than short-term solutions.

QUALITY ASSURANCE IN HEALTH CARE

History and evolution of health care quality assurance

Quality management is relatively new to health care. Historically, the delivery system has lacked standardization, relying instead on tradition, intuition, experience and the individual qualities of those who provided care. Until the introduction of standards, health care was plagued with care delays and inconsistencies, rising costs, unacceptable errors, and poor quality in some facilities. The adoption by health care organizations of more overt quality assurance practices drawn from industry has pushed health care toward accountability and patient-focused quality, that is: '... patient care that meets the valid needs as perceived by the customer' (Gallagher 1997).

In the UK, the current framework for helping clinicians to continuously improve quality and safeguard standards is termed 'clinical governance' (RCN 1998). It is an umbrella term for all activities that help to maintain and improve standards of patient care and embraces evidence-based practice, clinical effectiveness, clinical audit, risk management and assessment of competence. The focus is on continuous professional development and the aim is to assure that the culture, systems and ways of working at all levels within an organization facilitate clinical effectiveness, efficiency and equity. Underlying principles include a focus on the needs of patients, user–patient involvement, partnerships between clinicians, clinicians and patients, and clinicians and managers, and an open, enabling culture which complements professional self-regulation and individual professional accountability (Morison et al 1997).

Quality assurance includes three categories of activities:

- structure/systems – resources allocated to support care delivery

- processes – actual care delivery
- outcomes – assigning value to results
  (Berwick et al 1990, JCAHO 1990).

Health care QA requires coordination of activities, employee involvement and quality tools to identify and strengthen opportunities for growth and improvement. The process uses audit of clinical functions and the impact on patient outcomes. Conditions that are high volume, costly and characterized by variations in both practice and outcomes are ripe for quality assurance activities.

JCAHO credits health care quality assurance with providing a foundation for overall quality improvement; however, quality assurance 'implies that a specific level of quality is high and can be guaranteed' (JCAHO 1992). Current thinking is that quality can always be improved and cannot be guaranteed; therefore the term 'quality assurance' is no longer used by JCAHO. Because quality assurance has a generic meaning in other health care settings, it is used in that sense for this chapter.

As the health care delivery system has focused on high-quality clinical outcomes, managed care has emphasized increasing profits and cost control (Ennis & Meneses 1996). Managed care refers to prepaid health services or managed fees for service provided by health maintenance organizations (HMO) or preferred provider organizations (PPO). Corporations/payer sources strive to reduce hospitalization, discount fees, enrol the healthy and increase profits, in some instances, without addressing quality outcomes. Consumers expect care that is excellent, accountable, efficient, cost-effective, affordable and meets their needs. Public pressure is one force moving managed care organizations to add value and quality concepts, and to adopt a public health focus.

Quality management can succeed for health care facilities when it is the primary operating strategy. Health care organizations have been slow to accept that quality is driven by processes not people (Berwick et al 1990), and that health care QA is not merely meeting legal requirements and expectations of accrediting bodies. QA is ineffective when it concentrates on surveillance,

review and citation – a common approach for some regulatory agencies and facilities (Xakellis 1997). QA is best used to make a difference in outcomes, not to blame others. Benchmarking provides the opportunity for comparison with other similar facilities and encourages best practice (Bankett et al 1996, Department of Health 1997)

Nursing and quality

The profession of nursing has a history of commitment to quality. While the term 'quality assurance' emerged later, Florence Nightingale collected epidemiological data and introduced nursing standards to mid-nineteenth century practice (Phillips 1986). Over the next 150 years, nursing publications regularly promoted evaluation and improvement of care.

During the post-World War II era, nursing standards led efforts to upgrade practice. Progress was aided by development of the nursing process (Box 15.3), which applies the scientific method of problem solving to nursing practice (Eliopoulos 1987). Evaluation, the final step in addressing clinical problems, has often been overlooked but, without evaluation, effectiveness of interventions and quality of outcomes cannot be determined.

Early nursing research studies to address quality were first conducted in the 1950s. During the next decade, professional organizations recommended that nursing adopt self-regulation and expand quality management. In 1965, standards for organized nursing services were first published by the American Nurses' Association. An early model of nursing quality assurance was developed in 1974. In 1985 the 'Standards of Care

---

BOX 15.3 STEPS OF THE NURSING PROCESS

1 Assessment

2 Diagnosis and planning

3 Implementation

4 Evaluation

Project' was published by the Royal College of Nursing, which heralded a renewed interest in the dynamic process of standard setting by nurses in the UK (RCN 1990). Nursing quality assurance has evolved to include problem-focused evaluation studies as well as retrospective structure and process audits. QA on individual nursing units involves audits of unit-specific practice problems, data collection, analysing and reporting findings, then solving problems. Unit-based QA increases nursing autonomy and accountability while advancing practice.

Audits identify both past and current practice. Retrospective chart audits commonly review how care has been delivered. Indicators of quality include completed assessments, compliance with standards and documentation. Data are retrieved during the actual chart review; then data analysis identifies outcomes and compliance with current criteria. Variance from expected outcomes suggests remedial action, such as the development of new or updated standards of care, guidelines, critical pathways, protocols, and related structure or systems standards (Figs 15.1 and 15.2).

Concurrent audit provides immediate feedback. Tools and indicators include prevalence and incidence of clinical conditions, assessment processes/patient observation and documentation tools. Data may also be retrieved from patient or nurse interviews. Whatever the method, QA projects are most effective when indicators are specific, easily measured and linked to outcomes. Nursing QA demonstrates the profession's contributions to optimum care.

APPLYING QUALITY MANAGEMENT TO THE PREVENTION AND TREATMENT OF PRESSURE ULCERS

The problem of pressure ulcers

Management of pressure ulcers further burdens a health care system challenged by increasingly scarce resources (Boynton & Paustian 1995). Pressure ulcers are a concern in all care settings and prevalence varies widely (Ch. 2). The overall acute care prevalence rate in the USA during 1995 was 10.1%, with a range of 1.4–36.4%. In long-term care, prevalence averaged 23% (Lesham & Skelsky 1994, Sideranko & Yeston 1994). More pressure ulcers are present on admission to long-term care facilities than develop after admission. Pressure ulcers that develop in long-term care are generally less severe than those that are hospital-acquired. The sacrum and the heels are common sites of breakdown in most settings (Barczak et al 1997).

The estimated financial burden of treating pressure ulcers in US hospitals is $2000 to $70 000 per wound (NPUAP 1989) and annual costs range from $1.3 to $3.5 billion a year (Granick & Ladin 1998). In the UK, the cost of preventing and treating pressure ulcers in a 600-bed large general hospital has been estimated at between £600 000 and £3 million per year (Touche Ross & Co. 1993). Costs are affected by pressure ulcer stage/severity, pain, suffering, functional declines, quality of life issues, prolonged lengths of stay and related increases in morbidity and mortality (Chs 4 and 5).

Advances in pressure ulcer prevention and treatment are driven by goals of consistent, quality health care as well as control of costs. While standards of care, protocols, pathways and guidelines are increasingly common tools for supporting delivery of care (Cullum et al 1995, Hastings 1995, Hitch 1995, Shipperley 1998), selecting measurable indicators of outcomes is also important. The National Pressure Ulcer Advisory Panel (NPUAP) suggests the use of prevention and treatment protocols that promote consistent care, and recommends pressure ulcer incidence as an indicator of quality care. Health care professionals in the UK share similar views (Dealey 1996). The Health Care Finance Administration's (HCFA) long-term care guidelines for surveyors direct that residents of (Medicare) nursing care facilities not develop pressure ulcers 'unless the individual's clinical condition demonstrates that it is unavoidable' (HCFA 1995). Pressure ulcers are among the top 10 reasons why nursing care facilities receive deficiency ratings. JCAHO, the Agency for Health Care Research and Quality (AHCRQ),

---

SKIN INTEGRITY AUDIT

OUTCOME: During a given episode of care, the patient will remain free of pressure ulcers

SAMPLE: $n = 25$
                Patients admitted with a Braden Scale score of 16 or less
                No actual skin breakdown present at admission

	YES	NO
1. Skin condition is assessed and documented at time of admission	☐	☐
2. Impaired skin integrity, actual or potential, is identified as a problem on the care plan	☐	☐
3. Interventions for reducing pressure are documented (at least two)	☐	☐

   • Support surface in place ☐

   • Repositioned in bed at least every 2h ☐

   • Repositioned in chair every 15–30 min ☐

   • Heels suspended off bed ☐

   • Plan to improve activity/mobility ☐

	YES	NO
4. Nutrition consult documented if nutrition subscale score is 1 or 2	☐	☐
5. Interventions to manage moisture exposure are documented as appropriate	☐	☐
6. Persons at risk have documented Braden Scale scores twice weekly	☐	☐
7. Skin condition is assessed and documented at discharge	☐	☐

8. Comments:

_____

_____

_____

_____

_____

_____

Figure 15.1 Skin integrity audit.

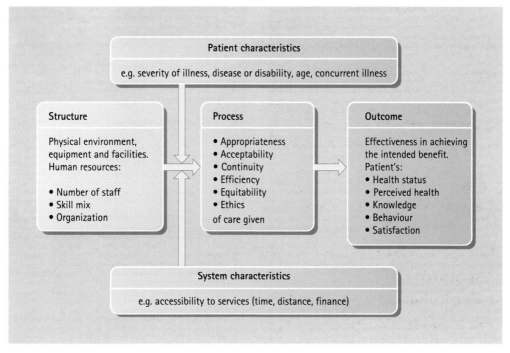

Figure 15.2   What to audit? Examples of factors to consider when developing a programme to measure the quality of care (after Donabedian 1969, Shaw 1986). Reproduced from Morison & Moffatt 1994, with permission.

managed care organizations, departments of health and the public also expect effective strategies for preventing pressure ulcers.

STRUCTURE/SYSTEMS ISSUES

Building quality into every aspect of pressure ulcer prevention and treatment is dependent upon a number of interacting systems, process and outcomes variables. Current quality management methodology assumes that quality fails when systems fail (JCAHO 1990). Administrative commitment to effective organizational support systems provides a foundation for practice innovations to advance the quality of pressure ulcer prevention and treatment (Box 15.4).

In the USA, reimbursement for pressure ulcer prevention and care represents an external systems issue. Payment depends largely on complete, accurate and timely documentation of care delivered (Motta 1996). Most third party payers cover 'reasonable and medically necessary care', but payment mechanisms do vary among geographical regions. Unfortunately, treatment decisions are often determined more by cost than effectiveness of therapy. Cost effectiveness is more than supply and labour expenses: it is the cost of producing desired outcomes (Bolton et al 1996, Dieter 1996).

Process/staff issues

Skin integrity and skin care are affected by staff knowledge of current risk assessment, prevention and treatment concepts (Chs 6–14). Staff generally want to perform well and make a difference for patients at risk of, or with pressure ulcers. Assessment of nursing knowledge, practice patterns and related staff issues suggest potential areas for improvement and tools to promote excellence in pressure ulcer prevention and treatment (Box 15.5).

237

BOX 15.4 SYSTEMS ISSUES

- Participative management that is dedicated to quality outcomes
- Support for teamwork and group participation
- Administrative support for standardizing a limited number of effective products that meet care needs, increase efficiency, reduce/ eliminate confusion in product selection and reduce waste/costs
- Processes for efficient and accurate ordering/charging of supplies
- Staffing systems that promote safe delivery of care, consider staff mix versus acuity, and assure appropriate assignments for level of education/experience
- Work environments that minimize staff turnover
- Work environments that empower employees to excellence
- Collaboration of multiple departments involved in pressure ulcer prevention and treatment, such as purchasing, central supply, linen services, nutrition, pharmacy, nursing and administration
- Time and resources to complete projects
- Systems that promote continuity of pressure ulcer prevention and treatment in the transition between acute and home care.

BOX 15.5 PROCESS ISSUES

- Staff awareness/understanding of existing standards and research for prevention and treatment of pressure ulcers
- Staff compliance with current standards of care
- Time constraints and interruptions that influence the efficiency and quality of care
- Documentation patterns
- Effectiveness of staff communication
- Staff morale/self-satisfaction/positive feedback.

Current care outcomes

The realization that pressure ulcers are a problem for a particular facility may begin with the subjective nursing opinion that too many pressure ulcers are developing in too many patients. Discussions with staff may uncover perplexing questions, common concerns, unmet care needs, or difficulties meeting current standards. Staff may be confused about appropriate prevention and management, leading to care that varies from shift to shift and person to person. While subjective opinions may be difficult to quantify, they can serve as the impetus for measuring more clearly identified outcomes and garnering support for change.

Preparing for change

Nursing is moving towards research-based practice. The process of research utilization represents expanded problem-solving and a means for transforming research into improved clinical practice. Research utilization is a good base point for critical thinking about pressure ulcers, and ensuring that risk assessment, prevention and treatment are based on reliable and valid research (Grinspun et al 1993). An application of research utilization to the problem of pressure ulcers is provided in Box 15.6. Research utilization is consistent with quality assurance and promotes improved patient care, increased nursing knowledge, professional growth, collaboration and cost containment.

Diagnose the problem

Specific problem diagnosis begins with data collection to document existing practice for risk assessment, prevention and treatment of pressure

BOX 15.6 THE PROCESS OF RESEARCH UTILIZATION

1 Diagnose the problem by developing a clear statement of concerns with current pressure ulcer practices

2 Organize a multidisciplinary skin team

3 Define current care outcomes through retrospective chart audit of pressure ulcer occurrence per total patient days; compliance with existing standards; and concurrent audits of prevalence, incidence and severity of pressure ulcers

4 Identify the current research base for pressure ulcers, concentrating on sources that speak to the specific concerns of facility practice

5 Develop and/or identify evidence-based standards, guidelines and protocols

6 Review, evaluate and select a limited number of appropriate support surfaces, skin cleansers, barriers, dressings, wound care products, etc.

7 Develop the implementation plan

8 Educate staff and others

9 Test the innovation in limited areas

10 Modify and monitor the plan

11 Implement the plan throughout the institution

12 Measure prevalence, incidence, severity and compliance with the new standards, guidelines and protocols

13 Maintain and refine improvements – ongoing

ulcers. Chart reviews may determine that skin assessments are not consistently performed/documented on admission and during the episode of care. Risk assessment for skin breakdown also may or may not be consistently performed/documented and clinicians may not accurately assess and document the extent of skin injury. Prevention and treatment interventions may lack standardization and reflect the opinions and judgement of individual caregivers rather than research. While audits can be helpful, inaccurate assessments and incomplete documentation often limit their usefulness (Gallagher 1997).

Measurable, longitudinal and event-specific indicators of quality include prevalence, incidence and severity of pressure ulcers. Studies of these indicators offer an alternative to chart audits. A baseline study determines the percentage of pressure ulcers present on admission (prevalence) and those that are facility acquired (incidence), in relation to the total number of persons assessed. The severity of pressure ulcers may be determined by summing the length and width of each wound, dividing by two, then multiplying by stage. Individual severity calculations for all facility-acquired pressure ulcers are summed to obtain an index for comparison with future measures. Prevalence, incidence and severity of incidence bear direct links to outcomes of pressure ulcer prevention and treatment strategies. These indicators gain importance as they are tracked over time (Gallagher 1997).

Prevalence and incidence studies are completed by teams of nurses trained in skin observations and pressure ulcer staging, who perform complete head-to-toe skin assessments and accurately document findings on standardized forms (Fig. 15.3). Standard data collection methods facilitate comparison of current statistics with those obtained after implementation of practice innovations (Lake 1999). Involving staff as auditors and data collectors promotes awareness of credible concerns and accountability for practice. Direct observation of care delivery and staff surveys or interviews also provide clues. Patient satisfaction questionnaires offer perceptions on how well care needs are met. Collectively, data form a baseline determination of existing concerns, the most problematic aspects of care, and the need for immediate/long-term practice change.

Organize the team

Advancing nursing practice is beyond the scope of one individual, no matter how capable.

SKIN ASSESSMENT TOOL

PATIENT: _____ AGE: _____ NURSING UNIT: _____

BED SURFACE: _____ AT RISK: ____ Y: _____ N: _____ Rm#: _____ MR#: _____

Assessment site	Skin condition	Documented on admission sheet

1. Back of head
2. Right ear
3. Left ear
4. Right scapula
5. Left scapula
6. Right elbow
7. Left elbow
8. Vertebrae (upper-mid)
9. Sacrum
10. Coccyx
11. Right iliac crest
12. Left iliac crest
13. Right trochanter (hip)
14. Left trochanter (hip)
15. Right ischial tuberosity
16. Left ischial tuberosity
17. Right thigh
18. Left thigh
19. Right knee
20. Left knee
21. Right lower leg
22. Left lower leg
23. Right ankle (inner/outer)
24. Left ankle (inner/outer)
25. Right heel
26. Left heel
27. Right toe(s)
28. Left toe(s)
29. Other (specify)

#1 site no. _____ ( )
    stage _____ ( )
    size _____ ( )
    depth _____ ( )

#2 site no. _____ ( )
    stage _____ ( )
    size _____ ( )
    depth _____ ( )

#3 site no. _____ ( )
    stage _____ ( )
    size _____ ( )
    depth _____ ( )

#4 site no. _____ ( )
    stage _____ ( )
    size _____ ( )
    depth _____ ( )

#5 site no. _____ ( )
    stage _____ ( )
    size _____ ( )
    depth _____ ( )

#1 Y_____ N _____

#2 Y_____ N _____

#3 Y_____ N _____

#4 Y_____ N _____

#5 Y_____ N _____

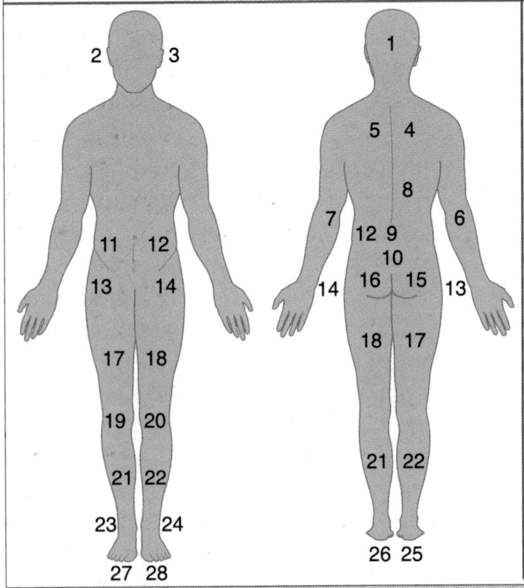

Patient had surgical procedure this admission   Y_____ N _____

If yes, name/type of surgery   _____

Care plan documents problem of skin integrity   Y_____ N _____

Care plan includes appropriate interventions   Y_____ N _____

Mark site(s) on diagram

Stage key

Stage 0   No redness or breakdown
Stage 1   Erythema only; redness does not disappear
Stage 2   Break in skin such as blisters or abrasions
Stage 3   Break in skin exposing subcutaneous tissue
Stage 4   Break in skin extending through tissue and subcutaneous muscle or bone
Stage 5   Dark necrotic tissue (use this rating until tissue sloughs, then continue staging)

Figure 15.3   Skin assessment tool.

BOX 15.7 SKIN COMMITTEE MEMBERSHIP

Staff nurses

Advanced practice nurses

Dietitians

Physical therapists

Physicians

Social workers

Discharge planners

Purchasing staff

Infection control and quality improvement practitioners

Staff from linen services

Staff from the supply department

Designating a group of change agents to develop and engineer the change brings consistency, order and control to the process (Granick & Ladin 1998). Forming a skin care team/committee begins with identifying persons from appropriate disciplines and departments who are committed to and responsible for skin care (Box 15.7). A team approach facilitates discussion, understanding and knowledge of processes and organizational culture, generates energy and enthusiasm, and encourages staff dedication to ongoing programme success (Lancellot 1996).

Meetings of the committee begin with team development and setting ground rules for meetings, division of work, leadership, authority and decision making. The group then moves to goal setting and brainstorming. Members of the skin care committee function as the champions for practice changes. The importance of administrative support for team activities cannot be overemphasized.

Determine the research base

The research literature for pressure ulcers is voluminous. Various sources identify pertinent literature for addressing specific practice con-cerns. Research studies, AHCRQ guidelines, and pressure ulcer prevention and treatment proto-cols are gathered and systematically assessed by the committee for quality, common themes and relevance to practice setting. Findings are subsequently summarized and used to select individual interventions. Advances in practice will more likely occur when the research base is adapted to the specific care setting, patients most at risk for pressure ulcers, staff mix and abilities.

Develop evidence-based practice

Research or evidence-based practice reflects the research from which it is derived. Practice based on science reduces dependence on tradition, intuition or a medical rationale as the major basis for making clinical decisions. Creating a new practice mode transforms the research base from general concepts to an organization-specific practice plan (Goode et al 1991). New or updated standards of care, guidelines, procedures and protocols serve as the underpinning of practice innovations.

Reducing pressure ulcer prevalence and incidence begins with prevention. Effective prevention of pressure ulcers depends upon identifying those at risk, determining the degree of risk and implementing appropriate interventions (Braden & Bergstrom 1996). Reliable and valid tools, such as the Braden Scale (Bergstrom et al 1987), assess risk and provide the basis for prevention. The six subscales of the Braden Scale measure sensory perception, activity, mobility, moisture, current nutritional status, friction and shear. Risk assessment is most effective when repeated in specific time-frames and when standards prompt staff to complete the assessments. Selected interventions relate to specific risk factors that can be diminished or eliminated.

The complex interaction of risk and aetiological factors makes both prevention and treatment challenging. Despite dedicated prevention efforts, pressure ulcers do develop. Complete and accurate assessment and documentation of existing pressure ulcers guide treatment decisions, evaluate progress and response to treatment, protect against litigation and support reimbursement. Photography facilitates documentation when proper equipment and procedures are available (Kutcher & Arnell 1992).

Review, evaluate and select products

Clinical decisions for prevention and treatment interventions are often hampered by the lack of standard products and supplies. A variety of interventions may be available for a single problem, leading to confusion and inconsistent care. The skin care committee makes a valuable contribution to quality when an extensive review of products is conducted. Support surfaces, dressings, barrier products and cleansing agents are among the items considered. A minimum number of products is selected, using criteria of performance, safety, cost and efficiency. Where research is not available to guide selection, or when more than one product meets the criteria, the selection process can be aided by piloting products in a representative variety of clinical settings (Bergstrom et al 1995). Once products and equipment are selected, they become part of a standard formulary to support clinical decisions.

The skin care committee also assumes responsibility for cost-effective management of therapeutic beds and support surfaces. An algorithm can guide decisions for initiating support surface use and selecting the most appropriate equipment. Consultation with a member of the skin care committee helps to match the appropriate surface with the specific patient need for pressure reduction/relief. Since interventions influence outcomes, patterns of use and costs of specific support surfaces serve as indicators of patient outcomes and cost-effective care. Members of the skin care committee collaborate to track these indicators and compare data over time.

Plan for change

The pace of planned change depends upon institutional culture and readiness for change. Members of the skin care committee meet with representatives of management and administration to negotiate support for minimizing or eliminating specific systems issues. To prepare

colleagues for advancing pressure ulcer prevention and treatment, skin care committee members make announcements and hold meetings to discuss the overall plan of action. The campaign for change includes newsletters, posters and bulletin boards that inform staff about proposed activities, the importance of practice changes, accomplishments to date and how staff will achieve excellence. Involving staff in pilot activities promotes acceptance of change.

Educate

Formal staff education communicates details of the innovation to be implemented. Standards and procedures for risk assessment, planning for prevention, and implementation of early treatment of pressure ulcers are conveyed through learning opportunities such as grand rounds, case studies, in-service education, practice sessions, committee meetings and computerized instruction. Committee members should explain existing practice problems and the research base, and respond to staff questions and concerns. Caregivers benefit from learning expectations and practical information that will promote successful implementation.

A manual of standards, guidelines, protocols, the products/equipment formulary and other important information combines a variety of tools that consider the different learning styles of adults. Equipment fairs display the armamentarium of products and encourage attendees to learn more about individual items, how they are used/not used, indications and operation. Education includes all levels of staff involved with and affected by change.

Implement the practice innovations

Implementation of change follows the skin care committee's structured action plan (van Etten et al 1990). Pilot implementation in stages and/or selected settings may precede institution-wide implementation. A pilot provides the opportunity to test and refine practice innovations and further the likelihood of successful change on a larger scale.

There are a number of barriers and challenges to change. A major challenge in establishing standardized pressure ulcer prevention and treatment is achieving agreement among professionals on protocols. Berwick et al (1990) stated that 'Outmoded practices, whose worth has long since been disproved by scientific evidence, tend to remain in practice for many years'. It can be difficult to convince staff not to use veterinary products on human skin, to avoid multiple layers of linen that can bunch up under patients, or that wet-to-dry dressings do not represent state of the science of wound care.

Convincing management, providers and payers to commit resources to prevention versus treatment of pressure ulcers is another challenge. Health care providers have been traditionally more interested in treating pressure ulcers than in preventing them. Enlisting physician support for change may also be difficult. Physicians often resist data collection that reflects on their practice. Standards may be viewed as cook-book medicine and a threat to autonomy. Hospitals may also experience conflict between the two lines of authority from administration and the medical staff (Berwick et al 1990). Collaboration is the key to success in implementing change.

Measure/evaluate outcomes

The final phase of planned change is to systematically evaluate outcomes of the practice innovations and ensure that evidence-based practice not only exists but can also be maintained. Specific indicators are measured, interpreted and reported for a selected time-frame after implementation of the new interventions. Comparisons with data collected prior to implementation determine the effectiveness of the practice innovations in achieving expected outcomes.

Structure/systems outcomes

The importance of systems variables to the success of quality improvement supports evaluation of specific systems issues addressed by the innovations for pressure ulcer prevention and treatment. Skin care committee members meet with management and administration to discuss issues, such as supplies, purchasing contracts and staffing, that have positively or negatively impacted outcomes. This process provides impetus for effective staff/management collaboration and problem resolution.

Process outcomes

Reviewing care delivery processes is the next step in determining the effectiveness of change. Chart reviews identify increases in staff knowledge of, and compliance with, new and updated standards of care. The nature and degree of improvement since the initial audits are evaluated. Documentation patterns are compared for changes in completeness, accuracy and consistency among providers, units and shifts. Current employee morale, attitudes and job satisfaction are determined through surveys and interviews.

Patient outcomes

The desired outcome of planned change in pressure ulcer prevention and treatment is that the maximum number of patients at risk of developing pressure ulcers will be free of skin breakdown at the completion of a given episode of care. Chart audits reveal specific patient outcomes such as the number of patients who had nutrition as a risk factor compared with those patients who received nutrition consultations. Patient surveys assess knowledge of prevention and care, and determine quality of life and satisfaction with care delivery and outcomes.

Repeat prevalence, incidence and severity of incidence studies directly reflect patient outcomes through comparisons with initial studies. Declines in any or all of these parameters suggest improved clinical practice. Over time, progressive decreases in prevalence and incidence can be expected, as well as lower severity of those pressure ulcers that do develop. One, midwestern, USA tertiary care facility documented progressive, positive impact on outcomes with evidence-based prevention and early treatment of pressure ulcers (Bergstrom et al 1995). Four years after implementation of practice innovations, the prevalence of pressure sores decreased from 22.9% to 10% and incidence fell from 18.7% to 6.4%. The initial severity index of 271 dropped to 56.5 during the same period. Seven years after implementation, research-based practice maintains its impact with a 12.2% prevalence rate, incidence of 5.2% and a severity index of 24.12. During the period that the number and severity of pressure ulcers declined, the use of expensive, therapeutic beds also decreased. By using an algorithm that matched the right surface with the right patient care needs, facility staff achieved and sustained a 65% reduction in equipment rental costs (C. Paustian, personal communication, 1999).

Celebrate

The ability of skin care committees and nursing departments to demonstrate reduced pressure ulcer prevalence, incidence and severity combined with reduced supply and support surface costs is a powerful statement of success. Changes of this magnitude require time, dedication and persistence, especially in an environment of scarce resources. Staff accomplishments in achieving quality outcomes deserve to be widely communicated and celebrated.

Refinements and future trends in pressure ulcer prevention and care

Advances in practice should be well established within 6–12 months of implementation. Mechanisms to sustain change address ongoing structure/systems, processes and outcomes. Ongoing attention to recalcitrant systems issues, such as time and resources, may be necessary to promote integration of practice innovations into daily care (Sacharok & Drew 1998). Innovations can be expanded to other clinical areas and successes multiplied. Sustained innovations may lead to higher levels of reimbursement through better documentation.

Staff benefit from ongoing feedback and recognition, as well as regular educational updates; designating and training unit-based experts in risk assessment, prevention and treatment sup-

ports ongoing staff competency and programme effectiveness. Programme supports such as manuals, tools and standards require updates as new information and research become available. Small group, problem-solving sessions are also helpful. Another effective educational avenue is the addition of pressure ulcer education to new employee orientation programmes. Education efforts should also extend to patients and their family caregivers. Repeated evaluations through chart audits and regularly scheduled prevalence, incidence and severity studies will highlight ongoing improvements. Repeated appraisals of indicators will uncover areas for future growth and practice advances.

Much of health care experience with individual pressure ulcer prevention and treatment interventions is subjective. Experience tends to guide decisions as clinicians compare past experiences with present situations, then predict whether specific interventions will succeed. One emerging trend is to ask clinicians to predict healing rates for pressure ulcers and other wounds. The complex aetiology and development of pressure ulcers currently makes it difficult to define a clinical path for healing (Bates-Jensen 1996). Ongoing research will address interventions and healing, refine existing, evidence-based practice and ensure quality outcomes for pressure ulcer risk assessment, prevention, treatment and healing.

KEY POINTS

- "Quality is not about control – it is about enabling people to succeed" (Deming 1986)
- Prevalence, incidence and severity bear direct links to outcomes of pressure ulcer prevention and treatment strategies.

SUMMARY AND CONCLUSIONS

Health care quality improvement has its roots in business and industry. Moving from quality control based on inspection of work, quality improvement initiatives now place the emphasis on managing systems and processes instead of people. As in business and industry, health care has lacked standards for promoting positive outcomes. Quality assurance and similar quality improvement models provide the foundation for reducing the problem of pressure ulcers.

Pressure ulcers are among the most common chronic health conditions, especially among frail, older adults. Ageing societies, prevalence of chronic disease and increasing patient acuity combined with health care restructuring and managed care demand action to control pressure ulcer prevalence, incidence, severity and costs. Development, implementation and maintenance of evidence-based practice positively affects structure, process and patient care outcomes. Research utilization promotes the move to evidence-based practice and skin care committee members and nursing staff serve as agents of change. Ongoing monitoring identifies variances from established standards, guidelines and protocols as well as opportunities for benchmarking with the best practices of similar facilities. It should be understood that change is continuous and quality can always be improved.

SELF-ASSESSMENT QUESTIONS

1 Head-to-toe skin assessments are essential to high-quality pressure ulcer risk assessment, prevention and care. Discuss the importance of performing and documenting complete skin assessments when persons are admitted to any health care facility. Identify patient factors to consider when performing these assessments.

2 Differentiate between prevalence and incidence. To what uses can prevalence and incidence data be put, in relation to pressure ulcers?

3 Develop an action plan for using pressure ulcer practice innovations to promote continuity of care between hospitals and home/community care agencies. Use concepts of planned change to create the plan.

4 Create a six-item questionnaire that measures patient satisfaction with pressure ulcer risk assessment, prevention and early treatment.

FURTHER READING

Bryant R A 1999 Acute and chronic wounds: nursing management, 2nd edn. Mosby, St Louis

Maklebust J, Sieggreen M 1996 Pressure ulcers: guidelines for prevention and management. Springhouse, Springhouse

REFERENCES

Bankett K, Daughtridge S, Meehan M, Colburn L 1996 The application of collaborative benchmarking to the prevention and treatment of pressure ulcers. Advances in Wound Care 9(2):21–29

Barr J, Cuzzell J 1996 Wound care clinical pathway: A conceptual model: Ostomy/Wound Management 42(7):18–26

Barczak C, Barnett R, Childs E, Bosley L 1997 Fourth annual pressure ulcer prevalence survey. Advances in Wound Care 10(4):18–26

Bates-Jensen B 1996 Wound care nurses' judgments on healing times in chronic wounds. Ostomy/Wound Management 42(4):36–42

Bergstrom N, Braden B J, Laguzza A, Holman V 1987 The Braden scale for predicting pressure sore risk. Nursing Research 36(4):205–210

Bergstrom N, Braden B, Boynton P, Bruch S 1995 Using a research-based assessment scale in clinical practice. Nursing Clinics of North America 30(3):539–551

Berwick D, Godfrey A, Roessner J 1990 Curing health care: new strategies for quality improvement. Jossey-Bass, San Francisco

Bolton L, van Rijswijk L, Shaffer F 1996 Quality wound care equals cost-effective wound care. Nursing Management 27(7):30–37

Boynton P, Paustian C 1995 Wound assessment and decision-making options. Critical Care Nursing Clinics of North America 8(2):125–139

Braden B J, Bergstrom N 1996 Risk assessment and risk-based programs of prevention in various settings. Ostomy/Wound Management 42(10A Suppl.):6S–12S

Cullum N, Deeks J, Fletcher A et al 1995 The prevention and treatment of pressure sores. Effective Health Care 2(1):1–16

Department of Health (DoH) 1997 Designed to care. Department of Health, Edinburgh

Dealey C 1996 Continuous quality improvement in pressure sores. British Journal of Nursing 5(16):1011–1015

Deming W E 1986 Out of the crisis. The W Edwards Deming Institute at Massachusetts Institute of Technology, Cambridge

Dieter D C 1996 Cost-effectiveness and quality nursing care. Clinical Nurse Specialist (10)3:153

Donabedian A 1969 Some issues in evaluating the quality of nursing care. American Journal of Public Health 39(10):1833–1836

Eliopoulos C 1987 A guide to the nursing of the aging. Williams & Wilkins, Baltimore

Ennis W J, Meneses P 1996 Clinical evaluation: outcomes, benchmarking, introspection and quality improvement. Ostomy/Wound Management 42(10 Suppl.):40S–47S

Gallagher S M 1997 Outcomes in clinical practice: pressure ulcer prevalence and incidence studies. Ostomy/Wound Management 43(1):28–35

Gawron C L 1993 Unit based quality assurance: a necessary component of E T nursing practice. Journal of E T Nursing 20:42–50

Goode C J, Butcher L A, Cipperly J A et al 1991 Research utilization, a study guide. Horn Video Productions, Ida Grove

Granick M S, Ladin D A 1998 The multidisciplinary in-hospital wound care team: two models. Advances in Wound Care 7:80–84

Grinspun D, MacMillan K, Nichol H, Shields D 1993 Using research findings in the hospital. Canadian Nurse 89(1):46–48

Hastings E (Chairman) 1995 Pressure area care: a report from a working party set up by the clinical resource and audit group. The Scottish Office, Department of Health, Edinburgh

Health Care Finance Administration (HCFA) 1995 Guidance to surveyors, state operations manual, provider certification, transmittal #274. Department of Health and Human Services, Health Care Finance Administration, Washington DC

Hitch S 1995 NHS executive nursing director of strategy for major clinical guidelines: prevention and management of pressure sores, a literature review. Journal of Tissue Viability 5(1):3–24

Joint Commission on Accreditation of Healthcare Organizations (JCAHO) 1990 Primer on indicator development and application: measuring quality in health care. Joint Commission of Healthcare Organizations, Oak Brook Terrace

Joint Commission on Accreditation of Healthcare Organizations (JCAHO) 1992 Using quality improvement tools in a health care setting. Joint Commission of Healthcare Organizations, Oak Brook Terrace

Kutcher J, Arnell I 1992 Documentation of skin using photography. Ostomy/Wound Management 38(9):23–28

Lake N 1999 Measuring incidence and prevalence of pressure ulcers for intergroup comparison. Advances in Wound Care 12(1):31–34

Lancellot M 1996 CNS combats pressure ulcers with skin and wound assessment team. Clinical Nurse Specialist 10(3):154–160

Lesham O A, Skelsky C 1994 Quality management, prevalence and severity in a long-term care facility. Advances in Wound Care 7(2):50–54

McGuckin M, Stineman M, Goin J, Williams S 1996 The road to developing standards for the diagnosis and treatment of venous leg ulcers. Ostomy/Wound Management 42(10A):62S–65S

Morison M J, Moffatt C J 1994 A colour guide to the assessment and management of leg ulcers. Mosby, London

Morison M, Moffatt C, Bridel-Nixon J, Bale S 1997 Nursing management of chronic wounds. Mosby, London

Motta G J 1996 Documentation and reimbursement in the clinical setting. Ostomy/Wound Management 42(4):18–23

National Pressure Ulcer Advisory Panel (NPUAP) 1989 Pressure ulcer prevalence, cost and risk assessment: consensus development conference statement. Decubitus 16(4):24–28

Phillips L 1986 A clinician's guide to the critique and utilization of nursing research. Appleton-Century-Crofts, Norwalk

Royal College of Nursing (RCN) 1990 Standards of care project: quality patient care: the dynamic standard setting system. RCN, London

Royal College of Nursing (RCN) 1998 Guidance for nurses on clinical governance. RCN, London

Sacharok C, Drew J 1998 Use of a total quality management model to reduce pressure ulcer prevalence in the acute care setting. Journal of Wound, Ostomy and Continence Nursing 25(2):88–92

Shaw C D 1986 Introducing quality assurance, paper no. 64. King's Fund, London

Shipperley T 1998 Guidelines for pressure sore prevention and management. Journal of Wound Care 7(b):309–311

Sideranko S, Yeston N 1994 Pressure sores no more: a quality improvement project. Journal of Nursing Quality 8(4):33–37

Touche-Ross & Co. 1993 The costs of pressure sores. Report to the Department of Health, UK. Department of Health, London

van Etten N K, Sexton P, Smith R 1990 Development and implementation of a skin care program. Ostomy/Wound Management 36:40–44

Webster's Seventh New Collegiate Dictionary 1976 G & C Merriam Company, Springfield

Xakellis G 1997 Quality assurance programs for pressure ulcers. Clinics in Geriatric Medicine 13(3):599–606

16

Moya J Morison, Yvonne Franks, Tim Kilner,
Linda Russell and Charlotte Woollaston

Advanced case studies

CASE STUDY 16.1

Karen Bates is 25 years old and is wheelchair-bound due to spina bifida. She is unmarried and lives alone in a flat where she is generally self-sufficient. However, she has developed a large sacral pressure sore (Fig. 16.1). She was referred to a plastic surgeon by her GP but the surgeon did not think that Karen was a suitable patient for a myocutaneous flap. She was then referred to the clinical nurse specialist who ran a 'problem wound clinic' at the hospital.

At this appointment, a week later, no dressing was found on the wound, Karen's reason for this

being that dressings did not stay in place because of her urinary incontinence. Initial assessment revealed a wound at the lower end of the sacrum of 10 cm², undermined by 4 cm distally. Her medical history included long-term steroid inhalers for asthma, urinary tract problems, including frequent infections, faecal incontinence and general tiredness.

At the appointment, Karen was very abrupt with the staff and critical of the nursing interventions over the years, in particular the number of different agency staff dispatched to change her dressings daily, and claimed that the dressing was usually off before they left the flat. The district nurses reported major problems with compliance. Past discussions about her lifestyle, smoking and dressings had been ignored. She was rude to staff and therefore they rotated the team for her visits. However, the relationship between the community nurses and the wound clinic staff in the hospital was good.

1 (a) What are the indications and contraindications for surgical closure of Karen's wound? (see Ch. 11)
   (b) Why might the surgeon have been reluctant to perform surgery in this case?
2 What tools would you use to assess this wound, and Karen's health and well-being more generally? (see Ch. 8)
3 The development of a care plan needs to be negotiated with Karen. What are likely to be the key components of the plan? (see Ch. 9)
4 (a) What are the goals of local wound management in this case?

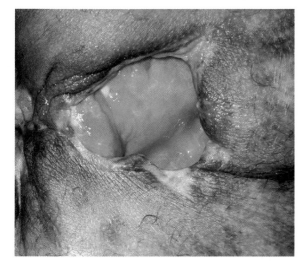

Figure 16.1 Longstanding sacral pressure ulcer, exuding large amounts of malodorous fluid.

(b) List the dressing regimens that could be appropriate for Karen. Give the advantages and disadvantages of each option. Which regimen would you try first, and why?

5 (a) The community nurses have identified Karen's 'non-compliance' as a major problem. How could you set about empowering Karen to enable her to take more control over her health and well-being?

(b) What teaching strategies might you use? (see Ch. 14)

CASE STUDY 16.2

Derek Brown is 77 years old and retired. He fell down the stairs at home, and was unable to move until a neighbour found him several hours later. He was admitted to a medical ward to investigate the reason for his fall and social assessments were made. He had sustained no broken bones, but had cuts and bruises on his head, right elbow, shoulder and left knee. There was a large bruise on his left thigh. He was reasonably fit prior to this accident but was awaiting bilateral hip replacements.

Ward nurses called the wound care specialist nurse 4 days after admission when the larger wounds were becoming very malodorous, necrotic and sloughy. On initial assessment the left thigh wound had brown necrotic tissue which was just starting to lift from the edges. The staff had not recognized at first that the patient's initial bruising was associated with deep dermal damage due to prolonged pressure while he was immobile following his fall. Thick yellow exudate was seeping from the edge of the wound and could be expelled with a little pressure. The surrounding skin was inflamed and oedematous. The wounds on his knee and shoulder contained softer yellow/green tissue and were also quite malodorous.

Sharp debridement was used on the thigh wound. This revealed necrotic fatty tissue (Fig. 16.2) that could be removed from the underlying tissue with ease. A hydrogel was used on the other wounds to soften and rehydrate the upper layers.

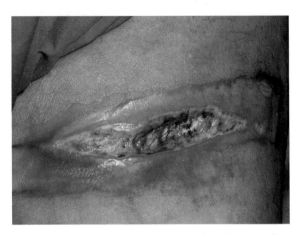

Figure 16.2 Thigh wound after sharp debridement of the dry necrotic cap.

The offensive odour from the wounds was the main issue for the patient, and the amount of exudate was increasing. The use of larval therapy was discussed with both patient and ward staff. The patient was very enthusiastic and had watched a television programme on its use. The ward staff had never used larvae before and the idea received a more mixed reception among them.

Larvae were ordered and were due to arrive the following day. The procedure attracted a large gathering, including ward staff and the Senior House Officer (SHO), with the patient's consent. He enjoyed being this centre of attention, joking that he was going to charge all observers. Following a detailed explanation of the procedure, the hydrocolloid border was placed at the wound edges, the larvae expelled from their container on to the mesh and placed over the wound. Safely secured with tape around the edges, a secondary dressing was applied with a bandage to hold it in place. The procedure was turned into a teaching session and many questions ensued. Staff made their plans to be on duty for the removal of the larvae in 3 days.

On removal of the dressing, both patient and staff were very aware of a change in the wound (Fig. 16.3). Its odour was greatly reduced and the wound appeared far deeper than before. The area was cleansed with saline and more larvae were applied.

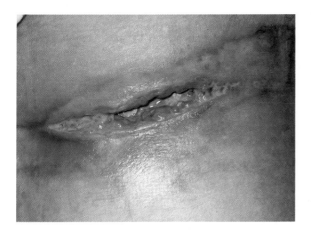

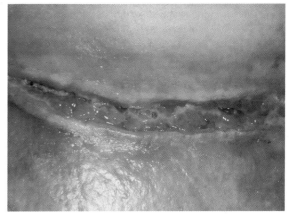

Figure 16.3 Three days after the first application of larvae. The wound appears deeper but already contracting from the sides.

Figure 16.4 Wound now filled with granulation tissue following the third application of larvae.

Because of the success of this strategy, some of the larval consignment was diverted to be used on the shoulder and knee wounds. One application on these more superficial wounds was found to be enough to clear these wounds of superficial slough and they progressed to healing within 1 week.

Three days later the final application of larvae to the thigh wound was performed by ward staff. All sloughy tissue had been removed. The wound edges had contracted significantly and the depth of the wound vastly reduced; granulation tissue formed bridges of new tissue across the wound (Fig. 16.4). Epithelialization was visible at the wound edges. The wound was dressed with a simple non-adherent (N/A) dressing and secondary padding was used to keep the wound warm and free from trauma. Two weeks from the start of larval therapy, the wound had continued to contract and epithelialize (Fig. 16.5), and the wounds were completely healed in 2.5 weeks; the patient regained his limited mobility and was fit enough to make his home visit for an assessment of his needs for the return home.

1 Discuss the aetiology of Mr Brown's pressure ulcer (see Ch. 3)
2 (a) What were the local problems at the wound site on his thigh and how would you have recorded them? (see Ch. 8)
  (b) What were the main treatment options? (see Ch. 10)
  (c) Why was the use of larval therapy so appropriate?
3 How could you set about auditing the use and effectiveness of larval therapy where you work? (see Ch. 15)
4 (a) What was the role of the clinical nurse specialist in this case?
  (b) How did she use the opportunities presented to facilitate learning among ward staff? (see Ch. 14)

CASE STUDY 16.3

Frank O'Brien is 95 years old and lives alone, since the death of his wife 15 years ago. He has suffered from congestive cardiac failure for the last 5 years, which is controlled with diuretics, cardiac glycosides and hypotensive drugs. More recently, he has developed chronic obstructive airways disease. He easily becomes breathless and now requires to sleep in a semi-upright position. So far, he has managed to remain at home, with the support of a home help. However, the home help became very concerned at the sudden and rapid deterioration in Mr O'Brien's physical and mental health and called the GP, requesting an urgent home visit.

On arrival, the GP found that Mr O'Brien was in very poor physical condition. From the way that his clothes hung upon him the GP suspected

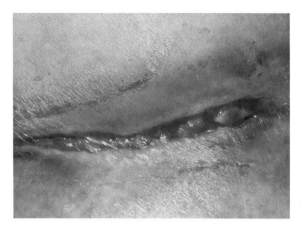

Figure 16.5   Wound contracted and epithelializing after just 2 weeks from the start of larval therapy.

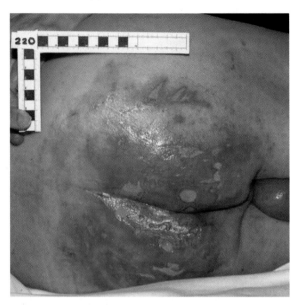

Figure 16.6   Mr O'Brien's sacral pressure ulcer on admission.

that he had lost a lot of weight. Mr O'Brien had lost all interest in living, although, when coaxed, he could talk lucidly and was able to retain information. On physical examination, the GP discovered superficial but extensive pressure ulcers on his sacrum (Fig. 16.6), and bilateral ulcers on his ankles. The GP organized an emergency admission to the local hospital.

Shortly after admission Mr O'Brien was incontinent of urine and faeces. Initial investigations revealed that his serum albumin concentration was 30 g/L and his haemoglobin was 12.7 g/dl. His body mass index (BMI) was 17. He had a very poor appetite.

1 (a) What are the indications that Mr O'Brien is malnourished?
   (b) List the methods that could be used to assess his nutritional status.
   (c) What are the immediate priorities in relation to his nutritional support? (see Ch. 13)
2 (a) What are the goals of local wound management in this case?
   (b) List the dressing regimens that could be appropriate for Mr O'Brien. Which regimen would you try first, and why? Give the rationale for your choice. (see Ch. 10)
3 Review the indications and contraindications for using low-level laser therapy and ultrasound to aid local wound healing (see Ch. 12). Might Mr O'Brien be a suitable candidate for either of these treatment approaches?
4 Devise a plan for Mr O'Brien's immediate care. (see Ch. 9)
5 Identify the health care professionals and other agencies with whom liaison and referral will be necessary to facilitate Mr O'Brien's immediate recovery, rehabilitation and long-term care.

CASE STUDY 16.4

Jeremy Hughes is 32 years old. He has made a written complaint to his local NHS Trust. He alleges that while in their care, following a road traffic accident, he developed pressure ulcers that resulted in his stay in hospital being longer than necessary. As a result he has had to take more time off work as a freelance journalist for the motoring press. The complaints manager has reviewed the nursing records in order to answer Mr Hughes' allegations.

Mr Hughes arrived at the Accident and Emergency (A&E) department by ambulance at

23.10 hours following a road traffic accident. In his examination, the doctor noted that Mr Hughes was a pedestrian crossing the road when a car collided with him. The examination revealed that he had bilateral femoral shaft fractures, a fracture of his left humerus and two fractured ribs on the left. Thomas traction splints were applied and Mr Hughes was admitted to the trauma ward.

Surgery could not be carried out immediately as Mr Hughes had eaten a large meal half an hour prior to his accident. Surgery was therefore planned for the following morning. The nursing assessment reports that Mr Hughes smokes 20 cigarettes per day, but has no obvious respiratory disease. Mobility is reported as being limited due to fractures and traction. The risk of pressure ulcer development is recognized and the care plan reflects this by requiring the use of a foam overlay mattress and regular position changes. However, in the evaluation of the care given there is little evidence to indicate that the positional changes had actually been carried out. When position changes had been attempted there is some suggestion in the records that they have been abandoned because the patient was experiencing too much pain, despite his analgesia having been reviewed.

The following day, the records indicated that Mr Hughes had developed a pyrexia of 40°C. Examination by the doctor revealed that Mr Hughes had developed a serious chest infection. As a consequence, surgery was delayed again until physiotherapy and antibiotics had taken effect. Evaluation of nursing care is documented for each shift over the next 4 days. Occasional reference is made to 'pressure areas relieved'; however, there is no indication of the frequency of this care nor is there reference to pressure area care in the report for each shift. Pain continued to be reported as an ongoing, unresolved issue in this preoperative period.

Surgery finally took place 4 days after admission by which time Mr Hughes had developed a grade II sacral pressure ulcer and several small areas of broken skin around the site of the rings of the Thomas splints.

1 What information would you expect to find incorporated into the nursing records relating to patient assessment, care planned, care given and the evaluation of care given, in this case?
2 What evidence is there that a 'duty of care' may have been breached?
3 What are the stages involved in resolving a complaint such as this?

CASE STUDY 16.5

Sylvia Shepherd is 69 years old, married and has two children. She is 1.7 m (5 ft 8 ins) tall and her normal weight is 73 kg (11½ stone). While on a shopping trip in London, she fell 8 m (26 ft) down a moving escalator and sustained several lumbar spinal fractures. Prior to this she had led an active life, which included hill walking and ballroom dancing.

Following prolonged but successful surgery in another hospital, she was initially cared for in an orthopaedic ward. The nurse who assessed her on arrival observed that she had been transferred with multiple pressure ulcers. She had been encased in a plaster 'jacket' to stabilize the surgical repairs. During the immediate postoperative period she had lost 8 kg (17 lbs) in weight and had developed a number of pressure ulcers, including one on the lateral aspect of her left heel (Fig. 16.7), and a large sacral pressure ulcer (Fig. 16.8). Pressure ulcers had also developed over her shoulder blades, where they were in contact with the plaster cast. The staff in the Spinal Unit were reluctant to take her for active rehabilitation until these wounds had healed.

1 (a) What are the 'grades' of the pressure ulcers illustrated in Figures 16.7 and 16.8? (see Ch. 8)
   (b) What are the local problems at the wound site, and how would you record them upon the patient's arrival from another hospital? (see Ch. 8)
   (c) Are there any potential legal implications for your hospital?
2 (a) What are the goals of local wound management in this case?

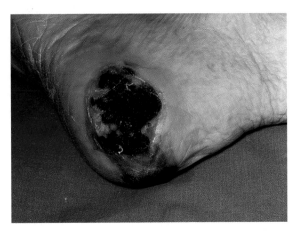

Figure 16.7 A necrotic pressure ulcer. (Reproduced with permission of Medical Illustration Group, Imperial College School of Medicine.)

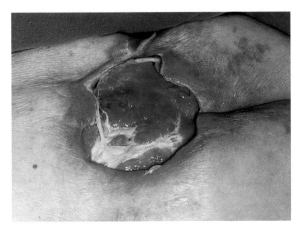

Figure 16.8 A large, sacral pressure ulcer. (Reproduced with permission of Medical Illustration Group, Imperial College School of Medicine.)

(b) List the dressing regimens that could be appropriate for Mrs Shepherd. Give the advantages and disadvantages of each option. Which regimen would you try first, and why? (see Ch. 10)

(c) What local and more general patient factors are likely to lead to delayed healing? (see Ch. 9)

3 The development of a care plan needs to be negotiated with Mrs Shepherd. What are likely to be the key components of the care plan? (see Ch. 9)

4 What strategies would you have used to relieve pressure from bony prominences, starting at the time when Mrs Shepherd entered the A&E department? (see Ch. 7)

5 (a) What impact may the development of these pressure ulcers have had on Mrs Shepherd's rehabilitation programme?

(b) What impact have they had on the quality of her life more generally? Plot the consequences over time. What are the possible consequences in the longer term? (see Ch. 4)

6 (a) What nutritional assessment methods would be most appropriate? (see Ch. 13)

(b) What effect does malnutrition have on wound healing?

(c) What methods of nutritional support might be considered in this case?

CASE STUDY 16.6

Yvonne Fletcher is 72 years old. She alleges that while in the care of the local acute NHS Trust she received negligent nursing care that resulted in her developing two sacral pressure ulcers, which now require surgical repair. She believes that if she had received adequate and reasonable care she would not have developed pressure ulcers. Her solicitor has commissioned a report from a nursing expert on the nursing care that Mrs Fletcher received while in the care of the NHS Trust. The nursing expert made the following observations.

Following a fall at home, Mrs Fletcher was taken by ambulance to the Accident & Emergency (A&E) department of the NHS Trust. The A&E record indicates that she arrived in the department at 10.20 hours, she was initially assessed by a nurse at 10.26 hours, and examined by a doctor at 10.57 hours. The A&E record indicates a fall as the chief complaint, with a diagnosis of 'confusion and dehydration'. A number of investigations were carried out at this time, including a 12-lead ECG, and X-rays of the chest, pelvis and hip.

The A&E record card has a box in which to record a Waterlow pressure ulcer risk score and the time when this was calculated. This box has not been completed. There is no record of any assessment of Mrs Fletcher's pressure ulcer risk, and no record of specific action being taken to relieve pressure. She left the A&E department at 13.40 hours and was admitted to a medical ward, once a bed had become available. The initial assessment by a nurse on the medical ward was based upon 'activities of living'. However, the assessment outlines previous health status rather than current health status.

When referring to eating and drinking, the assessment states: 'normally good appetite, eats and drinks normally'. The plan of care based upon this information does not outline any nursing action as being required, yet the evaluation of nursing care over subsequent days includes reports of diet being refused, small amounts of food being taken and diet not being tolerated.

The assessment referring to mobility reports that Mrs Fletcher is: 'slow to get going in the morning because of arthritis. Mobilizes reasonably well around the house but needs help with housework'. The care plan outlines the need for a nurse to assist Mrs Fletcher when mobilizing. An entry in the nursing evaluation on the day following admission reports that Mrs Fletcher had felt dizzy while returning to her bed from the bathroom. Her blood pressure was measured and found to be 90/60 mmHg. She returned to bed for the afternoon where she remained until the following morning. Regular measurements of her blood pressure were made and, generally, this improved over time. Her blood pressure the following morning was 110/80. However, the episodes of hypotension occurred on several subsequent occasions during her stay in hospital, each episode resulting in progressively longer times being spent on bed rest.

Pressure-relieving devices and pressure area care were not introduced into the nursing care plan until there was evidence of skin damage. At first, this manifested as redness over the sacrum and then broken skin. A grade III pressure ulcer rapidly developed.

The Waterlow pressure ulcer risk score on admission to the medical ward was recorded as 7 but there is no record of how this was calculated. It is reasonable to assume that the score was inaccurate as other evidence in the records for that time, such as age, medication and gender, suggest that the score would have been at least 10 and possibly higher. There is no evidence in the records that the Waterlow Score was recalculated at any time before skin damage was noticed.

1 What factors suggest that Mrs Fletcher was at particular risk of developing a pressure ulcer following her fall?

2 (a) What are the advantages and disadvantages of using pressure ulcer risk assessment tools? (see Ch. 6)

  (b) What part does clinical judgement play when assessing risk?

3 What information would you expect to find incorporated into the nursing records relating to patient assessment, care planned, care given and the evaluation of care given in this case?

4 (a) What is the role of nutrition in the aetiology of pressure ulcers? (see Chs 3 and 13)

  (b) What nutritional assessment methods would be most appropriate in Mrs Fletcher's case? (See Ch. 13)

  (c) What effect does malnutrition have on wound healing?

5 What strategies would you have used to relieve pressure from bony prominences, starting at the time when Mrs Fletcher entered the A&E department? (see Ch. 7)

6 (a) What evidence is there that a 'duty of care' may have been breached?

  (b) What are the points of similarity with Case Study 16.4, in this respect?

  (c) What role might a clinical audit play in highlighting the nature of the problems in these wards, and in developing local solutions? (see Ch. 15)

CASE STUDY 16.7

David Dawson is 71 years old and recently widowed. A former miner, he lives alone and is supported at home by a care assistant who calls once a day on weekdays to help with housework and shopping. He has had a grade III

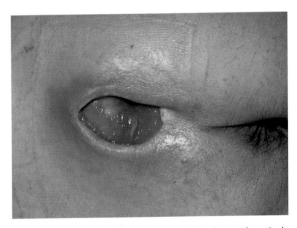

Figure 16.9 The pressure ulcer on admission to hospital. (Reproduced with permission of Medical Illustration Group, Imperial College School of Medicine.)

sacral pressure ulcer for over a year, which developed during a previous hospital admission; he is visited three times a week by the District Nurse to dress the wound. Despite her best efforts the wound shows no signs of improvement, but it has not enlarged in the last 3 months (Fig. 16.9).

Mr Dawson normally walks with a stick, but his mobility has been worsening recently, to the extent that he spends most of the day sitting by the fire in his small lounge, and he uses the furniture there as an aid to mobility. He suffers from benign prostatic hyperplasia (BPH) and has occasional incontinent episodes when he is unable to reach the bathroom in time. He also suffers from chronic obstructive airways disease. He requires a knee replacement, but the surgeons are reluctant to operate because of his other medical conditions. He is 1.52 m (5 ft) tall and weighs 51 kg (8 stone). He has been admitted to hospital following a fall at home, complaining of a very painful right knee. There is no referral letter from the District Nurse.

1 What information would you expect to find in the District Nurse's records relating to patient assessment, care planned, care given and the evaluation of care given, in this case?
2 (a) On admission, what strategies would you have used to relieve pressure from Mr Dawson's bony prominences? (see Ch. 7)
    (b) What factors mean that he is at considerable risk of developing further pressure area damage? (see Chs 2 and 6)
3 (a) The development of a care plan needs to be negotiated with Mr Dawson. What are the key components of the care plan while he is in hospital? (see Ch. 9)
    (b) What are likely to be the key components of a longer-term care plan for his return home?
4 (a) What are the goals of local wound management in this case? (see Ch. 10)
    (b) List the dressing regimens that could be appropriate for Mr Dawson and give the advantages and disadvantages of each option. Which regimen would you try first, and why?
5 (a) What nutritional assessment methods would be most appropriate? (see Ch. 13)
    (b) What effect does malnutrition have on wound healing?
    (c) What methods of nutritional support might be considered in this case?

CASE STUDY 16.8

Sheila Smith is 42 years old, married and registered disabled, following burns to her legs, torso and hands in 1975. She has had substantial skin grafting over the years since her accident. She has lost some fingers and the remaining ones are clawed and rigid. She has some shortening of the right leg and walks with a permanent limp on the outer aspect of her foot. She wears a heavy orthopaedic boot on this foot and walks only short distances. She drives an automatic car. She has no paid employment.

Two and a half years ago a pressure ulcer developed on the outer aspect of her right ankle, as a result of an ill-fitting boot. The surrounding scarred skin has broken down at times, reacting adversely to many dressings and topical applications. District nurses have tried all options available to them, including compression bandaging since Doppler assessment showed no arterial problems. She was referred to the prosthetist to ensure her boot was not applying pressure over the wound and routinely visits a chiropodist.

She was referred to a plastic surgeon by her GP, who applied a split-thickness skin graft to the ulcer. This graft failed and negative pressure was applied to encourage angiogenesis, reduce the bacterial count of the wound surface and to manage the large amount of exudate, which appeared to be irritating the surrounding skin. The plan was to re-graft when the wound bed was ready.

A second graft was applied 2 weeks later with negative pressure used over the graft. At the first dressing change only 50% of the skin was found to have adhered to the wound bed; the remaining area was raw, shiny and very wet (Fig. 16.10). A foam dressing was used to manage the exudate with a barrier cream liberally applied to the surrounding skin, which had become inflamed with superficial breaks, possibly as a reaction to the film dressing used with the negative pressure system. *Staphylococcus aureas* was isolated from the wound swab.

One week later the wound showed little evidence of the split-thickness skin graft. There were areas of slough and the wound surface had increased; therefore nurses suggested that low-level laser therapy be used. The therapy was used with the intention of reducing the bacterial growth, encouraging the removal of sloughy tissue and promoting epithelialization. Low-level laser therapy was commenced twice weekly while Mrs Smith was in hospital for 2 weeks and continued weekly at home.

Within 10 days, islands of epithelialization were apparent throughout the wound, and within 2 weeks 60% of the original area was epithelialized (Fig. 16.11). Slow but steady progress continued over several months (Fig. 16.12).

1 What are the most probable reasons for Mrs Smith's skin graft failing to take? (see Ch. 11)
2 What are the indications for the use of negative pressure and laser therapy to aid wound healing? (see Ch. 12)
3 (a) What are the goals of local wound management?
  (b) Review the dressing options. What dressing regimen would you choose for Mrs Smith and why? (see Ch. 10)
4 Although Mrs Smith is disabled, how might she become more involved in the care of her wound? (see Ch. 14)

CASE STUDY 16.9

Albert Thomson is 83 years old and lives with his 80-year-old sister. She is finding it increasingly difficult to cope with his frequent episodes of urinary incontinence and so he has been admitted to hospital for assessment and rehabilitation. His immediate problems include a suspected urinary tract infection and poor mobility. He is on medication for atrial fibrillation. Initial investigations reveal that his serum albumin level is

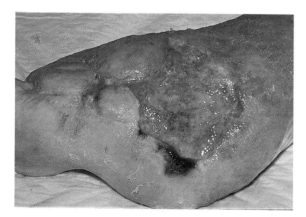

Figure 16.10   Only a few islands of skin are present post skin grafting. High levels of exudate are causing skin maceration.

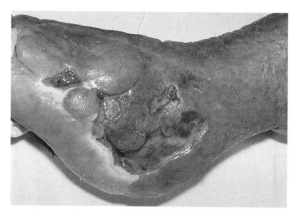

Figure 16.11   Large central area is now covered with skin, but the remaining areas would prove slow to heal.

255

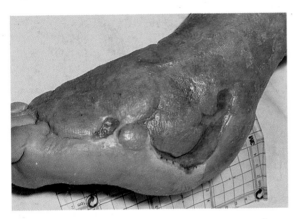

Figure 16.12 Whilst raw areas remain after 6 months, there is established skin here for the first time in 3 years.

33 g/L and his haemoglobin is 6.9 g/dl. His appetite is poor.

The nurses discover that he has developed a sacral pressure ulcer (Fig. 16.13), which his sister has been packing with gauze and an antiseptic cream obtained from the local chemist. Albert is deeply embarrassed that his sister has had to help him in this way, but neither has wanted to call in the District Nurses for fear that Albert is 'taken away' and placed in long-term care.

Mr Thomson's activity levels are assessed as poor, and he requires assistance to change his position both in bed and when sitting in a chair.

1 Discuss the aetiology of Mr Thomson's pressure ulcer. (see Ch. 3)
2 (a) What are the local problems at the wound site and how would you record them? (see Ch. 8)
   (b) Why may his sister's wound care regimen have contributed to delayed healing?
   (c) What are the main local treatment options and which would you choose? (see Ch. 10)
3 (a) What are the indications and contraindications for surgical closure of a pressure ulcer such as this? (see Ch. 11)
   (b) Why might the surgeons be reluctant to perform surgery in this case?
4 (a) What are the indications that Mr Thomson is malnourished?

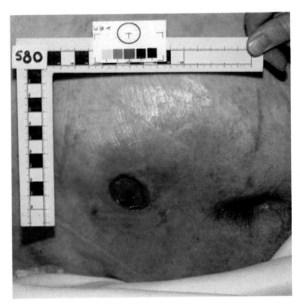

Figure 16.13 Mr Thomson's sacral pressure ulcer on admission.

   (b) List the methods that could be used to assess his nutritional status.
   (c) What are the immediate priorities in relation to his nutritional support? (see Ch. 13)
5 Devise a plan for Mr Thomson's immediate care (see Ch. 9)
6 How might both Mr Thomson and his sister be involved in his longer-term care? (see Ch. 14)
7 Identify the health care professionals and other agencies with whom liaison and referral will be necessary to facilitate Mr Thomson's immediate recovery, rehabilitation and long-term care.

CASE STUDY 16.10

Edward Gray is 84 years old and has been admitted to hospital from a local nursing home with an infected pressure ulcer over his right ischium (Fig. 16.14). His only son lives in South Africa and visits once a year. His wife died many years ago and he has few friends in the nursing home, preferring to 'keep himself to himself'. He particularly disliked any attempts at coercing him into taking

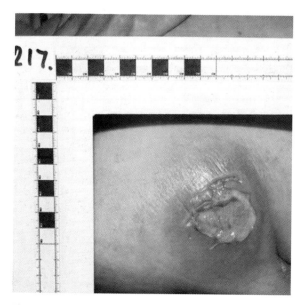

Figure 16.14 Mr Gray's sacral pressure ulcer on admission.

part in the social activities arranged by the nursing home staff, such as bingo and the gentle fitness programme ('music and movement') organized by the occupational therapist. He is a retired physics teacher. He blames the nursing home staff for the development of his pressure ulcer and complains that they are never about when he needs them. His son has written to him to say that he should sue the nursing home for negligence.

Recently, Mr Gray has had some episodes of confusion and he was disorientated by his admission to hospital. He has severely limited mobility and activity levels. He now smokes five cigarettes a day but he used to smoke many more. He has peripheral vascular disease and has already had a below-knee amputation to his left leg. His serum albumin level is 21 g/L and his haemoglobin is 10.5 g/dl. The microorganism *Proteus* sp. is isolated from the wound. Over a 3-week period his wound infection subsides and the necrotic tissue is debrided, revealing an extensive cavity (Figs 16.15 and 16.16).

1 What factors suggest that Mr Gray was at particular risk of developing a pressure ulcer? (see Chs 2 and 6)

2 (a) What are the advantages and disadvantages of using pressure ulcer risk assessment tools? (see Ch. 6)

   (b) What part does clinical judgement play when assessing risk?

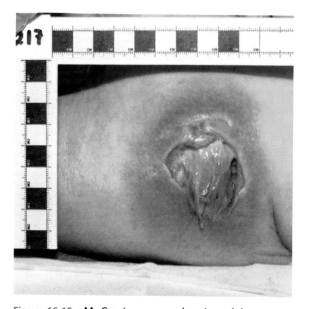

Figure 16.15 Mr Gray's pressure ulcer 1 week later.

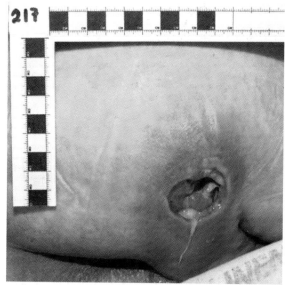

Figure 16.16 Mr Gray's pressure ulcer 3 weeks after admission.

3 (a) What is the role of nutrition in the aetiology of pressure ulcers? (see Chs 3 and 13)
   (b) What effect does malnutrition have on wound healing? (see Ch. 13)
4 What strategies would you have used to relieve pressure from Mr Gray's bony prominences? (see Ch. 7)
5 What information would you expect to find incorporated into the nursing home records relating to patient assessment, care planned, care given and the evaluation of care given in this case?

6 (a) What evidence is there that a 'duty of care' may have been breached in the nursing home?
   (b) What are the points of similarity with Case Studies 16.4 and 16.6, in this respect?
   (c) What role might a clinical audit play in highlighting the nature of any problems in the nursing home? (see Ch. 15)

The events and individuals in these case studies are entirely fictional. Any similarity with actual events or individuals is purely coincidental.

Index